Copyright © 2021 -All rights reserved.

No part of this book may be reproduced or transmitted in any form or by any means, electronic or mechanical, including photocopying and recording, or by any information storage and retrieval system, without permission in writing from the publisher. This is a work of fiction. Names, places, characters and incidents are either the product of the author's imagination or are used fictitiously, and any resemblance to any actual persons, living or dead, organizations, events or locales is entirely coincidental. The unauthorized reproduction or distribution of this copyrighted work is ilegal.

Please note the information contained within this document is for educational and entertainment purposes only. All effort has been executed to present accurate, up to date, reliable, complete information. No warranties of any kind are declared or implied. Readers acknowledge that the author is not engaged in the rendering of legal, financial, medical, or professional advice. The content within this book has been derived from various sources. Please consult a licensed professional before attempting any techniques outlined in this book. By reading this document, the reader agrees that under no circumstances is the author responsible for any losses, direct or indirect, that are incurred as a result of the use of the information contained within this document, including, but not limited to, errors, omissions, or inaccuracies.

CONTENTS

- INTRODUCTION 11
- WHAT TO EAT AND AVOID ON THE KETO DIET 13
  - Meat and poultry 13
- TOP 10 KETO DIET TIPS 17
- KETOGENIC RECIPES FOR BREAKFAST 20
  - Butter Eggs 20
  - Sausage Sandwich 20
  - Beef Bowl 20
  - Vanilla Pancakes 20
  - Eggs Bake 20
  - Coconut Smoothie 20
  - Mushroom Scramble 21
  - Bacon Muffins 21
  - Mozzarella Frittata 21
  - Eggs in Rings 21
  - Salmon Eggs 21
  - Creamy Omelet Roll 21
  - Asparagus Eggs 22
  - Bacon and Eggs Rolls 22
  - Avocado Boats 22
  - Cheese Baked Eggs 22
  - Cinnamon Eggs 22
  - Cauliflower Cakes 22
  - Seafood Mix 23
  - Dill Eggs 23
  - Chorizo Eggs 23
  - Herbed Eggs 23
  - Eggs and Beef Pie 23
  - Keto Coffee 23
  - Bok Choy Pan 23
  - Cheesy Fritatta 24
  - Pork Pan 24
  - Basil Scramble 24
  - Egg Casserole 24
  - Coconut Pancakes 24
  - Pork Cakes 25
  - Cauliflower Bowl 25
  - Keto Bake 25
  - Poached Eggs 25
  - Coconut Eggs 25
  - Chorizo Pizza 25
  - Jalapeno Bake 26
  - Parsley Eggs 26
  - Stuffed Avocado 26
  - Butternut Squash Spaghetti with Salami 26
  - Mozzarella Pancakes 26
  - Almond Porridge 26
  - Vanilla Chai 26
  - Blackberry Granola 27
  - Cauli Bowl 27
  - Coconut Chia 27
  - Cauliflower Cupcakes 27
  - Walnut Bowls 27
  - Kale Bake 27
  - Mug Bread 27
  - Cream Cheese Eggs 28
  - Scallions Muffins 28
  - Zucchini Latkes 28
  - Cauliflower Bread 28
  - Cream Muffins 28
  - Guacamole Sandwich 28
  - Brussel Sprouts with Eggs 29
  - Cayenne Muffins 29
  - Creamy Ramekins 29
  - Onion Cookies 29
  - Chia Smoothie 29
  - Chives and Bacon Muffins 29
  - Oregano Frittata 29
  - Thyme Muffins 30
  - Beef Casserole 30
  - Monterey Jack Muffins 30
  - Shrimps Pan 30
  - Chicken Scramble 30
  - Chia Drink 31
  - Strawberry Pudding 31
  - Egg Burrito 31
  - Egg Balls 31
  - Radish Hash 31
  - Chia Bowls 31
  - Bacon Mix 31
  - Basil Scotch Eggs 32
  - Hemp Bites 32
  - Fluffy Eggs 32
  - Coffee Porridge 32
  - Chia Oatmeal 32
  - Cinnamon Porridge 32
  - Garam Masala Bake 33
  - Macadamia Bowls 33
  - Parmesan Rings 33
  - Sweet Porridge 33
  - Egg Hash 33
  - Cream Pancakes 33
  - Rutabaga Pan 34
  - Cocoa Pancakes 34
  - Feta Pie 34
  - Chai Pancakes 34
  - Bacon Pancakes 34
  - Vanilla Toast 35
  - Lime Waffles 35
  - Butter Waffles 35
  - Chocolate Smoothie 35
  - Flax Meal Granola 35
  - Mushrooms Omelette 36
  - Cilantro Smoothie 36
  - Blue Cheese Quiche 36
  - Ginger and Parsley Smoothie 36
  - Sumac Shakshuka 36
  - Cocoa Mix 36
  - Flax Seeds Zucchini Bread 37
  - Breakfast Beef Mix 37
  - Seeds Granola 37
  - Spicy Bake 37
  - Coconut Souffle 37
  - Chicken Frittata 37

Ricotta Omelette 38
Raspberries Bowl 38
Chicken Meatballs 38
Pesto Fritatta 38
Mushroom Caps 38
Cheese Meatloaf 38
Matcha Bombs 39
Tuna Bowls 39
Almond Bowl 39
Tomatoes Salad 39
Garlic Bake 39

KETOGENIC RECIPES FOR LUNCH 40
Avocado and Chicken Salad 40
Chicken Stir-Fry 40
Beef Tacos 40
Salmon Bowl 40
Cauliflower Pizza 40
Broccoli and Bacon Bowls 40
Tomato Pan 41
Chicken Tortillas 41
Cheddar Pizza 41
Halloumi Salad 41
Ground Beef Salad 41
Zucchini Sandwich 42
Stuffed Bell Peppers 42
Shrimp and Avocado Salad 42
Beef Burgers 42
Savory Cauliflower Salad 42
Chili Burger 42
Tomato Cups 43
Garlic Zucchini Boats 43
Spinach Eggplant Sandwich 43
Cheese Zucchini Noodle 43
Mozzarella Burgers 43
Chicken Relish 43
Enchilada Mix 44
Steak Salad 44
Dill Bowls 44
Ricotta Chicken Salad 44
Pepper and Chicken Soup 44
Sardines Stuffed Avocado 45
Cauli Soup 45
Keto Tomato Salad 45
Onion and Chicken Bake 45
Mustard Salad 45
Marinara Chicken Tart 45
Crab Meatballs 46
Turmeric Pie 46
Cremini Mushrooms Muffins 46
Meatballs Soup 46
Scallions and Provolone Pork Pie 46
Cumin Pork Casserole 47
Sage Pâte 47
Tomato Cream 47
Chicken Soup with Basil 47
Cauliflower Risotto 47
Lemongrass Soup 47
Arugula Salad 48
Noodle Soup 48
Pork Dumplings 48

Turmeric Chicken 48
Halloumi Salad 48
Cream Cheese Rolls 49
Chicken Pockets 49
Cilantro Steak 49
Goat Cheese Pancakes 49
Lamb Meatballs 49
Pancakes Pie 49
Cauliflower Cream 50
Curry Soup 50
Green Bean Salad 50
Lettuce Tacos 50
Chipotle Cream 50
Bacon Salad 51
Parmesan Bake 51
Provolone Cream 51
Mayo Salad 51
Tuna Tartare 51
Brussels Sprout Bake 51
Clam Soup 52
Chili Asparagus 52
Beef Salad 52
Basil Shrimp Noodles 52
Bacon Zucchini Noodles 52
Tortilla Bake 53
Chia and Broccoli Soup 53
Garlic Pork Salad 53
Asparagus Pockets 53
Coconut Chicken Wings 53
Zucchini Stuffed Peppers 53
Portobello Skewers 54
Stuffed Eggplants 54
Tomato Cream Soup 54
Cardamom Chicken Cubes 54
Chorizo Wrap 54
Zucchini Baked Bars 54
Lobster Soup 55
Turnip Soup 55
Arugula and Halloumi Salad 55
Artichoke and Mushrooms Mix 55
Beef Stew 55
Seitan Salad 55
Shrimp and Spinach Mix 56
Coconut Mushroom Soup 56
Greens and Coconut Soup 56
Lettuce Salad 56
Cheddar Salad 56
Broccoli and Cucumber Bowl 56
Salmon Soup 57
Garlic Artichokes 57
Fish Soup 57
Lime Beef 57

KETOGENIC SIDE DISH RECIPES 58
Cabbage Mix 58
Italian Style Mushrooms 58
Cheddar Green Beans 58
Butter Asparagus 58
Cauliflower Puree 58
Sesame Brussel Sprouts 58
Tarragon Mushrooms 59

Spinach Mash	59
Pepper Brussels Sprouts	59
Chili Bok Choy	59
Spinach Sauce	59
Parmesan Broccoli Mix	59
Bacon Brussels Sprouts	59
Garlic Zucchini Noodles	60
Creamy Spinach	60
Dill Cabbage Mix	60
Chili Avocado	60
Cilantro Cauliflower Rice	60
Dill Cauliflower	60
Cayenne Green Beans	61
Onion Mushroom and Spinach	61
Herbed Spaghetti Squash	61
Bacon Okra	61
Cauliflower Tortillas	61
Onion Edamame	61
Coriander Eggplant Slices	62
Chili Collard Greens	62
Paprika Cauliflower Rice	62
Mozzarella Eggplant	62
Provolone Kale	62
Coconut Broccoli	62
Lemon Spinach	63
Cheesy Broccoli	63
Baked Parmesan Broccoli	63
Tender Onions	63
Cauliflower Puree	63
Baked Zucchini	63
Creamy Cabbage	64
Garlic Swiss Chard	64
Cauliflower Mix	64
Prosciutto Salad	64
Lime Cabbage Mix	64
Nutmeg Mushroom Mix	64
Keto Pesto	65
Basil Tomato Mix	65
Turmeric Eggplant	65
Cucumber Salad	65
Mozzarella Salad	65
Dill Tomatoes	65
Cinnamon Rutabaga	65
Fennel Salad	66
Artichoke Bake	66
Avocado Mix	66
Lemon Zucchini	66
Baked Eggplant	66
Cream Cauliflower Mix	66
Endive Salad	66
Cilantro Turnip Bake	67
Radish Salad	67
Curry Tofu	67
Mint Sauce	67
Baked Radishes	67
Jalapeno Sauce	67
Rosemary Zucchini Mix	68
Masala Fennel	68
Cardamom Eggplant	68
Dill Bell Peppers	68
Clove Carrots	68
Red Chard Stew	68
Bacon and Oregano Broccoli	68
Apple Cider Vinegar Kale	69
Cheesy Cauliflower Florets	69
Cabbage and Arugula Salad	69
Cheddar Kale	69
Pepper Cabbage	69
Zucchini Sticks	69
Scallions Green Beans	70
Lemon Cauliflower Shred	70
Cajun Zucchini	70
Onion Spinach	70
Oregano Olives	70
Zucchini Cakes	70
Cajun Zucchini Noodles	70
Broccoli Puree	71
Dijon Brussel Sprouts	71
Ricotta Cabbage	71
Monterey Jack Cheese Sauce	71
Dill Pickled Zucchini	71
Parsley Kohlrabi	71
Cheddar Jalapenos	72
Garlic Turnips Sticks	72
Cilantro Jalapenos	72
Butter Cauliflower Puree	72
Coconut Bread	72
Zucchini and Pancetta Mix	72
Cabbage Stew	72
Sausage Side Dish	73
Garlic Radicchio	73
Parsley Pilaf	73
Walnut Salad	73
Zucchini Noodle Salad	73
Taco Jicama	73
Broccoli and Spinach Bowl	74
Sriracha Slaw	74
Cauliflower Polenta	74
Mushroom Pan	74
Cheese and Peppers Bowl	74
Lime Salad	74
Nutmeg Mushrooms	75
Sweet Cranberry Sauce	75
Cumin Green Beans	75
Cauliflower Tots	75
Eggplant Sauce	75
Chili Zucchini Rounds	75
Cheese Ramekins	75
Harissa Turnip	76
Sweet Cauliflower Salad	76
Marinated Garlic	76
Spicy Risotto	76
Baked Okra	76

KETOGENIC SNACKS AND APPETIZERS RECIPES 77

Egg Balls	77
Pork Kebabs	77
Chorizo Dip	77
Chili Biscuits	77
Cauliflower Sauce	77

Jalapeno Stuffed Eggs	77
Cilantro Crackers	77
Oregano Mushroom Caps	78
Herbed Muffins	78
Spinach Dip	78
Seeds Chips	78
Crab Dip	78
Pork Rinds Balls	78
Paprika Wings	79
Pepperoni Balls	79
Cheese Plate	79
Pork Muffins	79
Cheddar Peppers	79
Cream Cheese Dip	79
Chicken Caps	79
Chorizo Muffins	80
Bacon Wraps	80
Fried Halloumi	80
Bacon Eggs	80
Energy Bars	80
Turmeric Eggs	80
Chia Crackers	81
Parmesan Chips	81
Thyme Cupcakes	81
Ham Bites	81
Garlic and Avocado Spread	81
Chorizo Tacos	81
Shrimp Bites	82
Roasted Cauliflower Florets	82
Zucchini Rolls	82
Broccoli Biscuits	82
Turmeric Sausages	82
Kalamata Snack	82
Peppers Nachos	83
Mozzarella Bites	83
Almond Bars	83
Almond Zucchini	83
Coated Zucchinis	83
Bacon Peppers	83
Zucchini Chips	83
Ham Bites	84
Zucchini Sauce	84
Cayenne Shrimp	84
Celery Boats	84
Fish Pancakes	84
Jerky	84
Paprika Beef Jerky	84
Crab Spread	85
Spinach Wraps	85
Nutmeg Balls	85
Kale Chips	85
Parsley Dip	85
Cucumber Bites	85
Mushrooms with Shrimps	85
Basil Bites	86
Cheese Cubes	86
Chili Caps	86
Turkey Meatballs	86
Escargot Ramekins	86
Italian Style Wings	86
Thyme Halloumi	86
Italian Sticks	87
Crispy Bites	87
Cauliflower Florets in Cheese	87
Eggplant Chips	87
Chocolate Bacon	87
Carrot Chips	87
Asparagus Chips	87
Sweet Bacon	87
Chicken Wraps	88
Garlic Rinds	88
Marinara Bites	88
Pepper Cucumbers	88
Jalapeño Bites	88
Baked Coconut Eggs	88
Stuffed Cucumber	88
Seaweed Chips	89
Eggs Salad	89
Berry Cubes	89
Peppers Kebabs	89
Pumpkin Bowls	89
Zucchini Rolls	89
Egg Sandwich	89
Basil Crackers	90
Monterey Jack Cheese Rolls	90
Ham Terrine	90
Chocolate Pecans	90
Jalapeno Salad	90
Rosemary Tomatoes	90
Egg Halves	90
Celery Skewers	90
Lemon Chips	91
Scallions Sandwich	91
Artichoke Dip	91
Coffee Cubes	91
KETOGENIC FISH AND SEAFOOD RECIPES	**92**
Tuna Pie	92
Wrapped Scallops	92
Lime Haddock	92
Salmon Boats	92
Cheddar Tilapia	92
Salmon Kababs	92
Soft Trout	92
Cod in Sauce	93
Lime Trout	93
Cod with Chives	93
Spicy Salmon	93
Tilapia Bowl	93
Salmon Meatballs	93
Cinnamon Hake	94
Oregano Salmon	94
Sage Cod Fillets	94
Herbed Oysters	94
Cod Curry	94
Parmesan Cod	94
Roasted Sea Eel	94
Cilantro Salmon	95
Italian Spices Seabass	95
Mustard Cod	95
Shrimp Chowder	95

Onion Salmon	95
Cheddar Pollock	95
Parsley Tuna Fritters	96
Clam Stew	96
Sour Cod	96
Fennel Seabass	96
Cheesy Tuna Bake	96
Parsley Sea Bass	96
Scallions Salmon Cakes	97
Tilapia with Olives	97
Cod Sticks	97
Halibut and Spinach	97
Coriander Cod	97
White Fish Stew	98
Crab Fritters	98
Lime Shrimp	98
Ginger Cod	98
Tomato Sea Bass	98
Scallions Salmon Spread	98
Tomato and Thyme Shrimps	98
Chili Cod	99
Shrimp Bowl	99
Tender Catfish	99
Cayenne Mahi Mahi	99
Sweet Salmon Steaks	99
Pepper Shrimp	99
Jalapeno Tilapia	100
Shrimp and Turnip Stew	100
Parmesan Tilapia Bites	100
Mushroom Shrimps	100
Creamy Cod	100
Shrimp Soup	100
Garlic Catfish	101
Lime Mussels	101
Salmon Kababs	101
Sriracha Calamari	101
Curry Cod	101
Turmeric Calamari	101
Parsley Cod	102
Lemon Octopus	102
Cod Packets	102
Clam Soup with Pancetta	102
Tuna Meatballs	102
Lemon Flounder	102
Creamy Halibut	103
Shrimp Salad	103
Salmon Quesadillas	103
Garlic Oysters	103
Onion Mahi Mahi	103
Spicy Salmon	103
Cod Sticks	104
Tuna Skewers	104
Turmeric Salmon Balls	104
Basil Shrimp	104
Cumin Seabass	104
Calamari Salad	104
Paprika Cod	105
Lettuce and Cod Salad	105
Marjoram Seabass	105
Sardine Salad	105
Garlic Mackerel	105
Rosemary Clams	105
Coconut Tilapia	105
Vinegar Salmon	106
Boiled Crab Legs	106
Salmon Sauce	106
Tuna Salad	106
Hot Salmon	106
Cod Casserole	106
Clams and Bacon	107
Taco Tilapia	107
Pomegranate Scallops	107
Tarragon Seabass	107
Spicy Marjoram Oysters	107
Pepper Tuna Cakes	107
Almond Squid	107
Dill Crab Cakes	108
Coated Shrimps	108
Tomato Mackerel	108
Stuffed Salmon with Spinach	108
Halibut with Mushrooms	108
Mustard Tilapia	108
Salmon Burger	109
Salmon and Radish Stew	109
Cardamom Shrimp	109
Oregano and Basil Scallops	109
Fennel Mussels	109
Cilantro Cod	109
Basil Clam Chowder	110
Chili Mussel Stew	110
Oysters Stir-Fry	110
Sweet Swordfish	110
Stuffed Calamari with Herbs	110
Greek-Style Tuna	110
Curry Crabs	111
KETOGENIC POULTRY RECIPES	**112**
Garlic Chicken	112
Chili Drumsticks	112
Sage Chicken Wings	112
Oregano Chicken Wings	112
Chicken Meatballs	112
Paprika Chicken Wings	112
Lime Chicken Wings	112
Coconut Chicken	113
Onion Chicken	113
Almond Chicken	113
Garlic and Dill Chicken	113
Cheese Chicken Casserole	113
Lemon Chicken	113
Italian Style Chicken	114
Paprika Chicken Fillet	114
Coconut Chicken Fillets	114
Chicken with Peppers	114
Chicken Pie	114
Tarragon Chicken	115
Masala Chicken Thighs	115
Chicken with Olives	115
Cheddar Chicken Thighs	115
Lemon Duck Breast	115
Parsley Chicken	115

Duck with Zucchinis	115
Oregano Meatballs	116
Duck Salad	116
Clove Chicken	116
Turkey Bake	116
Garlic and Curry Chicken	116
Turkey Soup	117
Cheese Pizza	117
Creamy Turkey	117
Cordon Bleu Chicken	117
Cumin Stew	117
Turkey Burgers	117
Chicken Curry	118
Chili Chicken	118
Turkey Salad	118
Rosemary Chicken	118
Stuffed Chicken	118
Chicken Tortillas	118
Dijon Chicken	119
Chicken and Cream	119
Arugula Chicken	119
Cheese Wrapped Chicken Wings	119
Grilled Chicken Sausages	119
Mushroom Chicken	119
Mozzarella Chicken	120
Vinegar Chicken	120
Fajita Chicken	120
Cajun Chicken	120
Chicken with Sauce	120
Lemon Chicken Breast	120
Chicken and Broccoli Casserole	121
Coconut Chicken	121
Dill Chicken Soup	121
Chicken Meatballs with Turmeric	121
Chicken Pancakes	121
Butter Chicken	122
Monterey Jack Cheese Chicken	122
Jalapeno Chicken Chowder	122
Bacon-Wrapped Chicken	122
Tender Chicken Fillets	122
Basil Chicken	122
Chicken Meatloaf	123
Orange Chicken	123
Sage Chicken	123
Crustless Chicken Pie	123
Coriander Chicken	123
Scallions Chicken	123
Seasoned Chicken	124
Sweet Chicken Wings	124
Sour Duck Breast	124
Cardamom Chicken	124
Garlic Duck Bites	124
Chicken in Parmesan Sauce	124
Saffron Duck	124
Chicken under Onion Blanket	125
Oregano Duck	125
Marjoram Chicken Breast	125
Turmeric Chicken Skin	125
Thyme Sausages	125
Strawberries Chicken	125
Parmesan Chicken Thighs	126
Chicken Spread	126
Macadamia Chicken	126
Duck Spread	126
Tomato Chicken	126
Cinnamon Chicken Drumsticks	126
Coated Chicken	127
Jalapeno Chicken	127
Chicken Calzone	127
Shredded Chicken Pancakes	127
Chicken Cream Soup	127
Crunchy Chicken Wings	128
Sriracha Chicken	128
Indian Style Chicken	128
Greens and Chicken Bowl	128
Chicken Roast	128
Cream Cheese Chicken	128
Chili Chicken Ground	129
Yogurt Chicken	129
Leek Chicken	129
Stuffed Chicken with Olives	129
Dill Chicken Muffins	129
Chicken with Crumbled Cheese	129
Chicken Lettuce Wraps	130
Chicken in Avocado	130
Duck Casserole	130
Mozzarella Chicken	130
Aromatic Cumin Chicken	130
Cilantro Chicken	130
Bacon Chicken	131
Herbed Ginger Chicken	131
Jalapeno Chicken with Cream Cheese	131
Chicken and Leek Stew	131
Fennel Chicken	131
Chicken with Asparagus Blanket	131
BBQ Shredded Chicken	132
KETOGENIC MEAT RECIPES	**133**
Lemon Pork Belly	133
Ground Pork Pie	133
Lemon Stuffed Pork	133
Beef and Vegetables Stew	133
Marinated Pork	133
Cheese and Pork Casserole	133
Pork and Cream Cheese Rolls	134
Leek Stuffed Beef	134
Garlic Pork Loin	134
Butter Pork	134
Almond Pork	134
Cumin Meatballs	135
Sweet Pork	135
Curry Meatballs	135
Thyme Pork Chops	135
Fajita Pork	135
Oregano Pork Chops	135
Chili Pork Skewers	136
Rosemary Pork Tenderloin	136
Paprika Pork Strips	136
Jalapeno Pork Chops	136
Beef Lasagna	136
Nutmeg Pork Chops	136

Chili Ground Pork	137
Thai Style Pork	137
2-Meat Stew	137
Pork and Vegetable Meatballs	137
Spring Onion Cubes	137
Pork and Mushrooms Roast	137
Turmeric Beef Tenders	138
Beef and Zucchini Muffins	138
Tomato Pork Ribs	138
Pork Balls Bake	138
Sage Pork Chops	138
Beef Stuffed Avocado	138
Tomato Pulled Pork	139
Beef with Pickled Chilies	139
Almond Meatballs	139
Scallions Beef Meatloaf	139
Bacon Beef	139
Beef Sauce with Broccoli	139
Parsley Taco Beef	140
Meatballs in Coconut Sauce	140
Pork Rolls	140
White Beef Soup	140
Cardamom Sausages	140
Spicy Ground Beef Casserole	140
Marjoram Pork Tenderloin	141
Beef with Noodles	141
Smoked Paprika Pork	141
Sweet Pork Belly	141
Dill Beef Patties	141
Beef Saute	141
Beef and Broccoli Stew	142
Cinnamon Beef Stew	142
Beef and Eggplant Stew	142
Beef Rolls	142
Mint Lamb Chops	142
Chipotle Lamb Ribs	143
Lamb and Pecan Salad	143
Lime Ribs	143
Hot Sauce Lamb	143
Paprika Beef Steaks	143
Mustard Lamb Chops	143
Masala Ground Pork	143
Ginger Lamb Chops	144
Parmesan Lamb	144
Clove Lamb	144
Carrot Lamb Roast	144
Lamb and Celery Casserole	144
Lamb in Almond Sauce	144
Sweet Leg of Lamb	145
Coconut Lamb Shoulder	145
Lavender Lamb	145
Dill Lamb Shank	145
Mexican Lamb Chops	145
Tender Lamb Stew	146
Lime Lamb	146
Basil Meatloaf	146
Lamb Saute with Mint and Lemon	146
Pancetta Lamb	146
Sweet Lamb with Oregano	146
Keto Pie	147

Veal and Cabbage Salad	147
Nutmeg Lamb	147
Thyme Beef	147
Sausage Casserole	147
Onion Beef Roast	147
Cajun Pork	148
Beef and Chili	148
Beef Loin in Parmesan Sauce	148
Coconut Pork Bowl	148
BBQ Pork Ribs	148
Sausage Stew with Turnip	148
Butter Beef	149
Spicy Beef	149
Tender Indian Pork	149
Keto Beef	149
Bergamot Pork	149
Wrapped Ham Bites	149
Avocado and Meat Salad	149
Tender Veal	150
Oil and Herbs Lamb	150
Sage Beef	150
Anise Beef	150
Spearmint Veal	150
Garlic Pork Ribs	150
Veal and Sorrel Saute	150
Creamy Pork Skewers	151
Grilled Pork Sausage	151
Allspice Pork	151
Hot Sauce Sausage	151
Tomato Beef Bake	151
Pork with Gouda Cheese	151
Sausage and Asparagus Bowl	152
Garlic Pork Ribs	152
Smoked Paprika Sausage Soup	152
Tomato Lamb Ribs	152
Beef Soup with Spinach	152
KETOGENIC VEGETABLE RECIPES	**153**
Bacon Broccoli Mash	153
Parsley Asparagus	153
Marinated Broccoli	153
Lemon Bell Peppers	153
Watercress Soup	153
Garlic Cauliflower Fritters	153
Coconut Mushroom Cream Soup	153
Rosemary Grilled Peppers	154
Roasted Bok Choy	154
Baked Rutabaga	154
Celery Cream Soup	154
Lettuce Sandwich	154
Fenugreek Celery Stalks	154
Cauliflower Cream	155
Celery Cream Soup	155
Broccoli Spread	155
Cheese and Spinach Cream	155
Brussel Sprouts Fritters	155
Lemon Greens	155
Garlic Mash	156
Buttered Onion	156
Broccoli Curry	156
Keto Tomatoes	156

Lime Green Beans	156
Mustard Asparagus	156
Baked Kale	156
Asparagus Soup	157
Parmesan Artichokes	157
Mustard Greens Soup	157
Rutabaga Cakes	157
Greens Soup	157
Cheese Edamame Beans	157
Cilantro Asparagus	158
Sauteed Collard Greens	158
Spinach Fritters	158
Oregano Eggplants	158
Yogurt Asparagus	158
Avocado and Walnut Bowl	158
Greens Omelette	159
Asparagus Masala	159
Monterey Jack Cheese Asparagus	159
Chives Fritters	159
Sprouts Salad	159
Cabbage Balls	159
Turmeric Radishes	159
Jicama Noodles	160
Rosemary Radish	160
Broccoli Slaw	160
Coated Radish	160
White Mushrooms Saute	160
Radish in Bacon Sauce	160
Sesame Broccoli	161
Garlic Soup	161
Cheese Mushrooms	161
Cilantro and Cabbage Salad	161
Cauliflower Pizza with Greens	161
Mustard Salad	161
Zucchini Ravioli	162
Lemon Salad	162
Broccoli Crackers	162
Avocado Spread	162
Paprika Okra	162
Spinach Soup	162
Lettuce and Mozzarella Salad	163
Thai Soup	163
Basil Bake	163
Marinated Broccoli Salad	163
Sesame Bok Choy	163
Scallions Soup	163
Eggplant Puree	163
Cumin Soup	164
Oregano Fennel	164
Zucchini Cream Soup	164
Mushroom Bake	164
Ginger Cream Soup	164
Butter Zucchini Pasta	164
Mozzarella Swiss Chard	165
Blue Cheese Cauliflower	165
Chard Salad	165
Flax Seeds Spinach	165
Oregano Chard Salad	165
Baked Broccoli	165
Apple Cider Vinegar Lettuce	165

Coconut Bok Choy	166
Mushroom Cream Soup	166
Parmesan Pancake	166
Brussel Sprouts Soup	166
Baked Asparagus	166
Keto Soup	166
Grilled Mushrooms	167
Grilled Garlic Eggplants	167
Parmesan Brussel Sprouts	167
Eggplant Saute	167
Cabbage Pancake	167
Vegetable Soup	167
Celery Root Puree	168
Green Cabbage Soup	168
Kale Soup	168

KETOGENIC DESSERT RECIPES 169
Butter Truffles	169
Pecan Brownies	169
Flaxseeds Doughnuts	169
Jelly Bears	169
Pecan Candies	169
Cocoa Pie	169
Cream Jelly	170
Vanilla Mousse	170
Cheese Pie	170
Avocado Mousse	170
Chocolate Pie	170
Coconut Panna Cotta	170
No-Baked Cheesecake	171
Coconut Cookies	171
Blackberries Bars	171
Cheesecake Bars	171
Cocoa Muffins	171
Coconut Pudding	171
Cream Cheese Mousse	172
Chocolate Bacon Strips	172
Cocoa Fudge	172
Coconut Cookies	172
Sweet Mousse	172
Lemon Pie	172
2-Ingredients Ice Cream	173
Berry Muffins	173
Cocoa Squares	173
Avocado Pie	173
Mint Brownies	173
Almond Bars	173
Coconut Chia Pudding	174
Matcha Muffins	174
Coconut Parfaits	174
Vanilla Shake	174
Lemon Pudding	174
Almond Biscotti	174
Peppermint Cream	174
Zucchini Pudding	175
Egg Pudding	175
Basil Cookies	175
Clove Pudding	175
Sweet Paprika Bars	175
Chia and Cocoa Biscuits	176
Pecan Fudge	176

Walnut Brownies	176
Cream Cheese Bombs	176
Blueberries Scones	176
Vanilla Donuts	176
Tender Cookies	177
Keto Caramel	177
Crustless Yogurt Cake	177
Almond Mousse	177
Cocoa Paste	177
Ricotta Bars	177
Stevia Pie	178
Lime Meringue	178
Cinnamon Buns	178
Coconut Pie	178
Coconut Custard	178
Almond Bun	178
Vanilla Topping	179
Vanilla Flan	179
Raspberry Cream	179
Vanilla Pancake Pie	179
Frozen Ice	179
Nutmeg Pies	179
Coconut Mascarpone	180
Seeds Bars	180
Lime Cheese	180
Egg Cake	180
Sorbet	180
Swerve Cookies	180
Vanilla Custard	181
Cardamom Shortcakes	181
Nutmeg Balls	181
Lime Cookies	181
Coffee Mousse	181
Butter Cookies	181
Pecan Granola	182
Sweet Bacon Bombs	182
Almond Pudding	182
Egg Clouds	182
Matcha Custard	182
Milk Sorbet	182
Salty Cookies	183
Fluffy Cookies	183
Vanilla Butter Bars	183
Peppermint Cookies	183
Cinnamon Marshmallows	183
Orange Ice Cream	183
Yogurt Pudding	184
Cream Popsicle	184
Keto Smoothie	184
Watermelon Sorbet	184
Sweet Ice Cubes	184
Peach Ice Cream	184
Strawberry Popsicles	184
Cantaloupe Sorbet	184
Carambola Jelly	185
Blueberry Ice Cream	185

APPENDIX : RECIPES INDEX 186

INTRODUCTION

The path to a perfect body and good physical health was very thorny for me. The only one wish which I was making for my birthdays for many years was to be a slim and beautiful girl. Alas, everything can't be as in fairy tales and the miracle didn't happen; my mirror was still showing the same fat, pimple girl. In childhood, the problem of overweight didn't bother me much; I can say that I didn't care about it at all, I didn't know that weight would be momentous for me. I was an ordinary smiling child, playing with my peers, going to school, and traveling with my parents. That time my chubby cheeks seemed very sweet to everyone. But that was then. At 11-year-old, I went to middle school. New people, new teachers, I had no friends at all. Mentally I was broken. I counted the minutes until the end of the last lesson, to quickly sit in my mom's car and leave school. I started to eat a lot. Now I see that in this way I stuck stress, but then the food served as my antidepressant. Dozens of hamburgers, fried potatoes, coke – they were "my best friends". In addition to everything, I started to have horrible skin problems, it seemed to me that there was no place on my face wherever they hadn't appeared yet. Time passed and I no longer loved my reflection in the mirror even in 1%. I couldn't wear the clothes that I liked. I usually wore oversized shorts and t-shirts. I couldn't afford to wear a short dress and high heels. At 15-year-old me was weighted more than 270lbs. I remember what I felt in those days, as it is happening now. I felt anger, irritation, hatred, and self-loathing. That prom party was the most terrible day of my life. Thank God it's over!

In those years, the keto diet was not very popular, fasting and drinking diets (which, as you already know, did not help me much) were more popular. Perhaps I wouldn't do anything, but my health problems were becoming more serious. It seemed that my body was simply screaming: please help me!

I remember the day that changed my life on a dime. I came to the clinic with pain in my stomach. But this time, I not only received painkillers but also found a mentor and friend. This was my physician. She had examined me and recommended to go on a diet. I didn't want to do something and was categorically against it. However, my mind changed when she said: love your body, care about it, and it will thank you. What was my surprise when the diet turned out to be very simple to follow. Is it so easy to love myself? As you could understand I am talking about my favorite keto diet. Every day I was eating a maximum of proteins and a minimum of carbohydrates. That meant to consume meat, poultry, and fish and make restrictions for vegetables, fruits, and sweets. After 2 weeks, I lost 83lbs, and further results were getting better and better. All this time I was under the supervision of a doctor and this yielded results. A year later, I completely changed all the clothes in my wardrobe and oh my God I was able to wear a short dress and skirts! Now I can say that I am the happiest person. It happened because I fall in love with myself and started treated my body as a diamond. My life was filled with bright colors, I have a beloved husband, children, work, friends, I am healthy and like myself in the mirror. I am telling this story a prove that the right diet can solve almost all problems with body and health. It is a fact that our body is capable to deal with dramatic changes, it is only worth loving it. Never rest on your laurels, never give up and forbid people to say that you cannot do something. You are already a great fellow that you bought this cookbook and decided to take a step ahead in the direction to your dream. Let this book become your ray of hope, a lifesaver on the way to your wonderful transformation. If you believe in yourself and love your body, believe me, the result won't be long in coming. You will see in the mirror a completely new version of yourself, updated physically and mentally! Just trust the keto diet and your inner voice. Set a goal today and start the way of achieving it right now. Don't try to do all in one time; let it be small step day by day. Exactly now, this is the right time to start creating a new version of you. If this diet was able to change my life, I'm sure it will help you too!

WHAT TO EAT AND AVOID ON THE KETO DIET

Meat and poultry

Actually, it is the primary type of food for the Keto diet. It contains 0% of carbs and is rich in potassium, selenium, zinc, and B vitamins. Grass-fed meat and poultry are the most beneficial. It caused by high omega 3 fats and antioxidants content. Bear in mind that Keto diet is a high-fat diet and high consumption of proteins can cause to harder getting of ketosis.

What to eat	Enjoy occasionally	What to avoid
• chicken • duck • goose • ground beef • lamb • ostrich • partridge • pheasant • pork • quail • turkey • venison	• bacon • ham • low-fat meat, such as skinless chicken breast • sausage	• breaded meats • processed meats

Dairy

High-fat dairy products are awesome for the keto diet. They are calcium-rich full-fat dairy product is nutritious and can make you full longer. Milk lovers should restrict or even cross out this product from the daily meal plan. It is allowed only 1 tablespoon of milk in your drink per day but doesn't abuse it daily.

What to eat	What to avoid
• butter • cheese (soft and hard) • full-fat yogurt • heavy cream • sour cream	• fat-free yogurt • low-fat cheese • milk • skim milk • skim mozzarella • sweetened yogurt

Eggs

This is the most wholesome food in the world. Use them everywhere you want! Containing less than one gram of carbohydrates, eggs are a wonderful food for the keto lifestyle. Eating eggs reducing the risk of heart disease and save your eyes health.
Note: free-range eggs are healthier options for the keto diet.

What to avoid	
• chicken eggs • duck eggs • goose eggs	• ostrich eggs • quail eggs

Fish and Seafood

Fatty fish as salmon is beneficial for the keto diet. Small fish like sardines, herring, etc. are less in toxins. The best option for a keto diet is wild-caught seafood; it has a higher number of omega 3 fats.
Scientifically proved that frequent eating of fish improves mental health.

What to eat		What to avoid
• catfish • clams • cod • crab • halibut • herring • lobster • mackerel • Mahi Mahi • mussels • oysters	• prawns • salmon • sardines • scallops • shrimp • snapper • swordfish • tilapia • trout • tuna	• breaded fish

Nuts and Seeds

These products are heart-healthy and fiber-rich. Nevertheless, eat nuts and seeds as a snack is a bad idea. As usual, the amount of eaten food can be much more than allowed. Nuts like cashews are very insidious and contain a lot of carbohydrates. Replace them with macadamia or pecan.

What to eat		What to avoid
- almonds - chia seeds - flaxseeds - hazelnuts - nut butter (unsweetened)	- peanuts - pecans - pumpkin seeds - walnuts - macadamia nuts	- cashews - pistachio - chocolate-covered nuts - nut butter (sweetened)

Oils and fats

It is the main component of the keto-friendly sauces and dressings.
Olive oil and coconut oil are highly recommending for everyone who decided to follow the keto diet. They are almost perfect it their fatty acid composition. Avoid artificial trans fats which are poison for our body. This type of fats, as usual, used in French fries, margarine, and crackers.

What to eat	What to avoid
- avocado oil - coconut oil - hazelnut oil - olive oil - pumpkin seed oil - sesame oil - walnut oil	- grapeseed oil - canola oil - cottonseed oil - hydrogenated oils - margarine - peanut oil - soybean oil - safflower oil - processed vegetable oils

Vegetables

Keto diet cannot work without vegetables, but their usage should be in moderation. Starchy vegetables such as potatoes, sweet potatoes, etc. are deadly for our body and will not bring anything more than overweight. At the same time, vegetables that are low in carbs, are rich in antioxidants and can protect the body from free radicals that damage our cells.

What to eat		What to avoid
- asparagus - avocado - broccoli - cabbage - cauliflower - celery - cucumber - eggplant - leafy greens - lettuce	- mushrooms - olives - onions - tomatoes - peppers - spinach - zucchini - other nonstarchy vegetables	- carrots - corn - beets - butternut squash - parsnips - potatoes (both sweet and regular) - pumpkin - turnips - yams - yuca - other starchy vegetables

Fruits

This type of food is high in carbs that's why they should be limited while keto diet. Besides this, almost all fruits are high in glucose and can enhance blood sugar.

Enjoy occasionally	What to avoid	
- lemons - pomegranates - limes	- apples - bananas - grapefruits - limes - mango - oranges	- peaches - pears - pineapple - plums - dried fruits

Berries
If you are looking for how to substitute fruits, this is your godsend. Berries contain up to 12 grams of net carbs per 3.5 ounces serving. They are high in fiber and can maintain the health of your body and fight with diseases. Note consumption of a huge amount of berries can be harmful.

Enjoy occasionally	What to avoid
- blackberries	- cherries
- blueberries	- grapes
- raspberries	- melon
- strawberries	- watermelon

Beans and legumes
There are no ingredients in this food group that would be healthy for a keto diet. Beans and legumes contain fewer carbs in comparison with root vegetables such as potatoes; nevertheless, this type of carbohydrates fastly adds up.

What to avoid	
- black beans	- navy beans
- chickpeas	- peas
- kidney beans	- pinto beans
- lentils	- soybeans

Condiments
Condiments can make any type of meal awesome. Even a piece of meat will turn into the masterpiece with them. There are only a few products which are better to avoid; nevertheless, nowadays, you can find keto-friendly substitutors in a supermarket.

One more hot tip: putting hot pepper in your meal will reduce the amount of salt you need and make the taste of the dish more saturated.

What to eat	What to avoid
- herbs and spices	- BBQ sauce
- lemon juice	- hot sauces
- mayonnaise with no added sugar	- ketchup
- salad dressings with no added sugar	- maple syrup
- salt and pepper	- salad dressings with added sugar
- vinegar	- sweet dipping sauces
	- tomato sauce

Grain products
Actually, it is needless to say that all grains are forbidden and can't be eaten if you want to achieve ketosis. Grains contain complex carbohydrates that have a feature to be absorbed slower than simple carbohydrates. For better understanding, if the food has keto-friendly carbs, look at the number of starch and sugar. Their number should be minimum.

What to avoid	
- baked goods	- muesli
- bread	- oats
- cereal	- pasta
- corn	- pizza
- crackers	- popcorn
- flour	- rice
- granola	- wheat

Beverages

A variety of keto drinks may shock you. Probably you know that the best beverage for a keto diet is water. Nevertheless, in order to brighten up a little gray everyday life of keto lovers, the consumption of alcoholic beverages is allowed in moderation. For instance, pure forms of alcohol, such as gin, vodka, or tequila can be drunk once per week. They contain zero amounts of carbs. Avoid all sweetened beverages; they are a priori high carbohydrate.

What to eat	Enjoy occasionally	What to avoid
- almond milk - bone broth - coffee (unsweetened) - flax milk - tea (unsweetened) - water (still and sparkling)	- dry wine - hard liquor - vodka - other low carb alcoholic drinks	- alcoholic drinks (sweetened) - beer - cider - coffee (sweetened) - fruit juice - soda - sports drinks - smoothies - tea (sweetened) - wines (sweet)

Sweets

Cakes and cookies cannot help in losing weight in any diet. As for keto, here everything is strict with this. You should try to avoid sugar and sweeteners in any form. Moreover, sweets negatively affect blood sugar and insulin levels.

Enjoy occasionally	What to avoid
- erythritol - stevia - sucralose	- artificial sweeteners - buns - candy - cakes - chocolate - cookies - custard - ice cream - pastries - pies - pudding - sugar - tarts

Others

Fast food and processed food contain a huge amount of stabilizers and harmful carbohydrates. The main rule of the Keto diet is avoiding sugar. 99,9% of such food contains harmful sugars. The existence of which in the body negates the achievement of ketosis.

What to avoid
- fast food - processed foods

TOP 10 KETO DIET TIPS

1. Combine together Keto and Intermittent fasting.

Intermittent fasting (IF) is the right way to get ketosis. It gives your body additional benefits. Scientists showed that connection keto diet and intermittent fasting can up the results which can give only strict following of the keto diet.

IF means not eating and drinking during a determined amount of time. It is recommended to separate your day into a building phase (BP) and cleansing phase(CP); where the building phase is the time between the first and last time of eating (first-last); and cleansing is the opposite time (last-first). Start from 14-hours CP and 11-hours BP. Continue like this till your body adapts to the new daily plan. It can take 2-3 days. The first days will be the hardest but then you will feel relief and you can safely proceed to the next stage where BP turns into 5 hours and CP - into 19 hours.

According to research, women get the highest benefits of IF. It is possible to get rid of adrenal fatigue, hypothyroid, and hormonal imbalance.

2. Staying hydrated is essential.

Our body is 60% water. Water ensures the normal digestion of food and the absorption of nutrients from the intestines. If there is not enough water in the body, there will be discomfort in the abdomen and constipation. Drinking water is important even if you are not on keto.

The kidneys filter 5,000 ounces of blood per day so that the result is 50 ounces of urine. For the normal elimination of toxins and waste substances, you need to drink at least 50 ounces of water per day, but preferably more.

Many people face the problem of unwillingness to drink water. The best way to prevent dehydration and all its unpleasant consequences is to put a bottle or cup of water on the table and take a sip every time you look at the water. If you realize that you are thirsty, then eliminate thirst in time.

Regular drinking of the right amount of water for 1 week will become a habit and you will not be able to live differently.

3. Salt isn't harmful.

Salt plays an important role in complex metabolic processes. It is part of the blood, lymph, saliva, tears, gastric juice, bile - that is, all the fluids of our body. Any fluctuations in the salt content in the blood plasma lead to serious metabolic disorders

When fewer carbohydrates enter the body, insulin levels drop. Less insulin circulating in the body leads to secrete excess water in the kidneys instead of holding it. It means that salt and other important minerals and electrolytes are washed out of the body.

Replenish salt is possible by eating bone broths, cucumbers, celeriac, salty keto nuts, and seeds.

The best salts for keto diet are 2 types of salt. Pink salt has a more saturated, saltier taste, and contains calcium, magnesium, and potassium. Sea salt is simply evaporated seawater. The crystals of sea salt are slightly larger than iodized salt, and it has a stronger aroma. It contains potassium, magnesium, sulfur, phosphorus, and zinc.

4. Sport is important.

It is proved that physical activity improves the health of the whole body in general and accelerates metabolism. When we do sport, the first thing is we get rid of carbohydrates, and only then we burn fats.

On a keto diet, even minimal physical activity contributes to the rapid decomposition of fats. You simply don't have glucose (carbohydrates) and any load breaks down fats. The most effective workouts on an empty stomach. Sports during keto are very comfortable. You do not feel hungry and can play sports without breakdowns and overeating. Your stamina is significantly increased. If the protein is correctly calculated, you don't lose muscle mass with a calorie deficit.

The combination of three types of workouts gives the best result for health, weight dynamics, and even mood! These are workouts, aerobic, and stretching. Start with small loads every day and increase it as you can. Do not forget to take measurements of your body to monitor the result!

5.   Reduce stress.

Sometimes, observing all the postulates of the keto lifestyle, ketosis does not occur or occurs very slowly. In 99 cases, it happens due to the level of stress in your life. Thus, the hormone cortisol rises, the sympathetic nervous system is stimulated.

Cortisol is produced in response to any stress, even the most minor. How does it happen?

Cortisol "eats" our muscles to turn them into glucose, it catabolizes bones, which is fraught with osteoporosis, causes increased appetite, and suppresses immunity. It also causes increased production of glucose and insulin, and exactly this stops ketosis.

During keto-adaptation (the first 3 weeks), increased cortisol is produced, because the usual energy, glucose, ceases to flow into the body, and it turns on the "self-preservation mode".

It is very important at first to minimize stress from the outside, then everything will normalize.

You should be able to switch from stimulation of the sympathetic nervous system to parasympathetic. Stimulation of the parasympathetic nervous system contributes to the restoration and accumulation of energy resources. This can be achieved by a simple 15 minutes' meditation. The time when you cannot be interrupted.

6.   Sleep above all!

Sleep and stress are two interconnected components. Lack of sleep leads to increased stress. Consequently, stress hormone levels and blood sugar levels rise and we gain weight very fast.

Doctors recommend an 8-9 hour sleep every day. The best time to fall asleep is before 11 pm. An hour before bedtime, try not to use any gadgets. It is better to spend this time in silence, meditation, listening to calm music or reading a paper book. Thus, we calm the nervous system and set it to sleep. If your stress level per day was high, try to spend more time sleeping. it is the sleep that contributes to our weight loss and getting rid of all diseases. There are some tips to improve your sleep comfort:

- Keep cool in the room. The optimum temperature should not exceed 65-70F.
- Use a black mask for sleeping and earplugs.
- Provide good room ventilation.

7.   Don't forget about vegetables.

It is obvious that the main resource of vitamins and minerals is vegetables. You can't cross out them totally from daily meals. Consuming them during the keto diet is very important, but should be in moderation. Starchy vegetables such as sweet potatoes and potatoes are not allowed. Nevertheless, at the same time, you can safely substitute them with broccoli, kale, spinach, white cabbage, Brussels sprouts to your diet. Such vegetables are not only low-carb, but also low-calorie and have a huge number of vitamins, antioxidants, and minerals. They will help you stay full for a long time and protect from eating an extra serving of nuts.

One of the tips of keto coaches is to pamper yourself with low-carb berries once a week. At the same time, it is very important to increase physical activity during this day. Cycling will be just right. All this will fill your body with useful antioxidants and will not add extra pounds.

8.   MCT oil is a treasure for a keto diet.

MCT oil is medium-chain triglyceride oil. It practically doesn't require splitting in the small intestine and is absorbed already in the duodenum, going directly to the liver. MCT oil is used by the body as an energy source, which leads to an increase in fat loss. On the other hand, MCT oil isn't deposited in body fat like fatty tissue in comparison with other fatty acids, and it has been shown that it improves thermogenesis, that is, the process during which the body creates heat using excess energy.

MCT oils are good for cooking, especially for baking, frying or grilling. This is due to their high point of "smoke", which means that they are very difficult to oxidize from heat and can withstand high temperatures without losing their original chemical structure at room temperature (losing their useful properties). You can also add MTC oil in keto shakes, coffee, tea, and other keto drinks.

9.   Do a kitchen audit

The key to getting ketosis is proper low-carb nutrition. Nevertheless, our brain, knowing that somewhere in the fridge or freezer are a bar of chocolate or a package of vanilla ice cream. So it unconsciously creates situations in which we are obliged to eat them. That's why there are no doubts that one of the best tips is to clean your kitchen and all the shelves from the "seducers". Firstly, write a list of food that is not allowed during the diet, and then one by one throw away everything that is on your list. It may seem too radical right away. But just know that all this will help you completely switch to keto life faster and less stressfully for your body. Also, you can make a list of all you have in the fridge and stick this sheet of paper on the fridge. Doing this you will not eat extra snacks during the day.

10.   Keep food near you.

Our life is full of events and sometimes we just don't have time to cook. We have a choice to buy high carbohydrate food in the shop or cook the right food by ourselves. All of this needs extra time. That's why you should always have a "healthy snack" with you. No matter what it is. It can be fat bombs, seeds, or nuts. If you have more time, make the keto salads, or find the keto fruits such as avocado and cook the spreads and dips. But bear in mind, you shouldn't cook much in advance. Their expired date is very short. Follow the rule to purchasing all ingredients for snacks in advance, so that they are always in your fridge. This way you can less likely break your diet and get rid of unnecessary overeating. If you don't know what to cook, use the recipe generator which can help you with the meal for your certain list of food.

KETOGENIC RECIPES FOR BREAKFAST

Butter Eggs

Prep time: 10 minutes
Cook time: 15 minutes
Servings: 4
Ingredients:
- 1 teaspoon garlic powder
- 2 tablespoons butter
- 1 teaspoon ground paprika
- 6 eggs, hard-boiled

Method:
1. Peel and cut the eggs into halves.
2. Then melt butter in the skillet and add egg halves and roast them for 1 minute.
3. Sprinkle the eggs with garlic powder and ground paprika.

Nutritional info per serve: Calories 149, Fat 8.6, Fiber 0.3, Carbs 1.3, Protein 8.6

Sausage Sandwich

Prep time: 10 minutes
Cook time: 15 minutes
Servings: 4
Ingredients:
- 4 eggs
- 1 tablespoon butter
- 1 teaspoon ground black pepper
- 8 lettuce leaves
- 4 sausages

Method:
1. Toss the butter in the pan and melt it.
2. Crack the eggs inside and add sausages.
3. Close the lid and cook the ingredients for 5-8 minutes.
4. Then put the eggs and sausages on the lettuce leaves.

Nutritional info per serve: Calories 135, Fat 8.2, Fiber 0.2, Carbs 1, Protein 8.2

Beef Bowl

Prep time: 15 minutes
Cook time: 10 minutes
Servings: 1
Ingredients:
- 4 ounces ground beef
- 1 oz avocado, chopped
- 1 tomato, chopped
- 1 tablespoon butter
- 1 teaspoon chili powder
- 2 oz fresh cilantro, chopped

Method:
1. Put butter in the pan and melt it.
2. Add ground beef and add chili powder and cilantro.
3. Cook the ground beef for 10 minutes on medium heat.
4. Transfer the meat in the bowls and top with tomato and avocado.

Nutritional info per serve: Calories 403, Fat 25, Fiber 5.1, Carbs 8.4, Protein 37.1

Vanilla Pancakes

Prep time: 10 minutes
Cook time: 10 minutes
Servings: 4
Ingredients:
- 1.5 cups almond flour
- 1 teaspoon vanilla extract
- 3 eggs, beaten
- 1 teaspoon baking powder
- 1 teaspoon Erythritol
- 2 tablespoons avocado oil

Method:
1. Pour avocado oil in the skillet and heat it well.
2. Meanwhile, mix all remaining ingredients in the bowl and whisk until smooth.
3. Pour the small amount of almond flour mixture in the hot skillet and flatten in the shape of the pancake.
4. Roast the pancakes for 1 minute per side on medium-low heat.

Nutritional info per serve: Calories 313, Fat 13.2, Fiber 4.8, Carbs 11.6, Protein 13.2

Eggs Bake

Prep time: 10 minutes
Cook time: 15 minutes
Servings: 4
Ingredients:
- 8 eggs, beaten
- 1 cup Cheddar cheese, shredded
- 1 teaspoon chili flakes
- 1 cup spinach, chopped
- 4 teaspoons butter
- ½ teaspoon onion powder

Method:
1. Grease the ramekins with butter.
2. Then mix cheese with eggs, chili flakes, spinach, and onion powder.
3. Pour the mixture in the ramekins and cover with foil.
4. Bake the meal at 365F for 15 minutes.

Nutritional info per serve: Calories 276, Fat 18.4, Fiber 0.2, Carbs 1.6, Protein 18.4

Coconut Smoothie

Prep time: 5 minutes
Servings: 2
Ingredients:
- 1 cup of coconut milk
- 1 cup fresh spinach
- 2 pecans, grinded
- 1 cup fresh parsley

Method:
1. Put all ingredients in the food processor and blend until smooth.

2. Ladle the smoothie in the glasses.
Nutritional info per serve: Calories 388, Fat 5.6, Fiber 5.5, Carbs 11.1, Protein 624

Mushroom Scramble
Prep time: 10 minutes
Cook time: 15 minutes
Servings: 2
Ingredients:
- 1 cup cremini mushrooms, chopped
- 5 eggs, beaten
- 2 tablespoons butter
- 1 teaspoon salt
- ½ teaspoon ground black pepper

Method:
1. Put butter in the pan and melt it.
2. Add mushrooms, salt, and ground black pepper. Roast the mushrooms for 5-10 minutes on medium heat.
3. Then add beaten eggs and carefully stir the mixture.
4. Cook the scramble for 3 minutes.
Nutritional info per serve: Calories 270, Fat 14.9, Fiber 0.4, Carbs 2.7, Protein 14.9

Bacon Muffins
Prep time: 10 minutes
Cook time: 12 minutes
Servings: 4
Ingredients:
- 4 bacon slices, cooked, chopped
- 4 eggs, beaten
- 4 tablespoons almond flour
- 1 teaspoon salt
- 1 teaspoon ground turmeric
- 1 tablespoon avocado oil

Method:
1. Brush the muffin molds with avocado oil.
2. After this, in the mixing bowl, mix eggs with almond flour, salt, ground turmeric, and bacon.
3. Pour the batter in the muffin molds (fill ½ part of every mold) and bake at 365F for 12 minutes.
Nutritional info per serve: Calories 214, Fat 16.1, Fiber 1, Carbs 2.7, Protein 14.2

Mozzarella Frittata
Prep time: 10 minutes
Cook time: 25 minutes
Servings: 4
Ingredients:
- 8 eggs, beaten
- ½ teaspoon ground nutmeg
- ½ cup Mozzarella, shredded
- 1 tablespoon coconut cream
- ½ teaspoon ground black pepper
- 1 tablespoon butter

Method:
1. Melt the butter in the skillet.
2. After this, mix eggs with all remaining ingredients.
3. Pour the egg mixture in the hot butter and close the lid.
4. Cook the frittata on low heat with the closed lid for 20 minutes.
Nutritional info per serve: Calories 172, Fat 12.2, Fiber 0.2, Carbs 1.3, Protein 12.2

Eggs in Rings
Prep time: 10 minutes
Cook time: 10 minutes
Servings: 4
Ingredients:
- 1 sweet pepper
- 4 eggs
- 1 teaspoon butter
- ½ teaspoon olive oil
- ¼ teaspoon chili powder

Method:
1. Slice the sweet pepper into 4 rings.
2. Then put butter in the skillet. Add olive oil.
3. After this, add sweet pepper rings and roast them for 1 minute.
4. Flip the pepper rings on another side.
5. Crack the eggs inside pepper rings and sprinkle with chili powder.
6. Cook the eggs for 4 minutes on medium heat.
Nutritional info per serve: Calories 86, Fat 6, Fiber 0.5, Carbs 2.7, Protein 5.9

Salmon Eggs
Prep time: 10 minutes
Cook time: 10 minutes
Servings: 2
Ingredients:
- 4 eggs, whisked
- 4 oz salmon fillet, chopped
- 1 tablespoon butter
- 1 teaspoon salt
- 1 tablespoon chives, chopped

Method:
1. Melt the butter in the skillet.
2. Add salmon and sprinkle with salt and chives.
3. Roast the fish for 2-3 minutes.
4. Then add whisked eggs and close the lid.
5. Cook the meal on medium heat for 4-5 minutes or until the eggs are set.
Nutritional info per serve: Calories 252, Fat 18g, Fiber 0, Carbs 0.8, Protein 22.2g

Creamy Omelet Roll
Prep time: 15 minutes
Cook time: 7 minutes
Servings: 4
Ingredients:
- 8 eggs, whisked
- ¼ cup cream
- 2 oz scallions, chopped
- 1 teaspoon ground paprika
- 1 teaspoon ground black pepper
- 2 oz Cheddar cheese, shredded
- 2 tablespoons avocado oil

Method:
1. Pour avocado oil in the skillet. Heat it well.

2. In the mixing bowl, mix eggs with cream.
3. Pour the egg mixture in the skillet and flatten in the shape of pancake (make 4 egg pancakes).
4. Then sprinkle every egg pancake with scallions, ground paprika, ground black pepper, and cheese.
5. Roll the egg pancakes.
Nutritional info per serve: Calories 209, Fat 15.3, Fiber 1, Carbs 3.4, Protein 15.2

Asparagus Eggs

Prep time: 10 minutes
Cook time: 7 minutes
Servings: 2
Ingredients:
- 3 oz asparagus, chopped, boiled
- 4 eggs, beaten
- 1 tablespoon butter
- ½ teaspoon salt

Method:
1. Melt the butter in the skillet.
2. Add chopped asparagus and eggs.
3. Sprinkle them with salt and close the lid.
4. Cook the eggs in medium heat for 5-6 minutes.
Nutritional info per serve: Calories 185, Fat 14.6, Fiber 0.9, Carbs 2.3, Protein 12.1

Bacon and Eggs Rolls

Prep time: 10 minutes
Cook time: 10 minutes
Servings: 4
Ingredients:
- 8 oz bacon, sliced
- 2 eggs, beaten
- 1 teaspoon coconut oil
- ½ teaspoon salt
- ¼ teaspoon ground paprika
- ½ teaspoon dried parsley

Method:
1. Toss the coconut oil in the skillet.
2. Melt it and add sliced bacon. Roast the bacon on medium heat for 1 minute per side.
3. After this, mix eggs with salt, ground paprika, and parsley.
4. Pour the egg mixture over the bacon and close the lid.
5. Cook it on medium heat for 7 minutes.
6. Roll the cooked egg mixture into the roll and cut into serving.
Nutritional info per serve: Calories 348, Fat 27, Fiber 0.1, Carbs 1.1, Protein 23.8

Avocado Boats

Prep time: 10 minutes
Cook time: 15 minutes
Servings: 2
Ingredients:
- 1 avocado, cut in half and pitted
- 2 eggs
- 1 teaspoon butter, softened
- ½ teaspoon ground black pepper

Method:
1. Put the butter in the avocado holes.
2. Crack the eggs inside and sprinkle with ground black pepper.
3. Bake the avocado boats for 15 minutes.
Nutritional info per serve: Calories 286, Fat 25.9, Fiber 6.9, Carbs 9.3, Protein 7.5

Cheese Baked Eggs

Prep time: 15 minutes
Cook time: 10 minutes
Servings: 4
Ingredients:
- 4 eggs
- ½ cup Mozzarella, shredded
- 1 tablespoon butter, softened
- ½ teaspoon chili powder

Method:
1. Grease the ramekins with butter.
2. Then crack the eggs inside.
3. Add chili powder and Mozzarella.
4. Bake the eggs at 365f for 15 minutes
Nutritional info per serve: Calories 99, Fat 6.6, Fiber 0.1, Carbs 0.7, Protein 6.6

Cinnamon Eggs

Prep time: 8 minutes
Cook time: 7 minutes
Servings: 2
Ingredients:
- 4 eggs, hard-boiled, peeled
- 1 teaspoon ground cinnamon
- 1 tablespoon butter
- 1 teaspoon heavy cream

Method:
1. Melt the butter in the skillet.
2. Then cut the eggs into halves and put in the melted butter.
3. Sprinkle them with ground cinnamon and heavy cream and cook for 2-3 minutes more.
Nutritional info per serve: Calories 188, Fat 11.2, Fiber 0.6, Carbs 1.7, Protein 11.2

Cauliflower Cakes

Prep time: 15 minutes
Cook time: 12 minutes
Servings: 3
Ingredients:
- 1 cup cauliflower, shredded
- 5 oz Parmesan, grated
- 3 eggs, beaten
- 1 teaspoon white pepper
- 1 tablespoon coconut flour

Method:
1. In the mixing bowl mix cauliflower with parmesan, eggs, white pepper, and coconut flour.
2. Make the cauliflower cakes and put them in the tray.
3. Bake the cauliflower cakes for 10-12 minutes at 365F.
Nutritional info per serve: Calories 235, Fat 14.8, Fiber 2, Carbs 5.9, Protein 21.8

Seafood Mix

Prep time: 10 minutes
Cook time: 15 minutes
Servings: 3
Ingredients:
- 4 bacon slices, chopped, cooked
- 4 ounces salmon, chopped
- 4 ounces shrimp, peeled
- 1 cup heavy cream

Method:
1. Pour heavy cream in the pan and bring it to boil.
2. Add bacon, salmon, and shrimps.
3. Close the lid and cook the meal on medium heat for 10 minutes.

Nutritional info per serve: Calories 370, Fat 28.4, Fiber 0, Carbs 2.1, Protein 26.1

Dill Eggs

Prep time: 10 minutes
Cook time: 7 minutes
Servings: 2
Ingredients:
- 2 eggs
- 1 teaspoon butter
- 1 tablespoon fresh dill, chopped
- ¼ teaspoon jalapeno pepper, diced

Method:
1. Melt the butter in the skillet and crack eggs inside.
2. Sprinkle them with dill and jalapeno.
3. Close the lid and cook the eggs for 5 minutes on medium heat.

Nutritional info per serve: Calories 84, Fat 6.4, Fiber 0.2, Carbs 1.2, Protein 5.9

Chorizo Eggs

Prep time: 10 minutes
Cook time: 12 minutes
Servings: 4
Ingredients:
- 4 eggs
- 6 oz chorizo, chopped
- 1 tablespoon avocado oil
- 1 tomato, chopped
- 1 teaspoon chili powder

Method:
1. Put the chorizo in the skillet.
2. Add avocado oil and roast for 4 minutes.
3. Then stir the chorizo and crack eggs.
4. Add tomato and chili powder.
5. Cook the eggs on medium heat for 7 minutes.

Nutritional info per serve: Calories 266, Fat 21.2, Fiber 0.6, Carbs 2.3, Protein 16.1

Herbed Eggs

Prep time: 10 minutes
Cook time: 12 minutes
Servings: 4
Ingredients:
- 4 eggs, beaten
- ¼ cup coconut cream
- 1 cup spinach, chopped
- 1 tablespoon butter
- ½ teaspoon salt
- 3 oz Mozzarella, shredded
- 1 teaspoon dried oregano

Method:
1. In the mixing bowl mix eggs with coconut cream, spinach, salt, and dried oregano.
2. Melt the butter in the skillet and add egg mixture.
3. After this, add mozzarella and close the lid.
4. Cook the meal on medium heat for 10 minutes.

Nutritional info per serve: Calories 156, Fat 10.9, Fiber 1.4, Carbs 2.4, Protein 12.2

Eggs and Beef Pie

Prep time: 15 minutes
Cook time: 40 minutes
Servings: 4
Ingredients:
- ½ spring onion, chopped
- 1 cup ground beef
- 1 teaspoon salt
- 3 tablespoons taco seasoning
- ½ cup fresh cilantro, chopped
- 8 eggs
- 1 teaspoon avocado oil

Method:
1. Brush the pie mold with avocado oil.
2. After this, in the mixing bowl mix chopped spring onion, ground beef, salt, taco seasoning, and cilantro.
3. Carefully mix the mixture and add cracked eggs. Mix it until homogenous.
4. Then transfer the mixture in the prepared mold and flatten.
5. Bake the beef pie for 40 minutes at 365F.

Nutritional info per serve: Calories 218, Fat 13, Fiber 0.4, Carbs 6.1, Protein 17.8

Keto Coffee

Prep time: 5 minutes
Cook time: 10 minutes
Servings: 2
Ingredients:
- 2 teaspoons instant coffee
- 1 cup of water
- 1/3 cup butter

Method:
1. Bring the water to boil and add instant coffee. Stir it well.
2. Then pour the coffee in the glasses and add butter.
3. Carefully mix the drink until butter is dissolved.

Nutritional info per serve: Calories 271, Fat 30.7, Fiber 0, Carbs 0, Protein 0.3

Bok Choy Pan

Prep time: 10 minutes
Cook time: 15 minutes

Servings: 2
Ingredients:
- 6 oz bok choy, sliced
- 1 tablespoon avocado oil
- 2 eggs, beaten
- 1 teaspoon chili powder

Method:
1. Heat the avocado oil in the pan.
2. Add sliced bok choy and sprinkle it with chili powder.
3. Roast the bok choy for 4-5 minutes. Stir it occasionally.
4. Then egg eggs and close the lid.
5. Cook the meal on medium heat for 4-7 minutes or until the eggs are set.

Nutritional info per serve: Calories 87, Fat 5.7, Fiber 1.6, Carbs 3.3, Protein 7.1

Cheesy Fritatta

Prep time: 10 minutes
Cook time: 15 minutes
Servings: 4
Ingredients:
- 5 eggs, beaten
- 1 tablespoon cream cheese
- 4 jalapeno pepper, sliced
- 3 oz Cheddar cheese, shredded
- ¼ cup cream
- 1 teaspoon avocado oil

Method:
1. Heat the avocado oil in the skillet.
2. Then mix eggs with cream cheese and cream.
3. Pour the liquid in the skillet and top with jalapeno peppers and cheddar cheese.
4. Close the lid and cook the frittata on medium heat for 15 minutes.

Nutritional info per serve: Calories 188, Fat 14.5, Fiber 0.4, Carbs 2.1, Protein 12.7

Pork Pan

Prep time: 10 minutes
Cook time: 15 minutes
Servings: 4
Ingredients:
- 1 teaspoon ground black pepper
- 1 pound minced pork
- 1 tablespoon avocado oil
- ½ teaspoon garlic powder
- 2 oz scallions, chopped

Method:
1. Heat the avocado oil in the pan.
2. Then add minced pork, ground black pepper, and garlic powder.
3. Roast the mixture for 10-15 minutes.
4. Transfer the cooked pork in the bowls and top with scallions.

Nutritional info per serve: Calories 174, Fat 4.5, Fiber 0.7, Carbs 1.8, Protein 30.1

Basil Scramble

Prep time: 10 minutes
Cook time: 15 minutes
Servings: 4
Ingredients:
- 1 teaspoon fresh basil, chopped
- 8 eggs, beaten
- 2 oz bacon, chopped
- ½ teaspoon salt
- 1 teaspoon olive oil

Method:
1. Heat the olive oil well.
2. Add bacon and roast it for 4-5 minutes or until it is cooked.
3. Add eggs, salt, and fresh basil.
4. Stir the eggs from time to time for 10 minutes or until they are set.

Nutritional info per serve: Calories 213, Fat 15.8, Fiber 0, Carbs 0.9, Protein 16.3

Egg Casserole

Prep time: 10 minutes
Cook time: 40 minutes
Servings: 4
Ingredients:
- 8 eggs, beaten
- 1-pound pork sausage, chopped
- 1 oz Parmesan, grated
- 1 tablespoon avocado oil

Method:
1. Brush the casserole mold with avocado oil.
2. After this, in the mixing bowl mix eggs with pork sausages.
3. Then pour the mixture in the prepared casserole mold.
4. Top it with Parmesan and bake in the preheated to 360F oven or 40 minutes.

Nutritional info per serve: Calories 538, Fat 42.9, Fiber 0.2, Carbs 1.1, Protein 35.4

Coconut Pancakes

Prep time: 10 minutes
Cook time: 15 minutes
Servings: 4
Ingredients:
- ½ cup almond flour
- ½ cup coconut flour
- 1 tablespoon coconut shred
- 1 tablespoon Erythritol
- 1 teaspoon baking powder
- ½ teaspoon vanilla extract
- 1 tablespoon avocado oil
- ½ cup heavy cream

Method:
1. Heat the skillet and pour avocado oil inside.
2. Then mix all remaining ingredients in the bowl, stir it until you get a smooth batter.
3. Pour the small amount of batter in the hot skillet and flatten it in the shape of a pancake.
4. Roast the pancake on medium heat for 1 minute per side.
5. Repeat the same steps with all remaining batter.

Nutritional info per serve: Calories 216, Fat 15.4, Fiber 7.9, Carbs 18.5, Protein 5.4

Pork Cakes

Prep time: 15 minutes
Cook time: 25 minutes
Servings: 4
Ingredients:
- 1 pound minced pork
- 1 teaspoon dried cilantro
- 1 teaspoon garlic powder
- 1 egg, beaten
- 1 tablespoon coconut oil

Method:
1. In the mixing bowl, mix minced pork with dried cilantro, garlic powder, and egg.
2. Then grease the casserole mold with coconut oil.
3. Make the small cakes from the pork mixture and put it in the casserole mold.
4. Cook the pork cakes in the oven at 365F for 25 minutes.

Nutritional info per serve: Calories 210, Fat 8.5, Fiber 0.1, Carbs 0.6, Protein 31.2

Cauliflower Bowl

Prep time: 15 minutes
Cook time: 30 minutes
Servings: 4
Ingredients:
- 1-pound cauliflower, head
- 1 scallion, diced
- 1 carrot, chopped
- 1 jalapeno pepper, chopped
- ¼ cup coconut cream
- 1 teaspoon ground black pepper

Method:
1. In the mixing bowl mix scallion, carrot, jalapeno pepper, and coconut cream. Add ground black pepper.
2. After this, chop the cauliflower into small pieces and mix with the carrot mixture.
3. Transfer the ingredients in the baking mold and bake at 365F for 30 minutes.
4. Transfer the cooked vegetables in the bowls.

Nutritional info per serve: Calories 83, Fat 3.8, Fiber 4.4, Carbs 11.5, Protein 3.1

Keto Bake

Prep time: 10 minutes
Cook time: 30 minutes
Servings: 6
Ingredients:
- 12 oz pork sausage, chopped
- ¼ cup heavy cream
- 1 tablespoon fresh dill
- 6 eggs, beaten
- 1 oz Parmesan, grated

Method:
1. Put the chopped pork sausages in the baking pan and flatten.
2. Then top them with fresh dill and parmesan.
3. In the mixing bowl, mix eggs with heavy cream. Pour the liquid over the pork sausages.
4. Bake the meal at 365F for 30 minutes.

Nutritional info per serve: Calories 289, Fat 23.3, Fiber 0.1, Carbs 0.9, Protein 18.3

Poached Eggs

Prep time: 10 minutes
Cook time: 10 minutes
Servings: 2
Ingredients:
- 4 eggs
- 1 tablespoon apple cider vinegar
- 1 teaspoon ground black pepper
- 1 cup water, for cooking

Method:
1. Pour water in the pan and make it hot but not boiling.
2. Add apple cider vinegar.
3. Then start to stir the water and crack the egg inside.
4. Cook it for 2 minutes. Then remove it from the water with the help of the ladle.
5. Repeat the same steps with remaining eggs.
6. Sprinkle the eggs with ground black pepper.

Nutritional info per serve: Calories 130, Fat 8.8, Fiber 0.3, Carbs 1.4, Protein 11.2

Coconut Eggs

Prep time: 10 minutes
Cook time: 20 minutes
Servings: 4
Ingredients:
- 1-pound sausage, chopped
- 8 eggs, beaten
- ¼ cup of coconut milk
- 1 tablespoon coconut shred
- 1 teaspoon garlic powder

Method:
1. Preheat the skillet well and add sausages.
2. Roast them for 5 minutes.
3. Then stir well and sprinkle with garlic powder and coconut shred.
4. Pour the eggs over the sausages and bake the meal at 365F for 10 minutes.

Nutritional info per serve: Calories 560, Fat 45.8, Fiber 0.7, Carbs 2.5, Protein 33.6

Chorizo Pizza

Prep time: 10 minutes
Cook time: 20 minutes
Servings: 4
Ingredients:
- 5 oz chorizo, chopped
- 4 oz Parmesan, grated
- 1 bell pepper, diced
- 1 tablespoon butter

Method:
1. Grease the pizza pan with butter.
2. Then mix chorizo with bell pepper and put over butter.
3. Top the mixture with Parmesan and bake the pizza at 360F for 20 minutes.

Nutritional info per serve: Calories 287, Fat 22.6, Fiber 0.4, Carbs 3.9, Protein 18

Jalapeno Bake

Prep time: 10 minutes
Cook time: 25 minutes
Servings: 4
Ingredients:
- 4 links chorizo, chopped
- 12 oz jalapeno, chopped
- 6 eggs, beaten
- 1 teaspoon olive oil
- 1 teaspoon dried oregano

Method:
1. Brush the ramekins with olive oil.
2. Then mix eggs with dried oregano and jalapenos.
3. Pour the liquid in the ramekins and top with chorizo.
4. Bake the meal at 360F for 25 minutes.

Nutritional info per serve: Calories 404, Fat 31.3, Fiber 2.5, Carbs 6.9, Protein 24

Parsley Eggs

Prep time: 10 minutes
Cook time: 8 minutes
Servings: 4
Ingredients:
- 8 eggs
- 1 oz fresh parsley, chopped
- 1 teaspoon ground paprika
- 1 tablespoon avocado oil

Method:
1. Preheat the skillet well.
2. Add avocado oil and heat it for 1 minute.
3. Then crack the eggs and sprinkle them with parsley and ground paprika.
4. Cook the meal on medium heat for 4-5 minutes or until the egg yolks are set.

Nutritional info per serve: Calories 135, Fat 9.3, Fiber 0.6, Carbs 1.6, Protein 11.4

Stuffed Avocado

Prep time: 10 minutes
Servings: 1
Ingredients:
- 1 avocado, halved, pitted
- 5 oz smoked salmon, chopped
- 1 garlic clove, diced
- 1 teaspoon olive oil
- ½ teaspoon lemon juice

Method:
1. In the mixing bowl, mix smoked salmon, garlic, olive oil, and lemon juice.
2. Then fill the halved avocado with salmon mixture.

Nutritional info per serve: Calories 621, Fat 50, Fiber 13.5, Carbs 18.3, Protein 29.9

Butternut Squash Spaghetti with Salami

Prep time: 10 minutes
Cook time: 45 minutes
Servings: 4
Ingredients:
- 4 tablespoons coconut oil
- 1 cup butternut squash, halved
- ½ cup tomatoes, cored and chopped
- ½ teaspoon Italian seasoning
- 3 ounces Italian salami, chopped, cooked
- 4 eggs

Method:
1. Put the butternut squash in the tray and bake at 365F for 30 minutes.
2. Then shred the squash with the help of the fork into the spaghetti and mix with Italian seasonings, tomatoes, and coconut oil.
3. Add salami.
4. Carefully mix the mixture and put it in the baking pan.
5. Crack the eggs over the butternut squash mixture and bake at 365F for 10 minutes.

Nutritional info per serve: Calories 237, Fat 19.6, Fiber 1.2, Carbs 9.5, Protein 7.7

Mozzarella Pancakes

Prep time: 10 minutes
Cook time: 10 minutes
Servings: 2
Ingredients:
- ½ cup Mozzarella, shredded
- 3 eggs, beaten
- ½ teaspoon salt
- 1 tablespoon olive oil
- 1 teaspoon dried oregano

Method:
1. Preheat the olive oil in the skillet well.
2. Then mix all remaining ingredients in the bowl.
3. Pour the small amount of the liquid in the hot skillet and make the pancake.
4. Cook it for 1 minute per side.
5. Repeat the same steps with the remaining pancake batter.

Nutritional info per serve: Calories 177, Fat 14.9, Fiber 0.3, Carbs 1.2, Protein 10.4

Almond Porridge

Prep time: 5 minutes
Cook time: 15 minutes
Servings: 2
Ingredients:
- 1 teaspoon ground nutmeg
- ½ cup almonds, ground
- 1 teaspoon Erythritol
- ¾ cup heavy cream

Method:
1. In the mixing bowl mix all ingredients and transfer in the ramekins.
2. Bake the porridge at 355F for 10-15 minutes.

Nutritional info per serve: Calories 298, Fat 28.9, Fiber 3.2, Carbs 9.4, Protein 6

Vanilla Chai

Prep time: 5 minutes
Cook time: 15 minutes
Servings: 2
Ingredients:
- 2 tablespoons chai tea

- 2 cups of water
- 1 teaspoon vanilla extract
- ¼ cup heavy cream

Method:
1. Bring the water to boil.
2. Add chai tea, vanilla extract, and heavy cream.
3. Simmer the mixture for 2-3 minutes.
4. Sift the chai and transfer in the serving glasses.

Nutritional info per serve: Calories 58, Fat 5.6, Fiber 0, Carbs 0.7, Protein 0.3

Blackberry Granola

Prep time: 7 minutes
Cook time: 0 minutes
Servings: 2
Ingredients:
- 2 pecans, chopped
- ¼ cup blackberries
- 1 oz dark chocolate, chopped

Method:
1. Mix all ingredients in the mixing bowl.
2. Transfer the mixture in the serving bowls.

Nutritional info per serve: Calories 181, Fat 14.3, Fiber 2.9, Carbs 12.2, Protein 2.8

Cauli Bowl

Prep time: 10 minutes
Cook time: 25 minutes
Servings: 4
Ingredients:
- 1 cup ground pork
- 1 cup cauliflower, chopped
- 1 teaspoon chili powder
- ½ cup coconut cream
- 1 tablespoon avocado oil

Method:
1. In the mixing bowl mix all ingredients and put in the casserole mold.
2. Bake it at 365F for 25 minutes.
3. Then stir the cooked meal and put it in the serving bowls.

Nutritional info per serve: Calories 314, Fat 24, Fiber 1.7, Carbs 3.6, Protein 21.4

Coconut Chia

Prep time: 15 minutes
Cook time: 0 minutes.
Servings: 2
Ingredients:
- 2 pecans, chopped
- 2 tablespoons flax seeds
- ½ full-fat milk
- 1 tablespoon chia seeds

Method:
1. Mix chis seeds with flax seeds.
2. Add milk and leave it for 10 minutes.
3. After this, add pecans, carefully mix the meal, and put in the serving glasses.

Nutritional info per serve: Calories 241, Fat 18.6, Fiber 8.3, Carbs 13, Protein 7.1

Cauliflower Cupcakes

Prep time: 10 minutes
Cook time: 13 minutes
Servings: 6
Ingredients:
- 6 tablespoons almond flour
- 1/3 cup cauliflower, chopped
- 6 eggs, beaten
- ½ teaspoon salt
- 3 teaspoons olive oil

Method:
1. In the mixing bowl mix almond flour with eggs, salt, and olive oil.
2. When the liquid is smooth, add cauliflower.
3. Put the mixture in the muffin molds and transfer it in the oven.
4. Bake the cupcakes at 365F for 13 minutes.

Nutritional info per serve: Calories 126, Fat 10, Fiber 0.9, Carbs 2.1, Protein 7.2

Walnut Bowls

Prep time: 5 minutes
Cook time: 0 minutes
Servings: 1
Ingredients:
- 1 pecan, chopped
- ½ cup heavy cream
- 1 teaspoon walnuts, chopped
- 1 tablespoon Erythritol
- 1 teaspoon vanilla extract

Method:
1. Put all ingredients in the mixing bowl. Carefully mix it.
2. Put the mixture in the serving bowls.

Nutritional info per serve: Calories 333, Fat 33.7, Fiber 1.7, Carbs 4.5, Protein 3.4

Kale Bake

Prep time: 10 minutes
Cook time: 8 minutes
Servings: 2
Ingredients:
- 4 eggs, beaten
- 3 oz Cheddar cheese, shredded
- 1 cup kale, chopped
- ½ teaspoon cayenne pepper
- 1 teaspoon olive oil

Method:
1. Brush the ramekins with olive oil.
2. After this, mix eggs with cheese, and cayenne pepper.
3. Put the kale in the bottom of the ramekins and top with egg mixture.
4. Bake the kale mixture for 8 minutes at 365F.

Nutritional info per serve: Calories 335, Fat 25.3, Fiber 0.6, Carbs 5, Protein 22.7

Mug Bread

Prep time: 10 minutes
Cook time: 18 minutes
Servings: 4
Ingredients:

- ½ teaspoon baking powder
- ⅓ cup coconut flour
- 2 eggs, beaten
- 1 teaspoon cream cheese
- 1 teaspoon coconut oil

Method:
1. Grease mugs with the coconut oil.
2. After this, in the mixing bowl, mix all ingredients.
3. Transfer the mixture in the prepared mugs.
4. Bake the bread at 360F for 18 minutes.

Nutritional info per serve: Calories 85, Fat 4.6, Fiber 4, Carbs 7.2, Protein 4.2

Cream Cheese Eggs

Prep time: 15 minutes
Cook time: 10 minutes
Servings: 2
Ingredients:
- 1 avocado, peeled, pitted, sliced
- 6 bacon slices
- 2 eggs, beaten
- 1 tablespoon cream cheese
- 1 tablespoon coconut oil

Method:
1. Melt the coconut oil in the skillet.
2. Then add bacon and roast it for 1 minute per side.
3. Add eggs and roast them for 4 minutes.
4. After this, cut the egg mixture into halves and transfer in the serving plates.
5. Top the eggs with cream cheese and avocado.

Nutritional info per serve: Calories 652, Fat 56.3, Fiber 6.7, Carbs 9.9, Protein 28.9

Scallions Muffins

Prep time: 10 minutes
Cook time: 12 minutes
Servings: 4
Ingredients:
- ¼ cup of coconut milk
- 4 eggs, beaten
- 1 tablespoon coconut oil
- 2 oz scallions, chopped
- 1 tablespoon coconut flour

Method:
1. Put all ingredients in the mixing bowl and stir until homogenous.
2. Then pour the mixture in the muffin molds.
3. Bake the muffins at 360F for 12 minutes.

Nutritional info per serve: Calories 139, Fat 11.6, Fiber 1.5, Carbs 3.5, Protein 138

Zucchini Latkes

Prep time: 10 minutes
Cook time: 15 minutes
Servings: 4
Ingredients:
- 1 zucchini, grated
- 1 egg, whisked
- 1 oz carrot, grated
- 1 teaspoon ground black pepper
- 1 tablespoon avocado oil

Method:
1. In the mixing bowl, mix grated zucchini, egg, carrot, and ground black pepper.
2. Then preheat the avocado oil well.
3. With the help of the spoon make the small latkes and transfer them in the hot oil.
4. Cook the latkes for 3 minutes per side on medium heat.

Nutritional info per serve: Calories 32, Fat 1.6, Fiber 1, Carbs 3, Protein 2.1

Cauliflower Bread

Prep time: 10 minutes
Cook time: 25 minutes
Servings: 7
Ingredients:
- 1 cauliflower head, shredded
- ½ cup coconut flour
- 5 eggs, beaten
- 1 tablespoon butter, melted
- 1 tablespoon cream cheese

Method:
1. In the mixing bowl, mix butter, cream cheese, eggs, and coconut flour.
2. When the mixture is smooth, add shredded cauliflower and transfer the mixture in the bread mold. Flatten it.
3. Bake the bread at 365F for 25 minutes.

Nutritional info per serve: Calories 108, Fat 6.2, Fiber 4.4, Carbs 8, Protein 6

Cream Muffins

Prep time: 10 minutes
Cook time: 13 minutes
Servings: 2
Ingredients:
- 4 eggs, whisked
- 1 tablespoon almond flour
- 1 tablespoon heavy cream
- ½ teaspoon chili powder

Method:
1. Put all ingredients in the mixing bowl and mix until you get a smooth batter.
2. Then pour the batter in the muffin molds.
3. Bake them at 360F for 13 minutes.

Nutritional info per serve: Calories 234, Fat 18.6, Fiber 1.7, Carbs 4.3, Protein 14.3

Guacamole Sandwich

Prep time: 10 minutes
Cook time: 7 minutes
Servings: 2
Ingredients:
- 1 egg, beaten
- 2 grain-free bread slices
- 1 teaspoon olive oil
- 1 tablespoon guacamole

Method:
1. Preheat the skillet well.
2. Add olive oil and egg. Flatten the egg in the shape of pancake and roast for 1.5 minutes per side.

3. Then cut the cooked egg pancake into halves.
4. Put every egg half on the bread slices.
5. Add guacamole.
Nutritional info per serve: Calories 145, Fat 8.7, Fiber 2.4, Carbs 12.6, Protein 3.9

Brussel Sprouts with Eggs
Prep time: 10 minutes
Cook time: 25 minutes
Servings: 4
Ingredients:
- 1 cup Brussel Sprouts, boiled, halved
- 4 eggs
- 1 tablespoon butter
- 1 teaspoon ground paprika

Method:
1. Grease the baking pan with butter.
2. Then mix Brussel sprouts with ground paprika and eggs.
3. Pour the mixture in the baking pan and cover with foil.
4. Bake the meal at 360F for 25 minutes.
Nutritional info per serve: Calories 99, Fat 7.4, Fiber 1, Carbs 2.6, Protein 6.4

Cayenne Muffins
Prep time: 10 minutes
Cook time: 14 minutes
Servings: 3
Ingredients:
- ½ cup ground chicken
- ½ teaspoon ground black pepper
- ½ teaspoon onion powder
- 1 tablespoon cayenne pepper
- 4 eggs, beaten
- 1 tablespoon coconut oil, melted

Method:
1. Mix all ingredients from the list above in the mixing bowl.
2. When the liquid is smooth, pour it in the muffin molds.
3. Bake the muffins at 360F for 14 minutes.
Nutritional info per serve: Calories 175, Fat 12.4, Fiber 0.6, Carbs 2, Protein 14.4

Creamy Ramekins
Prep time: 10 minutes
Cook time: 30 minutes
Servings: 2
Ingredients:
- 1 tablespoon coconut flakes
- 4 eggs, beaten
- 3 tablespoons coconut oil
- 3 tablespoons coconut flour
- ½ cup coconut cream

Method:
1. Mix coconut cream with coconut flour, coconut flakes, and eggs.
2. Then pour the liquid in the ramekins.
3. Bake them for 25 minutes at 350F.
4. Then add coconut oil and cook the meal for 5 minutes more.

Nutritional info per serve: Calories 545, Fat 50.1, Fiber 6.8, Carbs 13.5, Protein 14.4

Onion Cookies
Prep time: 15 minutes
Cook time: 12 minutes
Servings: 6
Ingredients:
- 6 tablespoons coconut oil
- 6 tablespoons almond flour
- 1 spring onion, minced
- 2 eggs, beaten
- 2 tablespoons heavy cream
- ½ teaspoon apple cider vinegar
- ¼ teaspoon baking soda

Method:
1. In the mixing bowl, mix coconut oil with almond flour, minced spring onion, eggs, heavy cream, apple cider vinegar, and baking soda.
2. Knead the dough and make the small balls.
3. Then press the dough balls gently to get the shape of cookies.
4. Bake them at 360F for 12 minutes.
Nutritional info per serve: Calories 323, Fat 30.9, Fiber 3.4, Carbs 8, Protein 8.2

Chia Smoothie
Prep time: 20 minutes
Servings: 2
Ingredients:
- 1 avocado, pitted
- ½ cup organic almond milk
- 1 tablespoon chia seeds
- 1 scoop protein powder

Method:
1. Blend the avocado until smooth and mix it with almond milk, chia seeds, and protein powder.
2. Leave the smoothie for 20 minutes and then transfer in the glasses.
Nutritional info per serve: Calories 437, Fat 37, Fiber 10.5, Carbs 16.8, Protein 15.5

Chives and Bacon Muffins
Prep time: 10 minutes
Cook time: 15 minutes
Servings: 4
Ingredients:
- 4 eggs, beaten
- 2 bacon slices, chopped, cooked
- ¼ cup heavy cream
- 1 teaspoon baking powder
- ½ cup coconut flour

Method:
1. In the mixing bowl, mix eggs with heavy cream, baking powder, and coconut flour.
2. After this, add chopped bacon and carefully mix the batter.
3. Transfer the egg mixture in the muffin molds and bake at 360F for 15 minutes.
Nutritional info per serve: Calories 201, Fat 12.6, Fiber 6, Carbs 11.3, Protein 11.2

Oregano Frittata

Prep time: 10 minutes
Cook time: 15 minutes
Servings: 2
Ingredients:
- ¼ cup coconut cream
- 4 eggs, beaten
- 6 oz shrimps, peeled
- 1 tablespoon dried oregano
- 1 tablespoon avocado oil

Method:
1. Preheat the skillet well and add avocado oil.
2. Then mix coconut cream with eggs, and dried oregano.
3. Pour the liquid in the hot skillet with oil.
4. Then top the egg mixture with shrimps and transfer in the preheated to 360F oven.
5. Bake the frittata for 15 minutes.

Nutritional info per serve: Calories 312, Fat 18.5, Fiber 1.9, Carbs 5.5, Protein 31.5

Thyme Muffins

Prep time: 10 minutes
Cook time: 15 minutes
Servings: 6
Ingredients:
- 1 teaspoon dried thyme
- ½ cup butter softened
- 3 cups coconut flour
- 1 teaspoon baking soda
- 4 eggs, beaten

Method:
1. In the mixing bowl, mix thyme with butter, coconut flour, baking soda, and eggs.
2. Stir the mixture until you get a smooth batter.
3. Then pour it in the muffin molds (fill ½ part of every mold) and bake at 360F for 15 minutes.

Nutritional info per serve: Calories 456, Fat 26.4, Fiber 28.1, Carbs 35.8, Protein 13.5

Beef Casserole

Prep time: 10 minutes
Cook time: 45 minutes
Servings: 6
Ingredients:
- 1 cup broccoli florets, chopped
- 3 oz Parmesan, grated
- 1 cup heavy cream
- 8 oz beef brisket, chopped
- 1 spring onion, sliced
- 1 tablespoon olive oil
- ½ teaspoon ground black pepper
- 1 teaspoon dried dill

Method:
1. Brush the casserole mold with olive oil.
2. After this, mix chopped beef with spring onion, ground black pepper, and dried dill.
3. Put the mixture in the casserole mold and flatten well.
4. After this, add the layer of broccoli and parmesan.
5. Add heavy cream and bake the casserole at 360F for 45 minutes.

Nutritional info per serve: Calories 218, Fat 15.2, Fiber 0.9, Carbs 4, Protein 17.1

Monterey Jack Muffins

Prep time: 10 minutes
Cook time: 14 minutes
Servings: 6
Ingredients:
- 2 tablespoons olive oil
- 1 egg, beaten
- 1 cup Monterey Jack cheese, shredded
- 1 cup almond flour
- ¼ teaspoon baking soda
- ½ cup of coconut milk

Method:
1. Brush the muffin molds with olive oil.
2. Then mix all remaining ingredients in the mixing bowl.
3. Fill ½ part of every muffin mold with batter and bake at 360F for 14 minutes.

Nutritional info per serve: Calories 193, Fat 18.2, Fiber 0.9, Carbs 2.3, Protein 7

Shrimps Pan

Prep time: 10 minutes
Cook time: 10 minutes
Servings: 4
Ingredients:
- 1 cup bell pepper, chopped
- 1-pound shrimps, peeled
- ½ teaspoon ground thyme
- ½ teaspoon paprika
- 1 tablespoon coconut oil

Method:
1. Melt the coconut oil in the pan.
2. Add bell pepper, ground thyme, and paprika.
3. Roast the vegetable for 4 minutes.
4. Add shrimps and stir well.
5. Cook the meal on medium heat for 5 minutes more.

Nutritional info per serve: Calories 175, Fat 5.4, Fiber 0.6, Carbs 4.2, Protein 26.2

Chicken Scramble

Prep time: 10 minutes
Cook time: 15 minutes
Servings: 1
Ingredients:
- ¼ cup ground chicken
- ¼ teaspoon ground black pepper
- 2 tablespoons avocado oil
- 2 eggs, beaten

Method:
1. Put the ground chicken in the pan and add avocado oil.
2. Roast the mixture for 5 minutes on medium heat.
3. Then add ground black pepper and eggs.
4. Cook the mixture for 10 minutes, stir it constantly.

Nutritional info per serve: Calories 231, Fat 14.9, Fiber 1.4, Carbs 2.6, Protein 21.6

Chia Drink

Prep time: 25 minutes
Cook time: 0 minutes
Servings: 4
Ingredients:
- 1 cup of coconut milk
- 2 tablespoons chia seeds
- ½ cup of water

Method:
1. Mix coconut milk with water and pour in the glasses.
2. Then add 1 tablespoon of chia seeds in every glass and leave for 25 minutes.

Nutritional info per serve: Calories 172, Fat 16.5, Fiber 3.8, Carbs 6.3, Protein 2.5

Strawberry Pudding

Prep time: 20 minutes
Cook time: 0 minutes
Servings: 4
Ingredients:
- 2 cups of coconut milk
- 1 tablespoon chia seeds
- 1 oz strawberries, sliced

Method:
1. Mix coconut milk with chia seeds and leave for 25 minutes in a warm place.
2. Then top the pudding with sliced strawberries.

Nutritional info per serve: Calories 296, Fat 29.7, Fiber 4, Carbs 8.7, Protein 3.4

Egg Burrito

Prep time: 10 minutes
Cook time: 20 minutes
Servings: 1
Ingredients:
- 1 teaspoon coconut oil
- 1 teaspoon garlic powder
- 2 oz ground beef
- ¼ spring onion, sliced
- 2 eggs, beaten

Method:
1. Melt the coconut oil in the skillet.
2. Then add ground beef and garlic powder.
3. Roast the mixture for 15 minutes on medium heat.
4. After this, remove the ground beef from the skillet.
5. Add beaten eggs and flatten them in the shape of the crepe. Roast the eggs for 1 minute per side or until they are solid.
6. Then fill the egg pancake with ground beef mixture and spring onion.
7. Roll it in the shape of buritto.

Nutritional info per serve: Calories 291, Fat 16.9, Fiber 0.9, Carbs 5.3, Protein 29

Egg Balls

Prep time: 10 minutes
Cook time: 0 minutes
Servings: 4
Ingredients:
- 4 oz bacon, chopped, cooked
- 4 eggs, boiled, peeled
- 1 tablespoon cream cheese
- 1 teaspoon onion powder
- 1 teaspoon butter, softened

Method:
1. Mix all ingredients in the mixing bowl.
2. Then make the small balls with the help of the scooper.
3. Store the egg balls in the fridge for up to 1 day.

Nutritional info per serve: Calories 236, Fat 18.1, Fiber 0, Carbs 1.3, Protein 16.3

Radish Hash

Prep time: 10 minutes
Cook time: 11 minutes
Servings: 2
Ingredients:
- 1 tablespoon butter
- ¼ teaspoon garlic powder
- 1 scallion, chopped
- 4 oz corned beef, chopped, cooked
- 2 cups radishes, cut in quarters

Method:
1. Toss the butter in the skillet and preheat it.
2. Add scallion and roast for 4 minutes.
3. Then add garlic powder, corned beef, and radishes.
4. Stir the ingredients well and close the lid.
5. Cook them for 5 minutes.

Nutritional info per serve: Calories 189, Fat 13, Fiber 3.1, Carbs 9.3, Protein 9.1

Chia Bowls

Prep time: 10 minutes
Cook time: 10 minutes
Servings: 4
Ingredients:
- 1 ½ cup of coconut milk
- 2 tablespoons chia seeds
- 3 oz Cheddar cheese, grated
- ½ teaspoon chili flakes
- ½ teaspoon salt
- 1 tablespoon coconut oil

Method:
1. In the mixing bowl mix all ingredients.
2. Make the small balls and refrigerate them for 10-15 minutes.

Nutritional info per serve: Calories 357, Fat 34.1, Fiber 4.4, Carbs 8.3, Protein 8.5

Bacon Mix

Prep time: 10 minutes
Cook time: 20 minutes
Servings: 3
Ingredients:
- 3 eggs, beaten
- 1 tablespoon coconut oil, melted
- 1 scallion, minced
- 1 cup Brussel sprouts, sliced
- 3 bacon slices, chopped
- 1½ chili powder

Method:
1. Put all ingredients in the big bowl and carefully mix.
2. Then transfer the mixture in the baking pan, flatten it if needed.
3. Bake the bacon mix for 20 minutes at 355F.
Nutritional info per serve: Calories 233, Fat 17.1, Fiber 2, Carbs 6.9, Protein 14

Basil Scotch Eggs

Prep time: 15 minutes
Cook time: 30 minutes
Servings: 4
Ingredients:
- 4 eggs, boiled
- 1 ½ cup ground pork
- ½ teaspoon white pepper
- ½ teaspoon dried basil
- 1 tablespoon butter

Method:
1. In the mixing bowl, mix ground pork with white pepper, and dried basil.
2. Then make 4 balls from the meat mixture.
3. Fill the meatballs with eggs.
4. Grease the baking tray with butter.
5. Put the stuffed pork balls in the tray and bake at 365F for 30 minutes.
Nutritional info per serve: Calories 147, Fat 11.3, Fiber 0.1, Carbs 0.5, Protein 10.6

Hemp Bites

Prep time: 10 minutes
Cook time: 15 minutes
Servings: 4
Ingredients:
- 4 tablespoons hemp seeds
- 1 cup of water
- 1 tablespoon vanilla extract
- 1 tablespoon psyllium powder
- 2 tablespoons butter
- 1 tablespoon Erythritol

Method:
1. Bring the water to boil and add hemp hearts. Remove it from the heat.
2. Then add all remaining ingredients and knead the dough.
3. Line the baking tray with baking paper.
4. Flatten the dough in the tray and cut into pieces.
5. Bake the hemp bites for 10 minutes at 360F or until they are light brown.
Nutritional info per serve: Calories 152, Fat 12.6, Fiber 2.2, Carbs 3.4, Protein 5.1

Fluffy Eggs

Prep time: 10 minutes
Cook time: 15 minutes
Servings: 2
Ingredients:
- 2 bacon slices
- 2 egg whites
- 1 teaspoon butter

Method:
1. Put the bacon in the skillet.
2. Add butter and roast the bacon for 2 minutes per side.
3. Meanwhile, whisk the egg whites until fluffy.
4. Pour the egg whites over the bacon and close the lid.
5. Cook the meal on low heat for 10 minutes.
Nutritional info per serve: Calories 137, Fat 9.9, Fiber 0, Carbs 0.5, Protein 10.7

Coffee Porridge

Prep time: 10 minutes
Cook time: 25 minutes
Servings: 2
Ingredients:
- 2 tablespoons instant coffee
- 2 cups of water
- 1 tablespoon chia seeds
- 1 tablespoon Erythritol
- 1 tablespoon vanilla extract
- ⅓ cup of coconut milk

Method:
1. Bring the water to boil and add instant coffee. Stir it well
2. Then add all remaining ingredients and pour in the glasses/bowls.
3. Leave the porridge for 15-20 minutes before serving.
Nutritional info per serve: Calories 145, Fat 11.7, Fiber 3.3, Carbs 6, Protein 2.1

Chia Oatmeal

Prep time: 10 minutes
Cook time: 15 minutes
Servings: 3
Ingredients:
- 1 cup organic almond milk
- 2 tablespoons chia seeds
- 1 tablespoon Erythritol
- 1 tablespoon almond flakes
- 2 tablespoons almond flour
- 1 tablespoon flax meal
- 1 pecan, chopped
- ½ teaspoon vanilla extract

Method:
1. Put all ingredients in the big pan and mix.
2. Then bring the mixture to boil.
3. Remove it from the heat and cool little before serving.
Nutritional info per serve: Calories 398, Fat 36.9, Fiber 8.5, Carbs 14.1, Protein 9

Cinnamon Porridge

Prep time: 10 minutes
Cook time: 15 minutes
Servings: 2
Ingredients:
- 1 tablespoon chia seeds
- 1 cup of coconut milk
- 2 tablespoons flaxseeds
- ½ cup hemp hearts
- ½ teaspoon ground cinnamon

- 1 tablespoon Erythritol
- ¼ cup coconut flour

Method:
1. Bring the coconut milk to boil and remove from the heat.
2. Add all remaining ingredients and whisk until smooth/homogenous.
3. Leave the porridge for 15 minutes in a warm place before serving.

Nutritional info per serve: Calories 646, Fat 52.8, Fiber 17.3, Carbs 25.1, Protein 21.6

Garam Masala Bake

Prep time: 10 minutes
Cook time: 30 minutes
Servings: 4
Ingredients:
- 1 cup ground pork
- 1 cup cauliflower, shredded
- ½ cup organic almond milk
- 1 spring onion, diced
- 1 teaspoon coconut oil
- ½ teaspoon salt
- ½ teaspoon paprika
- ½ teaspoon garam masala
- 1 tablespoon fresh cilantro, chopped
- 1 oz Parmesan cheese, grated

Method:
1. Put all ingredients in the mixing bowl and stir until homogenous.
2. Then transfer the mixture in the ramekins and cover with foil.
3. Bake the meal at 360f for 30 minutes.

Nutritional info per serve: Calories 352, Fat 26.1, Fiber 2, Carbs 6, Protein 23.9

Macadamia Bowls

Prep time: 10 minutes
Cook time: 5 minutes
Servings: 3
Ingredients:
- ½ cup coconut, shredded
- 4 teaspoons coconut oil
- 2 cups of coconut milk
- 1 tablespoon Erythritol
- ⅓ cup macadamia nuts, chopped
- ⅓ cup flaxseed

Method:
1. Bring the coconut milk to boil and remove it from the heat.
2. Add coconut oil, coconut shred, Erythritol, nuts, and flaxseeds.
3. Mix the mixture and put it in the serving bowls.

Nutritional info per serve: Calories 640, Fat 63.8, Fiber 9.4, Carbs 16.5, Protein 7.6

Parmesan Rings

Prep time: 10 minutes
Cook time: 17 minutes
Servings: 4
Ingredients:
- ½ cup almond flour
- 1 ½ teaspoon xanthan gum
- 1 egg, beaten
- 3 oz Parmesan, grated
- ½ teaspoon sesame seeds
- 1 teaspoon heavy cream
- 1 teaspoon coconut oil

Method:
1. In the mixing bowl mix all ingredients and knead the dough.
2. Line the baking tray with baking paper.
3. Then make the log from the dough and cut it into medium pieces.
4. Roll every piece of dough and make the bagels.
5. Put them in the baking tray and bake at 360F for 17 minutes.

Nutritional info per serve: Calories 150, Fat 9.2, Fiber 7.9, Carbs 9.2, Protein 9.1

Sweet Porridge

Prep time: 10 minutes
Cook time: 10 minutes
Servings: 2
Ingredients:
- 2 eggs, beaten
- 1 tablespoon Erythritol
- ⅓ cup coconut cream
- 2 tablespoons coconut oil
- 1 teaspoon vanilla extract

Method:
1. Mix eggs with coconut cream and coconut oil and bring to boil.
2. Remove it from the heat and add vanilla extract and Erythritol. Stir the porridge well and transfer in the serving bowls.

Nutritional info per serve: Calories 278, Fat 27.5, Fiber 0.9, Carbs 2.8, Protein 6.5

Egg Hash

Prep time: 10 minutes
Cook time: 20 minutes
Servings: 4
Ingredients:
- 4 eggs, beaten
- 1 spring onion, diced
- 6 oz turnip, chopped
- 1 chili pepper, sliced
- 5 oz Cheddar cheese, grated
- 1 tablespoon coconut oil
- ½ teaspoon Taco seasoning

Method:
1. Melt the coconut oil in the pan.
2. Then add all ingredients except cheese and eggs.
3. Roast them for 5 minutes.
4. Add eggs and carefully the mixture.
5. Then top it with cheese and close the lid.
6. Cook the egg hash for 10 minutes on low heat.

Nutritional info per serve: Calories 261, Fat 19.6, Fiber 1.4, Carbs 6.7, Protein 15.1

Cream Pancakes

Prep time: 10 minutes
Cook time: 12 minutes
Servings: 4
Ingredients:
- ½ teaspoon ground cinnamon
- 1 teaspoon Erythritol
- ¼ cup coconut flour
- 2 eggs
- ¼ cup heavy cream

Method:
1. Crack the eggs in the bowl.
2. Add all remaining ingredients and whisk until smooth.
3. Preheat the non-stick skillet.
4. Pour the small amount of pancake batter in the skillet and flatten it in the shape of a pancake.
5. Roast the pancakes for 1.5 minutes per side.

Nutritional info per serve: Calories 88, Fat 6, Fiber 2.7, Carbs 4.6, Protein 3.9

Rutabaga Pan

Prep time: 10 minutes
Cook time: 20 minutes
Servings: 4
Ingredients:
- 1 cup rutabaga, chopped
- 4 eggs, beaten
- ½ cup fresh parsley, chopped
- 4 oz chorizo, chopped
- ½ teaspoon chili powder
- 1 tablespoon avocado oil
- ¾ cup coconut cream

Method:
1. Pour avocado oil in the pan and preheat it.
2. Add rutabaga, parsley, chorizo, chili powder, and coconut cream.
3. Stir the mixture well and roast for 10 minutes.
4. Then add beaten eggs and mix well.
5. Close the lid and cook meal for 10 minutes on medium heat.

Nutritional info per serve: Calories 316, Fat 26.6, Fiber 2.4, Carbs 7.1, Protein 14.1

Cocoa Pancakes

Prep time: 10 minutes
Cook time: 15 minutes
Servings: 10
Ingredients:
- 6 eggs, beaten
- ½ cup almond flour
- 2 tablespoon Erythritol
- ⅓ cup coconut, shredded
- ½ teaspoon baking powder
- 1 cup of coconut milk
- 1 tablespoon coconut oil
- ¼ cup almonds, toasted
- 2 tablespoons cocoa powder

Method:
1. Melt the coconut oil in the skillet.
2. Then mix all remaining ingredients in the mixing bowl.
3. Laddle the small amount of cocoa batter in the preheated oil and flatten in the shape of the pancake.
4. Roast it for 1.5 minutes per side.
5. Then repeat the same steps with the remaining batter.

Nutritional info per serve: Calories 139, Fat 12.6, Fiber 1.6, Carbs 3.5, Protein 5

Feta Pie

Prep time: 10 minutes
Cook time: 35 minutes
Servings: 8
Ingredients:
- 8 oz Feta cheese, crumbled
- 6 eggs, whisked
- 2 cups spinach, chopped
- 1 teaspoon coconut oil
- 5 oz Mozzarella, chopped
- ½ teaspoon cayenne pepper
- 1 teaspoon paprika
- ½ teaspoon white pepper
- ½ cup coconut cream

Method:
1. Grease the pie pan with coconut oil.
2. After this, mix all remaining ingredients and pour them in the greased baking pan.
3. Flatten it well and bake at 365F for 35 minutes.

Nutritional info per serve: Calories 213, Fat 16.6, Fiber 0.5, Carbs 3.2, Protein 13.6

Chai Pancakes

Prep time: 10 minutes
Cook time: 15 minutes
Servings: 6
Ingredients:
- 1 egg, beaten
- 2 ounces coconut flour
- 2 ounces flaxseeds, ground
- 1 teaspoon baking powder
- 1 cup coconut cream
- 1 tablespoon chai masala
- 1 teaspoon vanilla extract
- 1 teaspoon Erythritol
- 1 teaspoon coconut oil

Method:
1. Melt the coconut oil in the skillet.
2. Then mix all remaining ingredients in the mixing bowl and stir until smooth.
3. Preheat the coconut oil well and ladle the small amount of batter in the hot skillet.
4. Flatten it in the shape of the pancake and cook for 2 minutes per side.
5. Repeat the same steps with the remaining pancake batter.

Nutritional info per serve: Calories 207, Fat 15.6, Fiber 7.3, Carbs 11.3, Protein 5.5

Bacon Pancakes

Prep time: 10 minutes
Cook time: 20 minutes
Servings: 2

Ingredients:
- 2 oz bacon, chopped
- ½ cup coconut flour
- ¾ cup heavy cream
- ½ teaspoon baking powder
- ¼ teaspoon salt
- 2 eggs, beaten

Method:
1. Roast the bacon in the hot skillet for 4-5 minutes or until the bacon is crunchy.
2. Then mix all remaining ingredients in the mixing bowl until smooth.
3. Add crunchy bacon and stir well.
4. Pour the small amount of the batter in the hot skillet and flatten in the shape of the pancake. Roast it for 2 minutes per side on medium heat.
5. Repeat the same steps with the remaining pancake batter.

Nutritional info per serve: Calories 493, Fat 35.9, Fiber 12, Carbs 22.6, Protein 21

Vanilla Toast

Prep time: 10 minutes
Cook time: 10 minutes
Servings: 4
Ingredients:
- 3 eggs, beaten
- 1 tablespoon cream cheese
- 4 grain-free bread slices
- ¼ cup heavy cream
- 1 teaspoon vanilla extract

Method:
1. Preheat the skillet well.
2. Meanwhile, mix eggs with cream cheese, vanilla extract, and heavy cream.
3. Dip the bread slices in the egg mixture well.
4. Then transfer the bread in the hot skillet and roast for 2-3 minutes per side or until the bread is light brown.

Nutritional info per serve: Calories 158, Fat 9.1, Fiber 1.9, Carbs 12.1, Protein 5.4

Lime Waffles

Prep time: 10 minutes
Cook time: 15 minutes
Servings: 4
Ingredients:
- 2 tablespoon coconut oil
- 4 eggs, beaten
- 1 teaspoon lime juice
- 1 cup coconut flour
- ½ teaspoon vanilla extract
- 1 tablespoon Erythritol
- ¾ cup organic almond milk

Method:
1. In the mixing bowl mix all ingredients and stir until smooth.
2. Then preheat the waffle maker well. When it shows hot, pour the needed amount of waffle batter inside and close it.
3. Bake the waffle for 2-3 minutes or as it is written in waffle maker directions.

Nutritional info per serve: Calories 249, Fat 15.7, Fiber 10.2, Carbs 16.8, Protein 9.7

Butter Waffles

Prep time: 10 minutes
Cook time: 15 minutes
Servings: 5
Ingredients:
- 5 eggs, beaten
- 3 tablespoons coconut milk
- 1 teaspoon baking powder
- 3 tablespoons Erythritol
- 4 tablespoons coconut flour
- 4 tablespoons butter, melted

Method:
1. Mix all ingredients in the bowl and whisk until smooth.
2. Preheat the waffle maker well.
3. Then ladle the needed amount of waffle batter in the waffle maker and cook the waffles.

Nutritional info per serve: Calories 190, Fat 16.5, Fiber 2.2, Carbs 4.5, Protein 6.7

Chocolate Smoothie

Prep time: 10 minutes
Servings: 4
Ingredients:
- 2 cups of coconut milk
- 2 tablespoons cocoa powder
- ½ avocado, peeled, chopped
- 2 tablespoons Erythritol
- ½ teaspoon vanilla extract

Method:
1. Put all ingredients in the food processor and blend until smooth.
2. Then transfer the smoothie in the serving glasses.

Nutritional info per serve: Calories 335, Fat 33.9, Fiber 5.1, Carbs 10.4, Protein 3.7

Flax Meal Granola

Prep time: 10 minutes
Cook time: 5 minutes
Servings: 4
Ingredients:
- 4 pecans, chopped
- 1 oz macadamia nuts, chopped
- ½ cup coconut shred
- ¼ cup flax meal
- ½ cup of coconut milk
- ¼ cup sunflower seeds
- 1 tablespoon Erythritol
- 2 tablespoons coconut oil

Method:
1. In the mixing bowl mix all ingredients and carefully stir.
2. Then transfer it in the lined with the baking paper tray and bake at 365F for 5 minutes.
3. Cool the granola and crush it into pieces.

Nutritional info per serve: Calories 448, Fat 45.8, Fiber 7.5, Carbs 12.2, Protein 6.1

Mushrooms Omelette

Prep time: 10 minutes
Cook time: 20 minutes
Servings: 4
Ingredients:
- 1 cup cremini mushrooms, chopped
- ½ teaspoon keto keto tomato paste
- 2 tablespoons water
- ½ teaspoon cayenne pepper
- ¾ teaspoon chili powder
- 4 eggs, beaten
- 1 tablespoon coconut oil

Method:
1. Put the coconut oil in the skillet.
2. Melt it and add cremini mushrooms. Roast the mushrooms for 5 minutes.
3. After this, add keto tomato paste, water, cayenne pepper, and chili powder. Stir the mixture well and cook for 5 minutes more.
4. Add eggs and close the lid. Cook the omelet for 10 minutes on low heat.

Nutritional info per serve: Calories 100, Fat 7.9, Fiber 0.4, Carbs 1.6, Protein 6.1

Cilantro Smoothie

Prep time: 5 minutes
Cook time: 0 minutes
Servings: 2
Ingredients:
- 2 macadamia nuts
- 1 cup of coconut milk
- ¼ cup almonds, chopped
- 2 cups fresh cilantro, chopped
- 1 teaspoon whey Protein
- 1 tablespoon erythritol

Method:
1. Put all ingredients in the food processor and blend for 5 minutes or until smooth.
2. Pour the drink in the glasses.

Nutritional info per serve: Calories 419, Fat 40.3, Fiber 5.1, Carbs 11.4, Protein 9.9

Blue Cheese Quiche

Prep time: 15 minutes
Cook time: 30 minutes
Servings: 6
Ingredients:
- 1/3 cup coconut oil, softened
- 1 cup coconut flour
- ½ teaspoon salt
- 1 spring onion, diced
- 1/3 cup coconut cream
- 5 oz Blue Cheese, crumbled
- 6 eggs, beaten

Method:
1. Mix coconut oil with coconut flour, salt, diced spring onion, coconut cream, and eggs.
2. When the mixture is homogenous, transfer it in the baking pan and flatten.
3. Top the quiche mixture with crumbled cheese and bake at 360F for 30 minutes. Cover the surface of the quiche with foil if needed.

Nutritional info per serve: Calories 369, Fat 29.1, Fiber 7.4, Carbs 14, Protein 13.8

Ginger and Parsley Smoothie

Prep time: 5 minutes
Cook time: 0 minutes
Servings: 2
Ingredients:
- 1 cup lettuce leaves
- 2 cups of water
- 2 tablespoons fresh parsley
- 1 teaspoon ground ginger
- 1 tablespoon Erythritol
- 1 cup cucumber, sliced

Method:
1. Put all ingredients in the food processor and blend until smooth.
2. Pour the smoothie in the glasses.

Nutritional info per serve: Calories 16, Fat 0.2, Fiber 0.7, Carbs 3.6, Protein 0.7

Sumac Shakshuka

Prep time: 10 minutes
Cook time: 15 minutes
Servings: 2
Ingredients:
- 1 tomato, diced
- 1 tablespoon keto keto tomato paste
- ¾ cup of water
- 1 teaspoon coconut oil
- 1 cup mushrooms, sliced
- 2 eggs
- ½ teaspoon sumac

Method:
1. Put the coconut oil in the pan and melt it.
2. Then add mushrooms and roast them for 7 minutes,
3. After this, stir the mushrooms carefully and add keto keto tomato paste and tomato.
4. Add water and sumac. Stir the mixture well.
5. Crack the eggs over the mixture and close the lid.
6. Cook shakshuka for 5 minutes on the medium heat.

Nutritional info per serve: Calories 102, Fat 6.8, Fiber 1.1, Carbs 4.2, Protein 7.3

Cocoa Mix

Prep time: 5 minutes
Cook time: 0 minutes
Servings: 3
Ingredients:
- 1 cup lettuce
- ¼ cup of cocoa powder
- 1 cup of coconut milk
- 1 cup blueberries, frozen
- 1 teaspoon ground turmeric

Method:
1. Put all ingredients and blend until smooth.
2. Serve the meal cold.

Nutritional info per serve: Calories 233, Fat 20.3, Fiber 5.3, Carbs 16.4, Protein 3.6

Flax Seeds Zucchini Bread
Prep time: 10 minutes
Cook time: 40 minutes
Servings: 8
Ingredients:
- 3 tablespoons flax seeds
- 1 teaspoon baking powder
- 1 tablespoon apple cider vinegar
- 1 ½ cup almond flour
- 1 zucchini, grated
- 1 teaspoon xanthan gum
- 1 tablespoon coconut oil, softened
- 3 eggs, beaten

Method:
1. In the mixing bowl, mix flax seeds with baking powder, apple cider vinegar, almond flour, zucchini, xanthan gum, and eggs.
2. Add coconut oil and mix the mixture until homogenous.
3. Then line the bread mold with baking paper and put the zucchini mixture inside.
4. Flatten it in the shape of bread and bake at 355F for 40 minutes.

Nutritional info per serve: Calories 188, Fat 14.2, Fiber 4.5, Carbs 7.8, Protein 7.4

Breakfast Beef Mix
Prep time: 10 minutes
Cook time: 15 minutes
Servings: 1
Ingredients:
- 4 ounces beef loin, sliced
- ½ avocado, sliced
- 1 egg
- 1 tablespoon coconut oil

Method:
1. Melt the coconut oil in the skillet.
2. Add sliced beef and roast it for 10 minutes.
3. Then stir the meat well and crack the egg.
4. Cook it for 5 minutes on medium heat more.
5. Serve the meal with sliced avocado.

Nutritional info per serve: Calories 592, Fat 47, Fiber 6.7, Carbs 9, Protein 37.8

Seeds Granola
Prep time: 15 minutes
Cook time: 10 minutes
Servings: 2
Ingredients:
- 1 pecan, chopped
- 1 oz walnuts, chopped
- 1 tablespoon chia seeds
- 2 tablespoons sunflower seeds
- 2 tablespoons flax seeds
- 1 tablespoon coconut shred
- 1 tablespoon Erythritol
- 2 tablespoons coconut oil

Method:
1. Mix all ingredients in the bowl.
2. Then line the baking tray with baking paper.
3. Put the granola mixture inside and flatten well.
4. Bake it at 350F for 10 minutes.
5. Then cool the granola well and crush into pieces.

Nutritional info per serve: Calories 359, Fat 34.5, Fiber 6.6, Carbs 8.6, Protein 7.4

Spicy Bake
Prep time: 10 minutes
Cook time: 30 minutes
Servings: 5
Ingredients:
- 5 eggs
- 1 cup coconut flour
- 1 tablespoon almond butter
- 1 zucchini, grated
- ½ cup coconut cream
- 1 teaspoon coriander seeds
- 1 teaspoon dried basil
- 2 cups ground chicken

Method:
1. In the mixing bowl, mix coconut flour, almond butter, grated zucchini, coconut cream coriander seeds, and dried basil.
2. Add ground chicken and carefully mix.
3. Then transfer the mixture into the ramekins.
4. Crack the eggs over the mixture and cover with foil.
5. Bake the meal at 360F for 30 minutes.

Nutritional info per serve: Calories 346, Fat 18.5, Fiber 10.9, Carbs 19.6, Protein 26.7

Coconut Souffle
Prep time: 10 minutes
Cook time: 20 minutes
Servings: 2
Ingredients:
- 2 oz Mozzarella, grated
- ½ teaspoon white pepper
- ½ cup of coconut milk
- ¼ teaspoon peppercorn
- 1 tablespoon coconut shred
- 2 teaspoon coconut oil
- 2 eggs, beaten

Method:
1. Grease the ramekins with coconut oil.
2. Then mix white pepper with coconut milk, peppercorn, coconut shred, and eggs.
3. Put the mixture in the ramekins and top with Mozzarella.
4. Bake the meal at 350F for 20 minutes.

Nutritional info per serve: Calories 371, Fat 33.2, Fiber 2.5, Carbs 7, Protein 15.5

Chicken Frittata
Prep time: 10 minutes
Cook time: 15 minutes
Servings: 2
Ingredients:
- 4 oz chicken fillet, cooked, shredded
- 1 tomato, chopped
- 1 bacon slice, cooked, chopped
- 2 eggs, beaten
- 1 oz chives, chopped

- 1 teaspoon avocado oil

Method:
1. Heat the avocado oil in the pan well.
2. Then add shredded chicken fillet, tomato, bacon, and chives.
3. Roast the mixture for 1 minute.
4. After this, add eggs and carefully mix them.
5. Close the lid and cook the frittata on medium heat for 10 minutes or until the eggs are set.

Nutritional info per serve: Calories 235, Fat 13, Fiber 0.8, Carbs 2.4, Protein 26.2

Ricotta Omelette

Prep time: 5 minutes
Cook time: 15 minutes
Servings: 2
Ingredients:
- 4 eggs, beaten
- 2 tablespoons ricotta cheese
- 1 bell pepper, diced
- 1 oz chives, chopped
- 1 tablespoon sesame oil

Method:
1. Preheat the sesame oil in the skillet well.
2. Meanwhile, mix all remaining ingredients in the bowl.
3. Pour the egg mixture in the hot skillet and close the lid.
4. Cook the omelet for 10-15 minutes on low heat.

Nutritional info per serve: Calories 231, Fat 17, Fiber 1.2, Carbs 6.6, Protein 13.9

Raspberries Bowl

Prep time: 10 minutes
Cook time: 0 minutes
Servings: 2
Ingredients:
- 1 cup spinach
- ½ cup of coconut milk
- 1 teaspoon Protein powder
- 4 raspberries
- 3 pecans, chopped
- 1 teaspoon chia seeds

Method:
1. Blend the spinach with coconut milk, protein powder, and pecans.
2. Then pour the smooth mixture in the glasses and add chia seeds and raspberries.

Nutritional info per serve: Calories 355, Fat 31.2, Fiber 7.6, Carbs 13.8, Protein 10.6

Chicken Meatballs

Prep time: 10 minutes
Cook time: 25 minutes
Servings: 4
Ingredients:
- 1-pound ground chicken
- 2 tablespoons coconut flour
- 1 egg, beaten
- 1 teaspoon dried oregano
- 1 teaspoon garlic powder
- 1 tablespoon coconut oil

Method:
1. Grease the baking tray with coconut oil.
2. Then mix ground chicken with coconut flour, egg, dried oregano, and garlic powder. Make the meatballs.
3. Put the meatballs in the prepared tray and bake at 365F for 25 minutes.

Nutritional info per serve: Calories 279, Fat 13.3, Fiber 1.7, Carbs 3.3, Protein 34.9

Pesto Fritatta

Prep time: 10 minutes
Cook time: 12 minutes
Servings: 1
Ingredients:
- 3 eggs, beaten
- 1 tablespoon coconut oil
- 1 oz Blue cheese, crumbled
- 1 tablespoon pesto sauce

Method:
1. Grease the baking pan with coconut oil.
2. Then mix pesto sauce with eggs and pour them in the baking pan.
3. Add cheese and bake it at 360F for 12 minutes.

Nutritional info per serve: Calories 474, Fat 41.4, Fiber 0.3, Carbs 2.7, Protein 24.2

Mushroom Caps

Prep time: 10 minutes
Cook time: 15 minutes
Servings: 2
Ingredients:
- 4 Portobello caps
- 4 quail eggs
- ½ teaspoon dried basil
- ¾ teaspoon ground black pepper
- 1 teaspoon coconut oil, melted

Method:
1. Brush the baking tray with coconut oil.
2. Then pur the Portobello caps inside.
3. Crack the eggs in the caps and sprinkle with dried basil and ground black pepper.
4. Bake the meal at 360F for 15 minutes or until eggs are set.

Nutritional info per serve: Calories 90, Fat 4.3, Fiber 2.2, Carbs 6.6, Protein 8.5

Cheese Meatloaf

Prep time: 10 minutes
Cook time: 30 minutes
Servings: 4
Ingredients:
- 1 teaspoon coconut oil
- 1 pound sausages, ground
- 2 eggs, beaten
- 1 cup Mozzarella cheese, shredded
- 1 teaspoon ricotta cheese
- 1 teaspoon chives, chopped

Method:
1. Grease the loaf mold with coconut oil.
2. Then mix ground sausages with eggs, mozzarella, ricotta cheese, and chives.

3. Put the mixture in the mold and flatten well.
4. Bake it at 360F for 30 minutes.
Nutritional info per serve: Calories 447, Fat 36.8, Fiber 0, Carbs 0.5, Protein 27

Matcha Bombs

Prep time: 15 minutes
Servings: 6
Ingredients:
- ½ cup almond butter
- 1 tablespoon matcha green tea
- ¼ teaspoon ground nutmeg
- ½ cup coconut shred

Method:
1. In the mixing bowl, mix the almond butter, matcha green tea, ground nutmeg, and coconut shred.
2. Make the small balls.

Nutritional info per serve: Calories 55, Fat 5.2, Fiber 1, Carbs 2.5, Protein 0.7

Tuna Bowls

Prep time: 10 minutes
Cook time: 0 minutes
Servings: 4
Ingredients:
- 2 tablespoons ricotta cheese
- 10 oz tuna, canned, shredded
- 2 tablespoons coconut shred
- 1 tablespoon scallions, chopped

Method:
1. In the mixing bowl mix all ingredients together.
2. Transfer the mixture in the serving bowls.

Nutritional info per serve: Calories 168, Fat 8.8, Fiber 0.5, Carbs 1.5, Protein 19.7

Almond Bowl

Prep time: 10 minutes
Servings: 3
Ingredients:
- 1 teaspoon flax seeds
- 1 teaspoon sunflower seeds
- ½ cup strawberries
- 1 cup organic almond milk
- 2 tablespoons Erythritol
- ½ teaspoon of cocoa powder
- 1 teaspoon vanilla extract

Method:
1. Put all ingredients except sunflower seeds and flax seeds in the blender and blend until smooth.
2. Pour the liquid in the serving glasses and top with sunflower seeds and flax seeds.

Nutritional info per serve: Calories 28, Fat 1.4, Fiber 1.1, Carbs 2.8, Protein 0.8

Tomatoes Salad

Prep time: 10 minutes
Cook time: 0 minutes
Servings: 1
Ingredients:
- 1 oz fresh spinach, chopped
- ¼ cup bell pepper, chopped
- ¼ cup cherry tomatoes halved
- 2 oz chicken fillet, boiled
- 1 tablespoon canola oil
- ½ teaspoon dried cilantro

Method:
1. Put all ingredients in the salad bowl and carefully mix.

Nutritional info per serve: Calories 256, Fat 18.5, Fiber 1.6, Carbs 5, Protein 17.9

Garlic Bake

Prep time: 10 minutes
Cook time: 10 minutes
Servings: 6
Ingredients:
- 1 cup coconut flour
- 1 teaspoon garlic powder
- ½ teaspoon baking powder
- 4 eggs, beaten
- 2 tablespoons cream cheese
- 1 tablespoon flax meal
- Cooking spray

Method:
1. Spray the baking pan with cooking spray from inside.
2. Then mix all remaining ingredients until you get a smooth mixture.
3. Put it in the baking pan and bake at 360F for 10 minutes.

Nutritional info per serve: Calories 71, Fat 4.8, Fiber 1.2, Carbs 2.5, Protein 4.6

KETOGENIC RECIPES FOR LUNCH

Avocado and Chicken Salad
Prep time: 10 minutes
Cook time: 0 minutes
Servings: 2
Ingredients:
- 1 avocado, pitted, peeled, and sliced
- 1 teaspoon chili powder
- 1 tablespoon cream cheese
- 1 chicken breast, grilled and shredded

Method:
1. In the salad bowl mix all ingredients.
2. Shake the salad before serving.

Nutritional info per serve: Calories 347, Fat 23.1, Fiber 7.2, Carbs 9.5, Protein 28.5

Chicken Stir-Fry
Prep time: 10 minutes
Cook time: 25 minutes
Servings: 4
Ingredients:
- 1-pound chicken fillet, sliced
- 3 oz Mozzarella, shredded
- ½ teaspoon white pepper
- 1 tablespoon avocado oil
- 1 bell pepper, sliced

Method:
1. Pour avocado oil in the skillet and heat well.
2. Then add chicken fillet and bell pepper.
3. Sprinkle the ingredients with white pepper and stir well.
4. Close the lid and cook the mixture for 10 minutes.
5. Then stir it well and top with Mozzarella. Close the lid and cook the meal for 10 minutes more on low heat.

Nutritional info per serve: Calories 290, Fat 12.7, Fiber 0.6, Carbs 3.4, Protein 39.2

Beef Tacos
Prep time: 10 minutes
Cook time: 25 minutes
Servings: 3
Ingredients:
- 1 cup Monterey jack cheese, shredded
- 1 teaspoon taco seasoning
- 7 oz beef loin, sliced
- 2 teaspoons keto riracha sauce
- 1 tomato, chopped
- 2 tablespoons coconut oil

Method:
1. Sprinkle the beef loin with taco seasonings.
2. Then melt the coconut oil in the pan.
3. Add beef loin and roast it on medium heat for 5 minutes.
4. Add sriracha sauce and chopped tomato. Carefully mix it.
5. Add Monterey jack cheese and transfer meat in the preheated to 360F oven.
6. Bake it for 20 minutes.

Nutritional info per serve: Calories 372, Fat 28.3, Fiber 0.3, Carbs 2.6, Protein 27.1

Salmon Bowl
Prep time: 10 minutes
Cook time: 10 minutes
Servings: 5
Ingredients:
- 12 oz salmon fillet
- ½ teaspoon ground nutmeg
- 1 tablespoon lime juice
- 1 tablespoon canola oil
- 2 cup fresh spinach, chopped
- ½ cup tomatoes, chopped
- 1 teaspoon sesame oil

Method:
1. Heat the sesame oil in the skillet.
2. Then chop the salmon fillet roughly and sprinkle with ground nutmeg.
3. Put it in the hot oil and roast for 2 minutes per side.
4. Then put the fish in the bowl.
5. Add lime juice, canola oil, tomatoes, and fresh spinach.
6. Shake the ingredients gently.

Nutritional info per serve: Calories 130, Fat 8.1, Fiber 0.5, Carbs 1.3, Protein 13.7

Cauliflower Pizza
Prep time: 15 minutes
Cook time: 10 minutes
Servings: 4
Ingredients:
- 1 tablespoon avocado oil
- 2 tablespoons coconut oil
- 2 cups Cheddar cheese, shredded
- ¼ cup mascarpone cheese
- 1⅓ cup cauliflower florets, steamed

Method:
1. Line the baking tray with cooking paper.
2. Then mash the cauliflower and mix it with avocado oil, coconut oil, and mascarpone.
3. Transfer the mixture in the baking tray and flatten in the shape of the pizza.
4. Top it with cheddar cheese and bake at 360F for 10 minutes.

Nutritional info per serve: Calories 341, Fat 28.1, Fiber 2.4, Carbs 6.3, Protein 17.7

Broccoli and Bacon Bowls
Prep time: 15 minutes
Cook time: 7 minutes
Servings: 4
Ingredients:
- 1 cup broccoli florets
- 1 spring onion, sliced
- 5 oz bacon, fried, chopped
- 5 oz Monterey Jack cheese, grated
- 1 tablespoon ricotta cheese
- 1 tablespoon fresh parsley, chopped
- ½ teaspoon chili powder
- 1 cup water, for cooking

Method:
1. Pour water in the pan and bring it to boil.
2. Add broccoli florets and boil them for 7 minutes.
3. After this, remove broccoli from the water and transfer it in the big bowl.
4. In the separated bowl, mix fresh parsley, chili powder, and ricotta cheese.
5. Melt the mixture and add in the broccoli.
6. Then add Monterey Jack cheese, spring onion, and bacon.
7. Shake the meal well and transfer in the serving bowls.

Nutritional info per serve: Calories 344, Fat 26, Fiber 1, Carbs 4, Protein 23.1

Tomato Pan

Prep time: 10 minutes
Cook time: 25 minutes
Servings: 6
Ingredients:
- ¼ cup bell pepper, chopped
- 2 cups Cheddar cheese, shredded
- 1 teaspoon taco seasoning
- 2 scallions, diced
- 1 tomato, chopped
- ½ cup ground sausages
- 1 tablespoon coconut oil

Method:
1. Melt the coconut oil in the pan and add bell pepper.
2. Roast it for 2 minutes and stir well.
3. Then add scallions and ground sausages.
4. Roast the ingredients for 10 minutes on medium heat.
5. Add all remaining ingredients except Cheddar cheese and roast the meal for 10 minutes.
6. Top the meal with Cheddar cheese.

Nutritional info per serve: Calories 188, Fat 14.8, Fiber 0.6, Carbs 3.3, Protein 10.6

Chicken Tortillas

Prep time: 10 minutes
Cook time: 20 minutes
Servings: 6
Ingredients:
- 1-pound chicken fillet, boiled, chopped
- 1 teaspoon ground black pepper
- ¾ cup coconut cream
- ½ teaspoon chili powder
- 1 teaspoon coconut oil
- 6 keto tortillas

Method:
1. Melt the coconut oil in the pan.
2. Then mix chopped chicken fillet with ground black pepper and chili powder.
3. Transfer the chicken in the melted coconut oil and roast for 5 minutes.
4. Then add coconut cream and cook the chicken for 10 minutes on medium heat.
5. Fill the tortillas with chicken and roll.

Nutritional info per serve: Calories 371, Fat 21.6, Fiber 4.8, Carbs 10, Protein 34.6

Cheddar Pizza

Prep time: 10 minutes
Cook time: 25 minutes
Servings: 6
Ingredients:
- 1½ cups cheddar cheese, shredded
- 1-pound ground beef, cooked
- 1 tomato, chopped
- 1 teaspoon avocado oil
- 1 teaspoon dried basil

Method:
1. Line the baking tray with baking paper.
2. Then mix dried basil with ground beef.
3. Sprinkle the tray with avocado oil and put the ground beef inside.
4. Flatten it in the shape of the pizza and bake at 360F for 15 minutes.
5. Then top the pizza with chopped tomato and cheese.
6. Cook it for 10 minutes more.

Nutritional info per serve: Calories 561, Fat 39.2, Fiber 0.2, Carbs 1.8, Protein 48.8

Halloumi Salad

Prep time: 10 minutes
Cook time: 3 minutes
Servings: 4
Ingredients:
- 4 oz Halloumi cheese
- 8 oz chicken breast, boiled, chopped
- 1 cup lettuce, chopped
- 1 pecan, chopped
- 2 tablespoons avocado oil
- 1 tablespoon lime juice

Method:
1. Preheat the grill to 400F.
2. Slice the halloumi cheese roughly and sprinkle with avocado oil.
3. Grill the cheese for 1 minute per side and put it in the salad bowl.
4. Add chopped chicken and all remaining ingredients.
5. Shake the salad.

Nutritional info per serve: Calories 203, Fat 13.3, Fiber 0.8, Carbs 2, Protein 18.7

Ground Beef Salad

Prep time: 10 minutes
Cook time: 15 minutes
Servings: 4
Ingredients:
- ¼ cup fresh parsley, chopped
- 1 avocado, pitted, peeled, chopped
- 1 tablespoon lemon juice
- ½ teaspoon garlic powder
- ¼ cup cherry tomatoes, halved
- 1 cup ground beef
- ½ cup coconut cream
- 1 teaspoon taco seasoning

Method:
1. Preheat the skillet well.

2. Then mix ground beef with taco seasonings and put in the hot skillet.
3. Roast the meat for 10-15 minutes on medium heat or until it is done.
4. Then mix all remaining ingredients in the big salad bowl.
5. Transfer the salad mixture in the serving plates and top with ground beef.
Nutritional info per serve: Calories 256, Fat 20, Fiber 4.3, Carbs 8, Protein 13.2

Zucchini Sandwich

Prep time: 10 minutes
Cook time: 10 minutes
Servings: 4
Ingredients:
- 1 zucchini, grated
- 4 keto bread slices
- 6 oz Cheddar cheese, grated
- 2 teaspoon coconut oil

Method:
1. Melt the coconut oil in the pan and add zucchini.
2. Cook it for 3 minutes on medium heat.
3. Then put the cooked zucchini on the bread slices.
4. Put the bread slices in the hot pan and top with cheese.
5. Close the lid and cook the sandwiches for 2 minutes on medium heat.
Nutritional info per serve: Calories 272, Fat 18.7, Fiber 2.4, Carbs 13.6, Protein 12.1

Stuffed Bell Peppers

Prep time: 10 minutes
Cook time: 30 minutes
Servings: 4
Ingredients:
- 4 bell peppers
- 1 tablespoon coconut oil
- 1 teaspoon herbs de Provance
- 10 oz ground sausages
- 1 teaspoon onion powder
- ½ cup of water

Method:
1. In the mixing bowl mix ground sausages, onion powder, and Herbs de Provance.
2. Then trim the bell peppers and remove the seeds.
3. Fill the peppers with ground sausages mixture and put them in the pan.
4. Add coconut oil and water.
5. Close the lid and cook the meal on medium heat for 30 minutes.
Nutritional info per serve: Calories 310, Fat 23.8, Fiber 1.6, Carbs 9.5, Protein 15

Shrimp and Avocado Salad

Prep time: 10 minutes
Cook time: 5 minutes
Servings: 4
Ingredients:
- 1-pound shrimps, peeled
- 1 avocado, chopped
- 1 tablespoon sesame oil
- 1 teaspoon sesame seeds
- ½ teaspoon chili powder
- ½ cup fresh spinach
- ½ teaspoon coconut oil

Method:
1. Melt the coconut oil in the skillet and add shrimps.
2. Sprinkle them with chili powder and roast for 2 minutes per side.
3. Then transfer the shrimps in the salad bowl and add all remaining ingredients.
4. Shake the salad well.
Nutritional info per serve: Calories 278, Fat 16.1, Fiber 3.7, Carbs 6.5, Protein 27.1

Beef Burgers

Prep time: 15 minutes
Cook time: 12 minutes
Servings: 6
Ingredients:
- 1-pound ground beef
- ½ teaspoon ground black pepper
- 1 tablespoon coconut oil
- 1 tablespoon garlic, minced
- 1 tablespoon Italian seasoning
- 1 onion, minced

Method:
1. In the mixing bowl, mix ground beef with ground black pepper, garlic, onion, and Italian seasonings.
2. Then melt the coconut oil in the skillet.
3. Make the 6 burgers and put them in the coconut oil.
4. Roast the burgers on medium heat for 5 minutes per side or bake them at 360F for 15 minutes.
Nutritional info per serve: Calories 177, Fat 7.7, Fiber 05, Carbs 2.6, Protein 23.3

Savory Cauliflower Salad

Prep time: 10 minutes
Cook time: 0 minutes
Servings: 2
Ingredients:
- 1 cup cauliflower, shredded
- 10 oz beef loin, boiled, chopped
- 1 jalapeno pepper, chopped
- 1 tablespoon ricotta cheese
- 2 spring onions, sliced

Method:
1. Put all ingredients in the salad bowl.
2. Shake the salad well.
Nutritional info per serve: Calories 330, Fat 14.1, Fiber 2, Carbs 6, Protein 42.8

Chili Burger

Prep time: 10 minutes
Cook time: 18 minutes
Servings: 5
Ingredients:
- 1 teaspoon minced garlic

- 1 teaspoon chili pepper
- 1 tablespoon coconut cream
- 1 tablespoon lemon juice
- 1½ pounds ground beef
- 1 scallion, minced
- ¼ teaspoon salt
- 1 tablespoon avocado oil

Method:
1. In the mixing bowl, mix minced garlic with chili pepper, ground beef, minced scallion, and salt.
2. Make the burgers.
3. Preheat the avocado oil in the skillet.
4. Put the burgers in the hot oil and roast for 4 minutes per side.
5. Then sprinkle the burgers with lemon juice and coconut cream and cook with the closed lid for 10 minutes on low heat.

Nutritional info per serve: Calories 944, Fat 32.2, Fiber 0.5, Carbs 1.7, Protein 151.7

Tomato Cups

Prep time: 10 minutes
Cook time: 0 minutes
Servings: 5
Ingredients:
- 5 tomatoes
- 12 oz salmon, canned, shredded
- 5 tablespoon ricotta cheese
- 1 oz Parmesan, grated

Method:
1. Remove the "caps" from the tomatoes.
2. Then remove the seeds and pulp from the tomatoes.
3. Mix shredded salmon with ricotta and Parmesan.
4. Fill the tomatoes with salmon mixture.

Nutritional info per serve: Calories 152, Fat 6.9, Fiber 1.5, Carbs 5.8, Protein 17.9

Garlic Zucchini Boats

Prep time: 15 minutes
Cook time: 35 minutes
Servings: 1
Ingredients:
- 1 zucchini, halved
- 1 teaspoon sesame oil
- 1 tablespoon garlic, minced
- ½ teaspoon dried basil
- ¼ cup ground chicken
- ¼ cup Asiago cheese, shaved

Method:
1. Scoop the zucchini flesh from the zucchinis.
2. After this, sprinkle the zucchinis with garlic, dried basil, and sesame oil. Fill the zucchini boats with ground chicken and Asiago cheese.
3. Bake the zucchini boats at 360F for 35 minutes.

Nutritional info per serve: Calories 351, Fat 23.5, Fiber 2.4, Carbs 9.4, Protein 27

Spinach Eggplant Sandwich

Prep time: 15 minutes
Cook time: 5 minutes
Servings: 4
Ingredients:
- 2 eggplants
- 1 cup fresh spinach
- 4 Monterey Jack cheese slices
- 1 teaspoon salt
- 1 tablespoon avocado oil

Method:
1. Slice the zucchini lengthwise and sprinkle with avocado oil and salt.
2. Then preheat the grill to 400F.
3. Put the zucchini slices in it and roast them for 1 minute per side.
4. Top every zucchini slice with spinach and cheese slices. Make sandwiches.

Nutritional info per serve: Calories 179, Fat 9.4, Fiber 10, Carbs 16.8, Protein 9.8

Cheese Zucchini Noodle

Prep time: 10 minutes
Cook time: 5 minutes
Servings: 2
Ingredients:
- 2 zucchinis, trimmed
- 6 oz Mozzarella, shredded
- ½ teaspoon ground black pepper
- 1 tablespoon butter

Method:
1. Make the noodles from zucchini with the help of the spiralizer.
2. Then toss the butter in the skillet and melt it.
3. Add zucchini noodles. Sprinkle them with ground black pepper.
4. Cook the vegetables for 2 minutes and add cheese. The meal is cooked.

Nutritional info per serve: Calories 324, Fat 21.1, Fiber 2.3, Carbs 9.9, Protein 26.5

Mozzarella Burgers

Prep time: 15 minutes
Cook time: 30 minutes
Servings: 4
Ingredients:
- 2 cups ground beef
- 1 teaspoon dried parsley
- 1 teaspoon dried basil
- ½ teaspoon salt
- ½ cup Mozzarella, shredded
- 1 tablespoon coconut oil

Method:
1. In the mixing bowl, mix ground beef, dried parsley, basil, salt, and Mozzarella.
2. Make the small burgers.
3. After this, grease the baking tray with coconut oil and put the burgers inside.
4. Bake them at 360F for 30 minuntes.

Nutritional info per serve: Calories 188, Fat 9.9, Fiber 0, Carbs 0.2, Protein 23.5

Chicken Relish

Prep time: 10 minutes
Cook time: 5 minutes

Servings: 4
Ingredients:
- 1 oz scallions, chopped
- 1 cup celery stalk, chopped
- 1 egg, hard-boiled, chopped
- 2 cups ground chicken, cooked
- ½ tablespoons dill relish
- 1 tablespoon butter
- 1 teaspoon ground paprika

Method:
1. Mix ground chicken with butter and ground paprika and put it in the skillet.
2. Preheat it for 5 minutes and add scallions, dill, and celery stalk. Mix well and put it in the serving bowl.
3. Add eggs.

Nutritional info per serve: Calories 182, Fat 9.3, Fiber 0.8, Carbs 1.7, Protein 22

Enchilada Mix

Prep time: 10 minutes
Cook time: 20 minutes
Servings: 2
Ingredients:
- ¼ cup ground beef
- 5 oz chorizo
- 1 tablespoon avocado oil
- 1 tablespoon Enchilada sauce
- 1 teaspoon taco seasoning
- 1 cup fresh parsley, chopped
- ½ cup fresh cilantro, chopped

Method:
1. Preheat avocado oil in the pan and add ground beef and chorizo.
2. Roast the ingredients for 15 minutes on medium heat. Stir them from time to time.
3. Then add taco seasonings and mix well.
4. Cook the mixture for 5 minutes more and add Enchilada sauce, parsley, and cilantro.
5. Carefully mix the meal and transfer in the serving bowls.

Nutritional info per serve: Calories 399, Fat 29.8, Fiber 2.3, Carbs 7.8, Protein 24.1

Steak Salad

Prep time: 10 minutes
Cook time: 15 minutes
Servings: 7
Ingredients:
- 1½ pound beef steak, sliced thin
- 3 tablespoons sesame oil
- 1 tablespoon lemon juice
- 2 cups lettuce, chopped
- 3 scallions, sliced
- 1 tablespoon avocado oil

Method:
1. Pour avocado oil in the skillet and make it hot
2. Add sliced beef steak and roast it for 7 minutes per side.
3. Then mix lettuce, scallions, and cooked beef in the salad bowl.
4. Sprinkle the ingredients with lemon juice and sesame oil.

Nutritional info per serve: Calories 725, Fat 28.4, Fiber 0.5, Carbs 2.1, Protein 108.4

Dill Bowls

Prep time: 10 minutes
Cook time: 7 minutes
Servings: 4
Ingredients:
- 4 eggs
- 2 tablespoon ricotta cheese
- ¼ cup fresh dill, chopped
- 1 teaspoon lemon juice
- ¼ teaspoon white pepper
- 1 cup water, for cooking

Method:
1. Put eggs in water and boil them for 7 minutes.
2. Then cool, peel, and chop the eggs. Transfer them in the salad bowl.
3. Add dill, lemon juice, and white pepper.
4. Then add ricotta and carefully mix.

Nutritional info per serve: Calories 82, Fat 5.1, Fiber 0.5, Carbs 2.5, Protein 7

Ricotta Chicken Salad

Prep time: 10 minutes
Cook time: 0 minutes
Servings: 4
Ingredients:
- 1-pound chicken breasts, boneless, skinless, cooked, chopped
- 2 tablespoons avocado oil
- 4 pecans, chopped
- 1½ cup fennel, chopped
- 2 tablespoons lime juice
- 3 tablespoons ricotta cheese
- ¼ teaspoon chili flakes

Method:
1. In the shallow bowl mix lime juice, ricotta cheese, chili flakes, and avocado oil. Melt the mixture until liquid.
2. Then put the chopped chicken breast in the salad bowl.
3. Add pecans, fennel, and liquid ricotta mixture.
4. Shake the salad well.

Nutritional info per serve: Calories 375, Fat 20.5, Fiber 5.5, Carbs 11.7, Protein 37.2

Pepper and Chicken Soup

Prep time: 10 minutes
Cook time: 25 minutes
Servings: 6
Ingredients:
- 4 cups of water
- 1-pound chicken breast, skinless, boneless, chopped
- 1 cup bell pepper, chopped
- ½ cup celery stalk, chopped
- 1 teaspoon avocado oil
- 1 teaspoon dried basil

Method:
1. Put the chicken in the saucepan and add water. Bring the chicken to boil and simmer for 10 minutes.
2. Add this roast the bell pepper in the avocado oil for 2 minutes and transfer in the chicken.
3. Add all remaining ingredients and simmer the soup on medium heat for 10 minutes.

Nutritional info per serve: Calories 95, Fat 2.1, Fiber 0.4, Carbs 1.8, Protein 16.3

Sardines Stuffed Avocado

Prep time: 10 minutes
Cook time: 0 minutes
Servings: 1
Ingredients:
- 1 avocado
- 4 ounces canned sardines, drained
- 1 green onion, peeled and chopped
- 1 tablespoon mayonnaise
- 1 tablespoon lemon juice
- Salt and ground black pepper, to taste
- ¼ teaspoon turmeric

Method:
1. Cut avocado in half, scoop out the flesh and put in a bowl.
2. Mix with the sardines and mash with a fork.
3. Mix with onion, lemon juice, turmeric, salt, pepper, and mayonnaise.
4. Stir everything, divide into avocado halves, and serve.

Nutritional info per serve: Calories 712, Fat 57.2, Fiber 13.8, Carbs 22.2, Protein 32.3

Cauli Soup

Prep time: 10 minutes
Cook time: 30 minutes
Servings: 4
Ingredients:
- ½ cup coconut cream
- 1 cup of water
- 2 cups broccoli florets
- ¼ cup spring onions, diced
- ½ teaspoon garlic powder
- 1 cup Cheddar cheese, shredded
- 3 oz bacon, chopped

Method:
1. Mix water and coconut cream and pour it in the saucepan.
2. Add broccoli florets, spring onion, bacon, and garlic powder. Simmer the soup on low heat for 20 minutes.
3. Add cheese and stir the soup until the cheese is dissolved.

Nutritional info per serve: Calories 317, Fat 25.6, Fiber 2, Carbs 6.3, Protein 17

Keto Tomato Salad

Prep time: 10 minutes
Cook time: 0 minutes
Servings: 4
Ingredients:
- 1-pound chicken breast, cooked and cubed
- ½ teaspoon dried basil
- 2 tomatoes, chopped
- 4 bacon slices, cooked, chopped
- 2 tablespoons cream cheese
- 1 tablespoon sesame oil

Method:
1. Put all ingredients in the salad bowl and carefully mix.

Nutritional info per serve: Calories 291, Fat 16, Fiber 0.7, Carbs 2.8, Protein 32

Onion and Chicken Bake

Prep time: 10 minutes
Cook time: 30 minutes
Servings: 4
Ingredients:
- 1-pound chicken fillet, boiled, shredded
- 2 spring onions, chopped
- ½ cup coconut cream
- 1 tablespoon olive oil
- ½ teaspoon ground nutmeg
- 1 cup Cheddar cheese, shredded

Method:
1. Brush the baking mold with olive oil.
2. In the mixing bowl mix chicken shred with spring onions, coconut cream, and ground nutmeg.
3. Put the mixture in the prepared baking mold, flatten well, and top with Cheddar cheese.
4. Cover the baking mold with foil and bake at 360F for 30 minutes.

Nutritional info per serve: Calories 441, Fat 28.5, Fiber 1.3, Carbs 4.7, Protein 40.9

Mustard Salad

Prep time: 10 minutes
Cook time: 15 minutes
Servings: 1
Ingredients:
- 1 beefsteak
- 1 cup fresh spinach, chopped
- 1 cup radish, chopped
- 1 tablespoon mustard
- 2 egg yolks, boiled
- 1 tablespoon heavy cream
- 1 teaspoon olive oil
- 1 teaspoon ground black pepper

Method:
1. In the shallow bowl, mix egg yolks with ground black pepper, mustard, and heavy cream.
2. Preheat the olive oil in the skillet, add beefsteak and roast it for 7 minutes per side.
3. Roughly chop the beefsteak and put it in the salad bowl.
4. Add spinach, radish, and mustard mixture.
5. Carefully mix the salad.

Nutritional info per serve: Calories 451, Fat 30.4, Fiber 4.7, Carbs 11.9, Protein 33.6

Marinara Chicken Tart

Prep time: 15 minutes
Cook time: 55 minutes
Servings: 4
Ingredients:

- 1-pound chicken breast, skinless, boneless
- ½ teaspoon avocado oil
- ½ teaspoon white pepper
- 2 oz Provolone cheese, grated
- 1 cup coconut flour
- 4 tablespoon coconut oil
- 1 egg, beaten
- 1 tablespoon fresh parsley, chopped
- 2 tablespoon marinara sauce

Method:
1. In the mixing bowl mix coconut flour with eggs, and avocado oil. Knead the dough.
2. Then place it in the non-stick baking pan and flatten in the shape of the pie crust.
3. Then chop the chicken breast and mix it with marinara sauce, parsley, cheese, and white pepper.
4. Put the mixture over the dough and flatten well.
5. Bake the tart at 355F for 55 minutes.

Nutritional info per serve: Calories 441, Fat 25.6, Fiber 10.3, Carbs 17.7, Protein 33.3

Crab Meatballs

Prep time: 10 minutes
Cook time: 7 minutes
Servings: 6
Ingredients:
- 1-pound crabmeat, canned, shredded
- ¼ cup fresh cilantro, chopped
- 1 egg, beaten
- 1 oz Parmesan
- 1 teaspoon coconut oil

Method:
1. In the mixing bowl, mix crabmeat with cilantro, egg, and grated Parmesan.
2. Then make the meatballs.
3. Preheat the coconut oil in the skillet well.
4. Add meatballs and roast them for 3 minutes per side.

Nutritional info per serve: Calories 104, Fat 2.9, Fiber 0.4, Carbs 11.6, Protein 8.2

Turmeric Pie

Prep time: 15 minutes
Cook time: 50 minutes
Servings: 6
Ingredients:
- 10 oz ground beef
- 1 teaspoon ground turmeric
- 1 teaspoon chili powder
- 1 tablespoon coconut oil
- 1/3 cup coconut cream
- 3 eggs, whisked

Method:
1. Mix all ingredients in the mixing bowl and stir until smooth.
2. Then transfer it in the non-stick round pan and flatten in the shape of a pie.
3. Bake the turmeric pie at 360F for 50 minutes.
4. Then cool it to the room temperature and cut into pieces.

Nutritional info per serve: Calories 172, Fat 10.7, Fiber 0.5, Carbs 1.4, Protein 17.5

Cremini Mushrooms Muffins

Prep time: 10 minutes
Cook time: 25 minutes
Servings: 8
Ingredients:
- 6 eggs, beaten
- ½ pound white mushrooms
- 4 tablespoons almond flour
- 1 cup cremini mushrooms, chopped
- 1 teaspoon coconut oil

Method:
1. Melt the coconut oil in the skillet.
2. Add cremini and white mushrooms and roast them for 10 minutes.
3. Then mix eggs with cooked mushrooms.
4. Add almond flour and transfer the mixture in the muffin molds.
5. Bake the muffins for 15 minutes at 360F.

Nutritional info per serve: Calories 141, Fat 10.9, Fiber 1.8, Carbs 4.6, Protein 8.3

Meatballs Soup

Prep time: 15 minutes
Cook time: 30 minutes
Servings: 4
Ingredients:
- 1 teaspoon avocado oil
- 2 spring onions, diced
- 1 cup ground beef
- ½ teaspoon ground black pepper
- 4 cups of water
- ½ cup of coconut milk
- 1 tablespoon fresh cilantro, chopped

Method:
1. In the mixing bowl, mix ground beef with ground black pepper.
2. Then heat the skillet with avocado oil.
3. Put the spring onions inside and roast it for 5 minutes.
4. Transfer the onion in the saucepan.
5. Add water and coconut milk.
6. Then make the small meatballs and add them in the soup too.
7. Add cilantro and boil the soup for 15 minutes on medium heat.

Nutritional info per serve: Calories 151, Fat 10.2, Fiber 1.1, Carbs 3.2, Protein 12.1

Scallions and Provolone Pork Pie

Prep time: 15 minutes
Cook time: 55 minutes
Servings: 6
Ingredients:
- 2 tablespoons coconut flour
- 1 tablespoon coconut oil
- ¼ teaspoon salt
- 3 oz provolone cheese, shredded
- 3 eggs, beaten
- 4 oz ground pork
- 1 teaspoon cream cheese

- 2 oz scallions, chopped

Method:
1. In the mixing bowl, mix coconut flour with cream cheese and salt. Knead the dough and place it in the non-sticky round pan. Flatten it in the shape of the pie crust.
2. Then mix ground pork with all remaining ingredients and transfer over the pie crust. Flatten it well.
3. Bake the pie at 360F for 55 minutes.

Nutritional info per serve: Calories 153, Fat 9.8, Fiber 1.9, Carbs 3.8, Protein 12.2

Cumin Pork Casserole

Prep time: 15 minutes
Cook time: 60 minutes
Servings: 6
Ingredients:
- 1 ½ cup coconut flour
- 3 eggs, beaten
- 3 tablespoon coconut cream
- 2 tablespoon coconut oil, melted
- 3 oz Mozzarella cheese, shredded
- 2 cups ground pork
- ½ teaspoon ground cumin
- ¼ teaspoon garlic powder
- 1 teaspoon ground coriander

Method:
1. In the shallow bowl mix ground coriander, garlic powder, and ground cumin.
2. Then mix ground pork with the spice mixture and put in the casserole mold. Flatten it.
3. Mix coconut cream with eggs, and coconut flour.
4. Put the mixture over the ground pork.
5. Then add Mozzarella and bake the casserole at 360F for 60 minutes.

Nutritional info per serve: Calories 143, Fat 9.4, Fiber 1.1, Carbs 2.5, Protein 11.9

Sage Pâte

Prep time: 10 minutes
Cook time: 0 minutes
Servings: 1
Ingredients:
- 4 ounces chicken livers, sautéed
- ½ teaspoon fresh sage, chopped
- ½ teaspoon dried basil
- 1 tablespoon coconut oil

Method:
1. Put all ingredients in the food processor and blend until smooth.
2. Transfer the pate in the serving bowl and store it in the fridge.

Nutritional info per serve: Calories 308, Fat 21, Fiber 0.1, Carbs 1.2, Protein 27.8

Tomato Cream

Prep time: 15 minutes
Cook time: 10 minutes
Servings: 2
Ingredients:
- 1 cup tomatoes
- ½ cup coconut cream
- 1 ½ cup water
- 1 garlic clove, peeled
- 1 teaspoon dried thyme

Method:
1. Put the tomatoes in the tray and sprinkle with thyme.
2. Bake them for 10 minutes at 365F.
3. Then transfer the baked tomatoes in the food processor.
4. Add all remaining ingredients and blend until smooth.

Nutritional info per serve: Calories 158, Fat 14.5, Fiber 2.6, Carbs 7.6, Protein 2.3

Chicken Soup with Basil

Prep time: 10 minutes
Cook time: 35 minutes
Servings: 4
Ingredients:
- 1-pound chicken breast, skinless, boneless
- 1 teaspoon dried thyme
- 1 cup broccoli, chopped
- 5 cups of water
- 1 teaspoon keto tomato paste

Method:
1. Pour water in the saucepan.
2. Add chicken and thyme. Boil the ingredients for 25 minutes.
3. Then add all remaining ingredients, carefully mix, and simmer the soup for 6 minutes more.

Nutritional info per serve: Calories 139, Fat 3, Fiber 0.7, Carbs 1.9, Protein 24.8

Cauliflower Risotto

Prep time: 10 minutes
Cook time: 25 minutes
Servings: 4
Ingredients:
- 3 oz bacon, chopped, cooked
- 2 cups cauliflower, shredded
- 1 tablespoon dried cilantro
- ½ cup fresh cilantro, chopped
- 2 oz white mushrooms, chopped
- 1 tablespoon coconut oil
- 2 cups of water

Method:
1. Melt the coconut oil in the pan.
2. Add mushrooms and roast them for 10 minutes.
3. Add all cilantro, bacon, and cauliflower.
4. Then mix the mixture well, add water, and close the lid.
5. Cook the risotto for 10 minutes on medium heat.

Nutritional info per serve: Calories 160, Fat 12.4, Fiber 1.4, Carbs 3.4, Protein 9.3

Lemongrass Soup

Prep time: 10 minutes
Cook time: 20 minutes
Servings: 3

Ingredients:
- 4 cups beef broth
- 1 teaspoon lemongrass
- ½ cup heavy cream
- 1-pound shrimps, peeled
- 1 cup broccoli, chopped
- 1 teaspoon chili powder

Method:
1. Pour beef broth and heavy cream in the saucepan. Bring the liquid to boil.
2. Add lemongrass, shrimps, broccoli, and chili powder.
3. Simmer the soup for 10 minutes on medium heat.

Nutritional info per serve: Calories 313, Fat 12, Fiber 1.1, Carbs 6.7, Protein 42.3

Arugula Salad

Prep time: 10 minutes
Cook time: 0 minutes
Servings: 2
Ingredients:
- 1 cup arugula, chopped
- 4 oz chicken fillet, boiled, chopped
- ½ avocado, chopped
- 1 tablespoon lime juice
- 1 teaspoon avocado oil
- 1 teaspoon almonds, toasted

Method:
1. Put all ingredients in the salad bowl.
2. Carefully mix the salad.

Nutritional info per serve: Calories 238, Fat 16.9, Fiber 3.7, Carbs 4.9, Protein 17.8

Noodle Soup

Prep time: 10 minutes
Cook time: 30 minutes
Servings: 6
Ingredients:
- 2 scallions, diced
- 1 jalapeño pepper, chopped
- 1 tablespoon avocado oil
- 1 teaspoon curry powder
- 6 cups chicken stock
- 1-pound chicken breasts, boneless, skinless, and sliced
- 1 zucchini, spiralized

Method:
1. Pour avocado oil in the saucepan and preheat it.
2. Add scallions and roast it for 3 minutes.
3. Then add jalapeno pepper, curry powder, chicken stock, and chicken breast.
4. Simmer the mixture for 15 minutes.
5. Then add spiralized zucchini and cook the soup for 10 minutes on low heat.

Nutritional info per serve: Calories 171, Fat 6.6, Fiber 1, Carbs 4, Protein 23.3

Pork Dumplings

Prep time: 15 minutes
Cook time: 30 minutes
Servings: 6
Ingredients:
- 2 zucchinis
- 1 cup ground pork
- 1 teaspoon onion powder
- ½ cup chicken stock
- 1 teaspoon avocado oil

Method:
1. Slice the zucchini lengthwise.
2. Then mix onion powder with ground pork, and make the small balls.
3. Wrap the meatballs in the slices zucchini.
4. Then brush the casserole mold with avocado oil.
5. Put the zucchini dumplings in the casserole mold. Add chicken stock.
6. Cook the meal at 360F for 30 minutes.

Nutritional info per serve: Calories 52, Fat 2.9, Fiber 0.8, Carbs 2.6, Protein 4.2

Turmeric Chicken

Prep time: 10 minutes
Cook time: 40 minutes
Servings: 4
Ingredients:
- 1 tablespoon coconut oil
- 1 tomato, chopped
- 2 cups of water
- 4 chicken thighs, skinless, boneless, chopped
- 1 teaspoon lemon juice
- 1 teaspoon ground turmeric
- 1 teaspoon fennel seeds

Method:
1. Put the coconut oil in the pan. Melt it.
2. Then add chicken thighs and roast them for 5 minutes per side on high heat.
3. Add all remaining ingredients and cook the chicken at 360F for 30 minutes.

Nutritional info per serve: Calories 313, Fat 14.4, Fiber 0.5, Carbs 1.3, Protein 42.5

Halloumi Salad

Prep time: 10 minutes
Cook time: 5 minutes
Servings: 4
Ingredients:
- 10 oz Halloumi cheese
- 1 teaspoon avocado oil
- ½ teaspoon chili powder
- 1 tablespoon lemon juice
- 1 cup lettuce, chopped
- 1 teaspoon sesame oil

Method:
1. Sprinkle the halloumi cheese with sesame oil and roast in the preheated skillet for 2 minutes per side.
2. Chop the cheese roughly and put it in the salad bowl.
3. Then add all remaining ingredients and shake the salad.

Nutritional info per serve: Calories 273, Fat 22.6, Fiber 0.3, Carbs 2.5, Protein 15.4

Cream Cheese Rolls

Prep time: 20 minutes
Cook time: 0 minutes
Servings: 4
Ingredients:
- 2 cups spinach leaves
- ½ cup cream cheese
- 1 oz Parmesan, grated
- 2 pecans, grinded
- 1 teaspoon minced garlic

Method:
1. In the mixing bowl, mix cream cheese, parmesan, pecans, and minced garlic.
2. Then spread the spinach leaves with cheese mixture and roll.

Nutritional info per serve: Calories 177, Fat 16.7, Fiber 1.1, Carbs 2.8, Protein 5.7

Chicken Pockets

Prep time: 15 minutes
Cook time: 10 minutes
Servings: 4
Ingredients:
- 2 eggs, beaten
- 1/3 cup coconut milk
- ½ teaspoon ground black pepper
- 1 teaspoon coconut oil
- 9 oz chicken breast, boneless, skinless, cooked
- 2 cups spinach
- 2 tablespoon heavy cream

Method:
1. Melt the coconut oil in the skillet.
2. Then mix eggs with coconut milk and ground black pepper.
3. Pour ¼ part of egg mixture in the skillet and make a crepe.
4. Roast the egg crepe for 1 minute per side.
5. Repeat the same steps with the remaining egg mixture. Make a total of 4 crepes.
6. After this, mix heavy cream with spinach, and blend until smooth.
7. Add chopped chicken and carefully mix the spinach mixture.
8. Put the chicken mixture on the egg crepes and roll them in the shape of pockets.

Nutritional info per serve: Calories 190, Fat 12.5, Fiber 0.8, Carbs 2.2, Protein 17.4

Cilantro Steak

Prep time: 10 minutes
Cook time: 20 minutes
Servings: 4
Ingredients:
- 4 beef steaks
- ½ cup cilantro, chopped
- 1 teaspoon ground black pepper
- 1 tablespoon coconut oil
- 1 tomato, chopped

Method:
1. Sprinkle the beef steaks with ground black pepper.
2. Then heat the coconut oil well.
3. Put the beef steaks in the skillet and roast for 5 minutes per side.
4. Add chopped tomato and cilantro.
5. Cook the steaks on medium heat for 10 minutes more.

Nutritional info per serve: Calories 192, Fat 8.8, Fiber 0.4, Carbs 1, Protein 26.1

Goat Cheese Pancakes

Prep time: 15 minutes
Cook time: 10 minutes
Servings: 4
Ingredients:
- 8 oz goat cheese, crumbled
- 1 cup coconut flour
- ¼ cup of coconut milk
- 1 teaspoon avocado oil
- ½ teaspoon dried parsley
- ½ teaspoon salt

Method:
1. Mix all ingredients in the mixing bowl and stir until smooth.
2. Then preheat the non-sticky skillet well.
3. Pour the small amount of batter in the skillet and flatten in the shape of the crepe. Cook it for 1 minute per side.
4. Repeat the same steps with the remaining batter.

Nutritional info per serve: Calories 307, Fat 24.4, Fiber 1.6, Carbs 4.1, Protein 18.2

Lamb Meatballs

Prep time: 15 minutes
Cook time: 30 minutes
Servings: 4
Ingredients:
- 1 cup cauliflower, shredded
- 1 egg, beaten
- 10 oz lamb fillet, ground
- 1 teaspoon dried mint
- 1 tablespoon coconut flour
- ½ teaspoon ground black pepper

Method:
1. In the mixing bowl, mix shredded cauliflower, egg, ground lamb, dried mint, coconut flour, and ground black pepper.
2. Make the meatballs and place them in the lined with baking paper tray.
3. Bake the meatballs for 30 minutes at 360F.

Nutritional info per serve: Calories 162, Fat 6.6, Fiber 1.4, Carbs 2.6, Protein 22.1

Pancakes Pie

Prep time: 25 minutes
Cook time: 10 minutes
Servings: 8
Ingredients:
- 2 cups almond flour
- ½ cup of coconut milk
- 1 teaspoon baking powder
- ½ teaspoon salt
- ½ cup cream cheese
- 1 teaspoon ground paprika

- 1 tablespoon fresh parsley, chopped
- 4 oz Mozzarella, shredded

Method:
1. Mix almond flour with coconut milk, baking powder, and salt.
2. Preheat the non-stick skillet well.
3. Then ladle the small amount of coconut batter in the skillet and flatten in the shape of pancakes.
4. Cook the pancake for 1 minute per side. Repeat the same steps with the remaining coconut mixture.
5. After this, mix Mozzarella, parsley, ground paprika, and cream cheese.
6. Spread the pancakes with cheese mixture and make the shape of the pie.

Nutritional info per serve: Calories 167, Fat 14.7, Fiber 1.2, Carbs 3.7, Protein 7

Cauliflower Cream

Prep time: 10 minutes
Cook time: 20 minutes
Servings: 4
Ingredients:
- 2 oz spring onions, chopped
- 1 tablespoon coconut oil
- 2 cups of water
- ½ teaspoon garlic powder
- 1 cup coconut cream
- 3 oz Provolone cheese, grated
- 2 cup cauliflower, chopped

Method:
1. Boil the cauliflower in water for 10 minutes.
2. Then blend the cauliflower and mix with all remaining ingredients.
3. Saute the mixture for 10 minutes on medium heat.

Nutritional info per serve: Calories 267, Fat 23.4, Fiber 3.2, Carbs 9.2, Protein 8.2

Curry Soup

Prep time: 10 minutes
Cook time: 35 minutes
Servings: 4
Ingredients:
- 1 cup of heavy cream
- 2 cups of water
- 1 teaspoon curry powder
- 1-pound chicken breast, skinless, boneless, chopped
- ½ teaspoon onion powder
- 1 teaspoon coconut oil
- 1 teaspoon chili flakes
- 1 tablespoon lemon juice

Method:
1. Pour water and heavy cream in the saucepan.
2. Add curry powder, chicken breast, and onion powder.
3. Boil the mixture for 20 minutes.
4. Then add coconut oil, chili flakes, and lemon juice.
5. Simmer the soup for 15 minutes more.

Nutritional info per serve: Calories 246, Fat 15.2, Fiber 0.2, Carbs 1.5, Protein 24.8

Green Bean Salad

Prep time: 10 minutes
Cook time: 15 minutes
Servings: 8
Ingredients:
- 2 tablespoons apple cider vinegar
- 1½ tablespoons mustard
- 2-pounds green beans
- 2 tablespoons coconut oil
- 2 oz celery stalk, chopped
- 4 oz goats cheese, crumbled
- 2 pecans, chopped

Method:
1. Melt the coconut oil in the pan.
2. Add green beans and roast for 15 minutes on medium heat.
3. Then transfer the green beans in the salad bowl.
4. Add all remaining ingredients and mix well.

Nutritional info per serve: Calories 169, Fat 11.6, Fiber 5.5, Carbs 12, Protein 7.2

Lettuce Tacos

Prep time: 15 minutes
Cook time: 5 minutes
Servings: 4
Ingredients:
- 4 lettuce leaves
- 1 bell pepper, sliced
- ½ jalapeno pepper, minced
- 1 tablespoon avocado oil
- 1-pound cod fillet
- 1 tablespoon lime juice
- ¼ teaspoon ground cumin

Method:
1. Heat the avocado oil in the skillet.
2. Then chop cod and sprinkle with ground cumin and lime juice.
3. Roast the fish in the oil for 5 minutes.
4. After this, fill the lettuce leaves with cod, bell pepper, and jalapeno pepper. Fold them in the shape of tacos.

Nutritional info per serve: Calories 107, Fat 1.6, Fiber 0.6, Carbs 2.8, Protein 20.7

Chipotle Cream

Prep time: 10 minutes
Cook time: 15 minutes
Servings: 6
Ingredients:
- ½ cup scallions, chopped
- 2 tablespoons coconut oil
- 1 tomato, chopped
- 1 tablespoon apple cider vinegar
- 1 teaspoon chipotle powder
- 1 teaspoon ground coriander
- 4 oz pumpkin puree
- ¼ cup coconut cream

Method:

1. Put all ingredients in the saucepan and simmer for 15 minutes on low heat.
2. Then blend the mixture until smooth and transfer in the bowls.
Nutritional info per serve: Calories 75, Fat 7, Fiber 1.1, Carbs 3.4, Protein 0.6

Bacon Salad

Prep time: 10 minutes
Cook time: 5 minutes
Servings: 2
Ingredients:
- 2 oz bacon, sliced
- 1 egg, boiled, peeled
- ½ cucumber, chopped
- 1 oz Feta cheese, crumbled
- 1 teaspoon scallions
- 1/3 cup lettuce, chopped
- 1 tablespoon heavy cream
- 1 tablespoon lemon juice

Method:
1. Roast the bacon in the skillet for 2 minutes per side.
2. Then chop the egg and put it in the salad bowl.
3. Add all remaining ingredients and shake well.
4. Add cooked bacon.
Nutritional info per serve: Calories 224, Fat 21, Fiber 3.3, Carbs 10.2, Protein 1.9

Parmesan Bake

Prep time: 10 minutes
Cook time: 40 minutes
Servings: 8
Ingredients:
- 1 pound green beans, halved
- 1 tablespoon coconut oil
- 2 scallions, chopped
- 1 cup of coconut milk
- 3 oz Parmesan cheese, grated

Method:
1. Mix green beans with coconut milk and scallions.
2. Then grease the casserole mold with coconut oil and add green beans mixture.
3. Top it with Parmesan and bake at 360F for 40 minutes.
Nutritional info per serve: Calories 141, Fat 11.2, Fiber 2.9, Carbs 7.4, Protein 5.3

Provolone Cream

Prep time: 10 minutes
Cook time: 15 minutes
Servings: 3
Ingredients:
- 2 spring onions, diced
- 5 oz provolone cheese, shredded
- ½ cup of coconut milk
- ½ cup of water
- 1 teaspoon ground black pepper
- 1 tablespoon coconut oil

Method:

1. Toss the coconut oil in the saucepan and melt it.
2. Add spring onions and roast it in the medium heat for 5 minutes.
3. Add all remaining ingredients and stir well.
4. Simmer the cream for 10 minutes on medium heat.
Nutritional info per serve: Calories 313, Fat 26.7, Fiber 1.9, Carbs 7.1, Protein 13.5

Mayo Salad

Prep time: 10 minutes
Cook time: 0 minutes
Servings: 4
Ingredients:
- 2 cups cauliflower florets, chopped, boiled
- 1 pecan, chopped, chopped
- 1 oz scallions, chopped
- 1 teaspoon flax seeds
- 1 teaspoon apple cider vinegar
- ¼ cup mayonnaise
- ½ teaspoon lemon juice

Method:
1. Mix cauliflower with pecan, scallions, flax seeds, and apple cider vinegar.
2. Then add lemon juice and mayonnaise,
3. Shake the salad.
Nutritional info per serve: Calories 100, Fat 7.7, Fiber 2, Carbs 7.4, Protein 1.7

Tuna Tartare

Prep time: 10 minutes
Servings: 4
Ingredients:
- 1-pound tuna, canned, chopped
- 1 tablespoon heavy cream
- 1 tablespoon lemon juice
- 2 oz avocado, chopped
- 1 teaspoon chili powder
- 1 tablespoon avocado oil

Method:
1. Put all ingredients in the mixing bowl and stir carefully.
2. Transfer the tuna tartare in the plates.
Nutritional info per serve: Calories 287, Fat 17, Fiber 1.2, Carbs 1.8, Protein 30.6

Brussels Sprout Bake

Prep time: 10 minutes
Cook time: 40 minutes
Servings: 4
Ingredients:
- 1-pound Brussel Sprouts
- ½ cup Cheddar cheese
- ½ cup of coconut milk
- 1 teaspoon Italian seasonings
- 1 teaspoon avocado oil
- 1 teaspoon dried oregano

Method:
1. Brush the casserole mold with avocado oil.
2. Then mix Brussel sprouts with Italian seasonings and dried oregano.

3. Grated the cheese and mix it with Brussel sprouts.
4. Put the mixture in the casserole mold. Add coconut milk and bake the meal at 360F for 40 minutes.
Nutritional info per serve: Calories 181, Fat 12.8, Fiber 5.1, Carbs 12.6, Protein 8.1

Clam Soup

Prep time: 10 minutes
Cook time: 20 minutes
Servings: 3
Ingredients:
- 1 cup of organic almond milk
- 1 cup of water
- 6 oz clam, chopped
- 1 teaspoon scallions
- ½ teaspoon ground black pepper
- ¾ teaspoon chili flakes
- ½ teaspoon salt
- 1 cup broccoli florets, chopped

Method:
1. Pour almond milk in the saucepan.
2. Add water and ground black pepper.
3. Then add chili flakes, salt, and broccoli florets. Simmer the liquid for 15 minutes.
4. Add clams and cook the soup for 5 minutes more.

Nutritional info per serve: Calories 223, Fat 19.3, Fiber 2.9, Carbs 13, Protein 3.1

Chili Asparagus

Prep time: 10 minutes
Cook time: 20 minutes
Servings: 4
Ingredients:
- 2 eggs, beaten
- 2 tablespoons coconut oil
- 1 tablespoon lemon juice
- ½ teaspoon chili powder
- 1-pound asparagus spears

Method:
1. Toss the coconut oil in the pan and preheat it.
2. Add asparagus spears and roast them for 10 minutes.
3. Then add all remaining ingredients and close the lid.
4. Cook the meal on medium heat for 10 minutes.

Nutritional info per serve: Calories 115, Fat 9.2, Fiber 2.5, Carbs 4.8, Protein 5.3

Beef Salad

Prep time: 10 minutes
Cook time: 40 minutes
Servings: 4
Ingredients:
- 14 oz beef brisket
- 1 teaspoon coriander seeds
- 1 tablespoon lemon juice
- 1 tablespoon sesame oil
- 1 spring onion, sliced
- 1 teaspoon ground black pepper
- 1 teaspoon coconut aminos
- 1 cup water, for cooking

Method:
1. Pour water in the pan and add beef brisket. Boil it for 40 minutes.
2. Then remove the meat from water and chop.
3. Put the chopped beef in the salad bowl.
4. Add coriander seeds, lemon juice, sesame oil, onion, ground black pepper, and coconut aminos.
5. Shake the salad.

Nutritional info per serve: Calories 239, Fat 10.8, Fiber 0.8, Carbs 3.2, Protein 30.5

Basil Shrimp Noodles

Prep time: 10 minutes
Cook time: 10 minutes
Servings: 4
Ingredients:
- 12 ounces Shirataki noodles
- 2 tablespoons olive oil
- Salt and ground black pepper, to taste
- 2 tablespoons butter
- 4 garlic cloves, peeled and minced
- 1 pound shrimp, peeled and deveined
- Juice of ½ lemon
- ½ teaspoon paprika
- ½ cup fresh basil, chopped

Method:
1. Put water in a saucepan, add some salt, bring to a boil, add the Shirataki noodles, cook for 2 minutes, drain and transfer to a heated pan.
2. Toast the noodles for a few seconds, take off the heat, and leave them aside.
3. Heat a pan with butter and olive oil over medium heat, add the garlic, stir, and brown for 1 minute.
4. Add shrimp, lemon juice, and cook for 3 minutes on each side. Add the noodles, salt, pepper, and paprika stir divide into bowls, and serve with chopped basil on top.

Nutritional info per serve: Calories 262, Fat 15.3, Fiber 2.2, Carbs 5.9, Protein 26.7

Bacon Zucchini Noodles

Prep time: 10 minutes
Cook time: 15 minutes
Servings: 6
Ingredients:
- 3 zucchini, trimmed
- ½ cup coconut cream
- 5 oz bacon, chopped
- 4 oz Provolone cheese, grated
- 1 tablespoon coconut oil

Method:
1. Put the bacon in the skillet and roast for 5 minutes. Stir it from time to time.
2. Then make the noodles from the zucchini.
3. Add them to the skillet.
4. Then add coconut oil and coconut cream.
5. Simmer the noodles for 5 minutes. Add Provolone cheese.

Nutritional info per serve: Calories 275, Fat 22.1, Fiber 1.5, Carbs 5.1, Protein 15.2

Tortilla Bake

Prep time: 10 minutes
Cook time: 40 minutes
Servings: 6
Ingredients:
- ½ cup bell pepper, chopped
- 2 jalapeños, chopped
- 1 tablespoon avocado oil
- ¼ cup coconut cream
- 1-pound chicken breast, skinless, boneless, chopped
- 4 keto tortillas, chopped

Method:
1. Brush the casserole mold with avocado oil.
2. Then mix bell pepper with jalapenos, chopped chicken.
3. Put the mixture in the casserole mold and flatten gently.
4. Add coconut cream and tortillas.
5. Bake the meal at 360F for 40 minutes.

Nutritional info per serve: Calories 217, Fat 10, Fiber 3.3, Carbs 7.1, Protein 24.5

Chia and Broccoli Soup

Prep time: 10 minutes
Cook time: 30 minutes
Servings: 4
Ingredients:
- 2 cups broccoli, chopped
- 1 tablespoon flax seeds
- 1 tablespoon chia seeds
- 1 teaspoon coconut oil
- 1 scallion, diced
- ½ cup heavy cream
- 1 cup of water
- 4 oz Provolone cheese, grated

Method:
1. Put the coconut oil in the saucepan and melt it.
2. Add scallion and roast it for 2 minutes.
3. Add broccoli, water, and heavy cream.
4. Boil the mixture for 10 minutes.
5. Then add all remaining ingredients and simmer the soup for 15 minutes.

Nutritional info per serve: Calories 206, Fat 16, Fiber 3, Carbs 6.7, Protein 9.8

Garlic Pork Salad

Prep time: 10 minutes
Cook time: 15 minutes
Servings: 4
Ingredients:
- 1-pound ground pork
- 2 tablespoons apple cider vinegar
- ½ teaspoon garlic powder
- 2 tablespoons avocado oil
- ½ cup celery stalk, chopped

Method:
1. Put the ground pork in the skillet.
2. Add avocado oil and garlic powder. Roast the meat for 15 minutes.
3. Then transfer it in the salad bowl.
4. Add celery stalk and apple cider vinegar. Mix the salad.

Nutritional info per serve: Calories 176, Fat 4.9, Fiber 0.5, Carbs 1.1, Protein 29.9

Asparagus Pockets

Prep time: 15 minutes
Cook time: 30 minutes
Servings: 6
Ingredients:
- 1-pound asparagus
- 4 oz prosciutto, sliced
- 1 tablespoon butter, melted
- 1 teaspoon chili powder
- ½ cup of water
- 1 tablespoon lemon juice

Method:
1. Pour water in the casserole mold.
2. Then wrap asparagus in the prosciutto and put in the casserole mold.
3. Add lemon juice, butter, and chili powder.
4. Bake the meal at 360F for 30 minutes.

Nutritional info per serve: Calories 61, Fat 3.2, Fiber 1.8, Carbs 3.5, Protein 5.7

Coconut Chicken Wings

Prep time: 10 minutes
Cook time: 30 minutes
Servings: 6
Ingredients:
- 2 tablespoons coconut oil
- 6 chicken wings
- ½ teaspoon onion powder
- 1 teaspoon chili powder
- 1 teaspoon coconut shred

Method:
1. Sprinkle the chicken wings with onion powder and chili powder.
2. Then put the chicken in the skillet, add coconut oil, and roast them for 5 minutes per side.
3. Sprinkle the chicken wings with coconut shred and put in the preheated to 360F oven.
4. Bake the chicken wings for 20 minutes.

Nutritional info per serve: Calories 205, Fat 15.8, Fiber 0.4, Carbs 6, Protein 9.8

Zucchini Stuffed Peppers

Prep time: 15 minutes
Cook time: 30 minutes
Servings: 4
Ingredients:
- 4 bell peppers
- 1 ½ cup ground pork
- 1 zucchini, grated
- ½ teaspoon ground cardamom
- 1 tablespoon sesame oil
- 1 teaspoon white pepper
- 3 oz Provolone, grated

Method:

1. Trim the bell peppers and remove the seeds.
2. Then mix zucchini with ground pork, ground cardamom, sesame oil, and white pepper.
3. Add Provolone cheese.
4. Fill the bell peppers with zucchini mixture and bake them for 30 minutes at 360F.
Nutritional info per serve: Calories 264, Fat 17.7, Fiber 2.4, Carbs 11.6, Protein 16.7

Portobello Skewers

Prep time: 10 minutes
Cook time: 25 minutes
Servings: 6
Ingredients:
- 1-pound Portobello mushrooms
- 6 bacon strips
- 2 tablespoons avocado oil
- ½ teaspoon ground cumin

Method:
1. String the mushrooms into the skewers and wrap them in the bacon strips.
2. Then sprinkle the mushrooms with avocado oil and ground cumin.
3. Bake the skewers at 360F for 25 minutes.
Nutritional info per serve: Calories 127, Fat 9.6, Fiber 1.2, Carbs 3.3, Protein 7.1

Stuffed Eggplants

Prep time: 20 minutes
Cook time: 20 minutes
Servings: 4
Ingredients:
- 1 large eggplant, trimmed
- 1 tomato, crushed
- 1 teaspoon onion powder
- 1 cup spinach, chopped
- 4 oz Feta cheese, crumbled
- 1 teaspoon coconut oil
- 2 oz Monterey Jack cheese, shredded

Method:
1. In the mixing bowl, mix crushed tomatoes, onion powder, spinach, and Monterey jack cheese.
2. Then cut the eggplants into halves and bake for 10 minutes.
3. Remove the eggplant flesh from the vegetables and fill them with tomato mixture.
4. Top the stuffed eggplants with Feta and bake for 10 minutes at 360F.
Nutritional info per serve: Calories 173, Fat 11.7, Fiber 4.4, Carbs 9.3, Protein 9

Tomato Cream Soup

Prep time: 10 minutes
Cook time: 25 minutes
Servings: 4
Ingredients:
- 1 cup ground beef
- 3 cups of water
- 1 tablespoon keto tomato paste
- 1 teaspoon Italian seasonings
- 2 scallions, diced
- 1 tablespoon coconut oil

Method:
1. Put the coconut oil in the saucepan and melt it.
2. Add ground beef and Italian seasonings.
3. Then add diced scallions and roast the mixture for 10 minutes.
4. After this, add keto tomato paste and water and cook the soup on medium heat for 15 minutes.
Nutritional info per serve: Calories 121, Fat 6.7, Fiber 0.8, Carbs 3.5, Protein 11.7

Cardamom Chicken Cubes

Prep time: 10 minutes
Cook time: 50 minutes
Servings: 6
Ingredients:
- 3-pound chicken breast, skinless, boneless
- 1 teaspoon garam masala
- 1 teaspoon curry powder
- 1 teaspoon ground cardamom
- 1 cup of coconut milk

Method:
1. Mix garam masala, curry powder, and ground cardamom in the bowl,
2. Add coconut milk and carefully mix.
3. Then chop chicken into the cubes and put in the coconut milk.
4. Transfer it in the casserole mold and bake at 360F for 50 minutes.
Nutritional info per serve: Calories 353, Fat 15.3, Fiber 1.1, Carbs 2.6, Protein 49.1

Chorizo Wrap

Prep time: 10 minutes
Cook time: 35 minutes
Servings: 4
Ingredients:
- 8 bacon strips
- 4 oz chorizo, roughly chopped
- 4 Cheddar cheese slices
- ¼ teaspoon ground black pepper
- ½ teaspoon ground paprika paprika

Method:
1. Mix chorizo with ground black pepper and ground paprika and wrap in the bacon strips.
2. Then put the wraps in the baking pan.
3. Add cheese and bake at 360F for 35 minutes.
Nutritional info per serve: Calories 442, Fat 38.1, Fiber 0, Carbs 1, Protein 21.8

Zucchini Baked Bars

Prep time: 15 minutes
Cook time: 25 minutes
Servings: 4
Ingredients:
- 3 zucchini, grated
- 2 teaspoons coconut oil
- 3 eggs, beaten
- 4 tablespoons almond flour
- 5 oz Feta cheese, crumbled
- 4 oz provolone cheese, shredded
- 1 teaspoon lime juice

Method:
1. In the mixing bowl, mix zucchini with almond flour, all cheese, and lime juice.
2. Line the baking tray with baking paper and grease with coconut oil.
3. Then put the zucchini mixture in the tray and flatten it well.
4. Bake it at 360F for 25 minutes.
5. Cook the bake and cut into bars.

Nutritional info per serve: Calories 443, Fat 34.9, Fiber 4.6, Carbs 13.2, Protein 24.2

Lobster Soup

Prep time: 10 minutes
Cook time: 15 minutes
Servings: 4
Ingredients:
- 1 teaspoon garlic powder
- 2 scallions, chopped
- 9 oz lobster meat, chopped
- 1 teaspoon keto tomato paste
- ½ cup celery stalk, chopped
- ½ cup coconut cream
- 1 teaspoon dried lemongrass
- ¼ teaspoon lemon zest

Method:
1. Put all ingredients in the saucepan and bring to boil.
2. Boil the soup for 10 minutes.
3. Then cool it to the room temperature.

Nutritional info per serve: Calories 143, Fat 7.8, Fiber 1.6, Carbs 5.5, Protein 13.4

Turnip Soup

Prep time: 10 minutes
Cook time: 25 minutes
Servings: 4
Ingredients:
- 1 cup of water
- 1 cup of organic almond milk
- 1 cup cremini mushrooms, chopped
- 1 tablespoon coconut oil
- 2 oz turnip, chopped
- 1 teaspoon dried parsley
- ½ teaspoon white pepper
- ¾ teaspoon ground paprika
- 1 oz celery stalk, chopped

Method:
1. Melt the coconut oil in the saucepan.
2. Add cremini mushrooms and turnip and roast for 10 minutes.
3. Stir the mixture well and add all remaining ingredients.
4. Close the lid and cook the soup on medium heat for 10 minutes.

Nutritional info per serve: Calories 179, Fat 17.8, Fiber 2, Carbs 5.6, Protein 2.1

Arugula and Halloumi Salad

Prep time: 10 minutes
Cook time: 0 minutes
Servings: 1
Ingredients:
- 3 oz halloumi cheese, sliced
- 1 oz macadamia nuts, chopped
- 1 teaspoon sesame oil
- 1 cup baby arugula, chopped
- 1 tablespoon apple cider vinegar

Method:
1. Cut the sliced halloumi into the strips and put it in the salad bowl.
2. Add macadamia nuts, sesame oil, baby arugula, and apple cider vinegar.
3. Shake the salad.

Nutritional info per serve: Calories 561, Fat 51.5, Fiber 2.8, Carbs 7, Protein 21.1

Artichoke and Mushrooms Mix

Prep time: 10 minutes
Cook time: 15 minutes
Servings: 4
Ingredients:
- 1 cup cremini mushrooms, chopped
- 1 cup spinach, chopped, steamed
- 2 oz artichoke hearts, drained, chopped
- ½ cup of coconut milk
- 1 teaspoon ground black pepper
- ½ teaspoon ground turmeric

Method:
1. Sprinkle the mushrooms with ground black pepper and turmeric and bake in the oven at 360f for 15 minutes. Stir them from time to time to avoid burning.
2. Then transfer the mushrooms in the bowl.
3. Add all remaining ingredients and carefully mix.

Nutritional info per serve: Calories 85, Fat 7.3, Fiber 1.9, Carbs 4.7, Protein 1.9

Beef Stew

Prep time: 10 minutes
Cook time: 50 minutes
Servings: 6
Ingredients:
- 1-pound beef loin, chopped
- 3 cups of water
- 3 oz spaghetti squash, chopped
- 1 teaspoon dried thyme
- 1 teaspoon keto tomato paste
- 3 oz fennel bulb, chopped

Method:
1. Put all ingredients in the saucepan and carefully mix.
2. Simmer the stew on medium heat for 50 minutes.

Nutritional info per serve: Calories 122, Fat 5.5, Fiber 0.5, Carbs 3.2, Protein 14.3

Seitan Salad

Prep time: 10 minutes
Servings: 1
Ingredients:
- 1 cup lettuce, roughly chopped
- 3 oz seitan, chopped
- 1 tablespoon sesame oil
- 1 teaspoon flax seeds

- 1 teaspoon lime juice
- 1 oz Parmesan, chopped

Method:
1. Put all ingredients in the salad bowl and carefully mix.

Nutritional info per serve: Calories 570, Fat 24.4, Fiber 4.6, Carbs 3.3, Protein 73.7

Shrimp and Spinach Mix

Prep time: 10 minutes
Cook time: 5 minutes
Servings: 2
Ingredients:
- 2 cups fresh spinach, chopped
- 1-pound shrimps, peeled
- 1 tablespoon coconut oil
- 1 teaspoon chili powder
- 1 tablespoon sesame oil

Method:
1. Melt the coconut oil in the skillet.
2. Add shrimps and sprinkle them with chili powder.
3. Roast the shrimps for 4 minutes.
4. Then put them in the bowl and add remaining ingredients. Shake the mixture.

Nutritional info per serve: Calories 399, Fat 17.8, Fiber 1.1, Carbs 5.2, Protein 52.7

Coconut Mushroom Soup

Prep time: 10 minutes
Cook time: 20 minutes
Servings: 6
Ingredients:
- 1 cup of coconut milk
- 4 cups of water
- 2 cups mushrooms, chopped
- 2 spring onions, chopped
- 1 tablespoon coconut oil
- 1 oz celery stalk, chopped
- 1 teaspoon ground paprika

Method:
1. Melt the coconut oil in the saucepan and add mushrooms and spring onions. Roast the vegetables for 10 minutes. Stir them from time to time.
2. Then add ground paprika, celery stalk, water, and coconut milk.
3. Simmer the soup for 6 minutes on medium heat.

Nutritional info per serve: Calories 126, Fat 12, Fiber 1.7, Carbs 5, Protein 1.9

Greens and Coconut Soup

Prep time: 10 minutes
Cook time: 30 minutes
Servings: 6
Ingredients:
- ½ cup fresh spinach, chopped
- 1 cup coconut cream
- 4 cups of water
- 1 cup leek, chopped
- 1-pound chicken breast, skinless, boneless, chopped

Method:
1. Bring the water to boil and add chopped chicken breast.
2. Then boil the chicken on medium heat for 20 minutes.
3. Add all remaining ingredients and cook the soup for 10 minutes more.

Nutritional info per serve: Calories 188, Fat 11.5, Fiber 1.2, Carbs 4.4, Protein 17.2

Lettuce Salad

Prep time: 10 minutes
Cook time: 5 minutes
Servings: 3
Ingredients:
- 10 oz asparagus, chopped, boiled
- 1 tablespoon sesame oil
- ½ teaspoon white pepper
- 4 oz goat cheese, crumbled
- 1 cup lettuce, chopped
- 1 tablespoon avocado oil
- 1 teaspoon apple cider vinegar

Method:
1. Preheat the avocado oil in the skillet.
2. Add asparagus and roast it for 5 minutes.
3. Then transfer it in the salad bowl, add white pepper, goat cheese, lettuce, sesame oil, and apple cider vinegar.
4. Shake the salad gently.

Nutritional info per serve: Calories 240, Fat 18.7, Fiber 2.4, Carbs 5.6, Protein 13.8

Cheddar Salad

Prep time: 5 minutes
Cook time: 0 minutes
Servings: 2
Ingredients:
- ½ cup Cheddar cheese, chopped
- 1 tomato, sliced
- ½ cup fresh spinach, chopped
- 1 tablespoon apple cider vinegar
- 1 tablespoon sesame oil

Method:
1. Put all ingredients in the salad bowl and carefully mix.

Nutritional info per serve: Calories 183, Fat 16.3, Fiber 0.5, Carbs 1.9, Protein 7.5

Broccoli and Cucumber Bowl

Prep time: 15 minutes
Cook time: 0 minutes
Servings: 4
Ingredients:
- 1-pound broccoli head, chopped, cooked
- 1 cucumber, chopped
- 2 tablespoons lime juice
- 2 tablespoons sesame oil
- ½ cup dill, chopped
- ½ teaspoon garlic powder
- 1 oz chives, chopped

Method:
1. Put all ingredients in the bowl and carefully mix.

2. Leave the mixture in the fridge for 10-15 minutes before serving.
Nutritional info per serve: Calories 94, Fat 7.2, Fiber 1.7, Carbs 7.4, Protein 2.3

Salmon Soup

Prep time: 10 minutes
Cook time: 15 minutes
Servings: 5
Ingredients:
- 4 leeks, trimmed and sliced
- 1 tablespoon sesame oil
- 4 cups of water
- 1 teaspoon ground paprika
- 1-pound salmon, cut into small pieces
- 1 cup of coconut milk

Method:
1. Pour coconut milk in the saucepan.
2. Add water, ground paprika, and sesame oil.
3. Bring the liquid to boil and add leeks and salmon.
4. Simmer the soup for 5 minutes.

Nutritional info per serve: Calories 299, Fat 20, Fiber 2.5, Carbs 13, Protein 19.8

Garlic Artichokes

Prep time: 10 minutes
Cook time: 15 minutes
Servings: 4
Ingredients:
- 4 artichokes
- 2 oz Monterey Jack cheese, grated
- 2 teaspoon coconut flour
- 1 teaspoon garlic powder
- 3 tablespoons cream cheese
- 1 teaspoon sesame oil
- 1 cup water, for cooking

Method:
1. Pour water in the saucepan, add artichokes and simmer them for 5 minutes.
2. Then remove the artichokes from the saucepan and transfer in the tray.
3. Mix coconut flour with garlic powder, cream cheese, and sesame oil.
4. Sprinkle the artichokes with garlic mixture and top with Monterey Jack cheese.
5. Bake the artichokes at 360F for 10 minutes.

Nutritional info per serve: Calories 172, Fat 8.4, Fiber 9.3, Carbs 18.7, Protein 9.6

Fish Soup

Prep time: 15 minutes
Cook time: 10 minutes
Servings: 4
Ingredients:
- 2 scallions, chopped
- 6 oz spaghetti squash, chopped
- 1 tablespoon sesame oil
- 1 teaspoon ginger powder
- 2 cups of water
- 1-pound salmon, cut into medium chunks

Method:
1. Put all ingredients in the saucepan and bring to boil.
2. Simmer the soup for 10 minutes.

Nutritional info per serve: Calories 206, Fat 10.7, Fiber 0.7, Carbs 5.8, Protein 22.6

Lime Beef

Prep time: 10 minutes
Cook time: 18 minutes
Servings: 2
Ingredients:
- 1-pound beef loin, sliced
- 2 garlic cloves, peeled, diced
- 2 tablespoons coconut oil
- 1 tablespoon cream cheese
- ½ teaspoon ground paprika
- 1 tablespoon lime juice
- 1 teaspoon lime zest, grated

Method:
1. Preheat the coconut oil in the pan and add sliced beef loin.
2. Sprinkle it with garlic cloves, cream cheese, ground paprika, lime juice, and lime zest.
3. Carefully mix the beef and close the lid.
4. Cook the meal on medium heat for 20 minutes, stir it from time to time.

Nutritional info per serve: Calories 554, Fat 34.4, Fiber 0.4, Carbs 1.6, Protein 61.3

KETOGENIC SIDE DISH RECIPES

Cabbage Mix

Prep time: 10 minutes
Cook time: 0 minutes
Servings: 6
Ingredients:
- 2 pounds white cabbage, shredded
- ½ cup turnip, chopped
- 2 tablespoons scallions, chopped
- 2 tablespoons chili powder
- 1 teaspoon garlic powder
- 1 teaspoon ginger powder

Method:
1. In the mixing bowl, mix white cabbage with turnip, scallions, and chili powder.
2. Add garlic powder and ginger powder.
3. Carefully mix the meal and leave for 10 minutes before serving.

Nutritional info per serve: Calories 52, Fat 0.6, Fiber 5, Carbs 11.5, Protein 2.5

Italian Style Mushrooms

Prep time: 10 minutes
Cook time: 30 minutes
Servings: 4
Ingredients:
- 2 cups cremini mushrooms
- 1 teaspoon Italian seasoning
- 2 tablespoons coconut oil
- ¼ cup coconut cream

Method:
1. Melt the coconut oil in the saucepan.
2. Add mushrooms and roast them for 10 minutes.
3. Then sprinkle them with Italian seasonings and coconut cream.
4. Bake the mushrooms at 360F for 15 minutes.

Nutritional info per serve: Calories 106, Fat 10.8, Fiber 0.6, Carbs 2.4, Protein 1.2

Cheddar Green Beans

Prep time: 10 minutes
Cook time: 20 minutes
Servings: 4
Ingredients:
- ½ cup Cheddar cheese, shredded
- 2 cups green beans, chopped
- 1 teaspoon ground black pepper
- 1 tablespoon olive oil

Method:
1. Sprinkle the green beans with ground black pepper and olive oil and put in the hot skillet.
2. Roast the green beans for 10 minutes on medium heat.
3. Stir them from time to time to avoid burning.
4. Then top the vegetables with cheese and close the lid.
5. Cook the meal on low heat for 10 minutes.

Nutritional info per serve: Calories 105, Fat 8.3, Fiber 2, Carbs 4.4, Protein 4.6

Butter Asparagus

Prep time: 10 minutes
Cook time: 25 minutes
Servings: 4
Ingredients:
- 1.5-pound asparagus
- 2 tablespoons lemon juice
- 1 teaspoon lemon zest, grated
- 4 tablespoons butter
- ¼ cup coconut cream
- ¼ teaspoon chili flakes

Method:
1. Chop the asparagus and put it in the baking tray.
2. Sprinkle the vegetables with lemon juice, lemon zest, butter, coconut cream, and chili flakes.
3. Shake the ingredients and bake at 360F for 25 minutes.

Nutritional info per serve: Calories 173, Fat 15.4, Fiber 4, Carbs 7.7, Protein 4.3

Cauliflower Puree

Prep time: 10 minutes
Cook time: 15 minutes
Servings: 2
Ingredients:
- ¼ cup coconut cream
- 1 cup cauliflower chopped
- 1 teaspoon salt
- 2 cups of water

Method:
1. Pour water in the saucepan.
2. Add cauliflower and boil it for 15 minutes.
3. Then drain water and mash the cauliflower with the help of potato masher.
4. Add all remaining ingredients and carefully mix the meal.

Nutritional info per serve: Calories 82, Fat 7.2, Fiber 1.9, Carbs 4.3, Protein 1.7

Sesame Brussel Sprouts

Prep time: 10 minutes
Cook time: 6 minutes
Servings: 4
Ingredients:
- 3 cups Brussel sprouts
- 1 teaspoon garlic, minced
- 1 teaspoon sesame seeds
- 1 tablespoon coconut oil
- ½ cup of water

Method:
1. Bring the water to boil.
2. Add Brussel sprouts and boil them for 1 minute.
3. Then transfer them in the hot skillet.
4. Add garlic, sesame seeds, and coconut oil.
5. Carefully mix and cook the meal for 5 minutes on medium heat. Stir it from time to time.

Nutritional info per serve: Calories 63, Fat 4, Fiber 2.6, Carbs 6.4, Protein 2.4

Tarragon Mushrooms

Prep time: 10 minutes
Cook time: 15 minutes
Servings: 4
Ingredients:
- 10 oz cremini mushrooms, sliced
- 2 tablespoons avocado oil
- ½ teaspoon tarragon, dried
- 2 tablespoons apple cider vinegar

Method:
1. Sprinkle the baking tray with avocado oil.
2. Then mix mushrooms with tarragon and apple cider vinegar.
3. Put them in the baking tray and flatten in the layer.
4. Bake the mushrooms at 360F for 15 minutes. Stir them from time to time to avoid burning.

Nutritional info per serve: Calories 30, Fat 1, Fiber 0.8, Carbs 3.4, Protein 1.9

Spinach Mash

Prep time: 5 minutes
Cook time: 5 minutes
Servings: 3
Ingredients:
- 3 cups fresh spinach, chopped
- 1 tablespoon ricotta cheese
- ¼ cup coconut cream
- 1 spring onion, diced
- 1 teaspoon coconut oil
- 1 oz Parmesan, grated

Method:
1. Melt the coconut oil in the saucepan.
2. Add chopped spinach and roast it for 3 minutes on medium heat.
3. Carefully mix the spinach and add ricotta cheese, coconut cream, spring onion, and Parmesan.
4. Carefully mix the spinach until the cheese is melted and remove it from the heat.

Nutritional info per serve: Calories 104, Fat 8.8, Fiber 1.1, Carbs 2.9, Protein 5

Pepper Brussels Sprouts

Prep time: 10 minutes
Cook time: 11 minutes
Servings: 4
Ingredients:
- 1-pound Brussels sprouts, trimmed and halved
- 1 teaspoon chili powder
- 1 teaspoon garlic powder
- 1 teaspoon avocado oil
- 1 tablespoon apple cider vinegar
- 1 cup of water

Method:
1. Put the Brussel sprouts in the pan and add water. Boil the vegetables for 10 minutes.
2. Then drain water and add all remaining ingredients.
3. Carefully mix the mixture and cook it on medium heat for 1 minute more.

Nutritional info per serve: Calories 56, Fat 0.7, Fiber 4.6, Carbs 11.3, Protein 4.1

Chili Bok Choy

Prep time: 10 minutes
Cook time: 7 minutes
Servings: 4
Ingredients:
- 1-pound bok choy
- 1 teaspoon chili flakes
- 2 tablespoons avocado oil
- 1 teaspoon lemon juice

Method:
1. Preheat the avocado oil in the skillet.
2. Slice the bok choy and put it in the hot oil.
3. Sprinkle it with lemon juice and chili flakes and roast for 2 minutes per side.

Nutritional info per serve: Calories 24, Fat 1.1, Fiber 1.5, Carbs 2.9, Protein 1.8

Spinach Sauce

Prep time: 10 minutes
Cook time: 10 minutes
Servings: 4
Ingredients:
- 1 tablespoon coconut oil
- 2 cups fresh spinach, chopped
- 1 pecan, chopped
- 2 oz Provolone, grated
- 1 teaspoon minced garlic

Method:
1. Melt the coconut oil and put spinach in it.
2. Add pecan, cheese, and minced garlic.
3. Carefully mix the mixture and cook it for 5 minutes.
4. Then blend it with the help of the immersion blender until smooth.

Nutritional info per serve: Calories 108, Fat 9.7, Fiber 0.7, Carbs 1.6, Protein 4.5

Parmesan Broccoli Mix

Prep time: 10 minutes
Cook time: 20 minutes
Servings: 4
Ingredients:
- 14 oz broccoli, roughly chopped
- 2 tablespoons coconut oil
- 1 teaspoon onion powder
- 3 oz Parmesan, grated
- ½ teaspoon white pepper
- ¾ teaspoon ground nutmeg

Method:
1. Grease the baking tray with coconut oil.
2. Then put the broccoli inside.
3. Sprinkle it with all remaining ingredients and bake at 360F for 20 minutes or until cheese is light brown.

Nutritional info per serve: Calories 172, Fat 13, Fiber 2.8, Carbs 7.9, Protein 8.3

Bacon Brussels Sprouts

Prep time: 10 minutes
Cook time: 15 minutes
Servings: 4
Ingredients:
- 3 oz bacon strips, chopped
- 1 pound Brussels sprouts, trimmed and halved
- 1 teaspoon ground coriander
- ½ teaspoon chili flakes
- 1 tablespoon coconut oil

Method:
1. Melt the coconut oil in the saucepan.
2. Then add bacon and roast it on medium heat for 1 minute per side.
3. After this, add all remaining ingredients and carefully mix the mixture.
4. Close the lid and cook the meal on medium heat for 10 minutes.

Nutritional info per serve: Calories 153, Fat 10.5, Fiber 4.3, Carbs 10.3, Protein 6.9

Garlic Zucchini Noodles

Prep time: 10 minutes
Cook time: 7 minutes
Servings: 2
Ingredients:
- 1 zucchini
- ½ cup heavy cream
- 1 teaspoon minced garlic

Method:
1. Spiralize the zucchini with the help of the spiralizer.
2. Then pour the heavy cream in the saucepan and bring it to boil.
3. Add minced garlic and remove the cream from the heat.
4. Add zucchini noodles and carefully mix them.
5. Leave the meal for 5 minutes to rest before serving.

Nutritional info per serve: Calories 121, Fat 11.3, Fiber 1.1, Carbs 4.6, Protein 1.9

Creamy Spinach

Prep time: 10 minutes
Cook time: 10 minutes
Servings: 2
Ingredients:
- ½ cup coconut cream
- 3 cups fresh spinach, chopped
- 1 teaspoon onion powder
- 1 teaspoon ground black pepper

Method:
1. Put all ingredients in the saucepan and bring to boil.
2. Then close the lid and remove from the heat.
3. Leave the spinach for 10 minutes to rest.

Nutritional info per serve: Calories 155, Fat 14.5, Fiber 2.7, Carbs 6.6, Protein 2.9

Dill Cabbage Mix

Prep time: 10 minutes
Cook time: 15 minute
Servings: 4
Ingredients:
- 1 oz bacon, chopped
- 1 tablespoon coconut oil
- 1 teaspoon dried dill
- 2 cups white cabbage, shredded
- ¼ cup of water

Method:
1. Mix cabbage with dried dill and bacon.
2. Then grease the baking tray with coconut oil.
3. Add water.
4. Put the cabbage mixture in the tray in one layer and flatten well.
5. Bake the cabbage at 355F for 15 minutes.

Nutritional info per serve: Calories 77, Fat 6.4, Fiber 0.9, Carbs 2.3, Protein 3.1

Chili Avocado

Prep time: 10 minutes
Cook time: 5 minutes
Servings: 2
Ingredients:
- 1 avocado, pitted, peeled, halved, and sliced
- 1 tablespoon avocado oil
- 1 teaspoon chili powder

Method:
1. Sprinkle the avocado slices with chili powder.
2. Then preheat the avocado oil in the skillet well.
3. Add the avocado slices and roast them for 2 minutes per side.

Nutritional info per serve: Calories 271, Fat 26.8, Fiber 7.2, Carbs 9.4, Protein 2.1

Cilantro Cauliflower Rice

Prep time: 10 minutes
Cook time: 10 minutes
Servings: 6
Ingredients:
- 3 cups cauliflower, shredded
- 1 cup fresh cilantro, chopped
- ¼ cup coconut cream
- ¾ cup of water
- 1 teaspoon salt
- ½ teaspoon coconut oil

Method:
1. Melt the coconut oil in the saucepan.
2. Add cauliflower, water, and salt.
3. Bring the mixture to boil.
4. Then add coconut cream and cilantro.
5. Carefully mix the meal and cook it for 2 minutes more.

Nutritional info per serve: Calories 39, Fat 2.8, Fiber 1.5, Carbs 3.3, Protein 1.3

Dill Cauliflower

Prep time: 10 minutes
Cook time: 25 minutes
Servings: 6
Ingredients:
- 1 cauliflower head, separated into florets

- ½ teaspoon ground black pepper
- 1 oz Parmesan, grated
- ½ cup fresh dill, chopped
- 1 tablespoon coconut oil

Method:
1. Sprinkle the cauliflower with ground black pepper and dill.
2. Then grease the tray with coconut oil.
3. Put the cauliflower in the tray and flatten it in one layer.
4. Top the vegetables with Parmesan and bake at 360F for 25 minutes.

Nutritional info per serve: Calories 56, Fat 3.5, Fiber 1.7, Carbs 4.9, Protein 3.2

Cayenne Green Beans

Prep time: 5 minutes
Cook time: 20 minutes
Servings: 4
Ingredients:
- 2 cups green beans
- 1 tablespoon sesame oil
- 1 teaspoon coconut oil
- ½ teaspoon cayenne pepper

Method:
1. Melt the coconut oil in the skillet.
2. Add green beans and roast them for 10 minutes on medium heat. Stir them from time to time.
3. After this, add sesame oil and cayenne pepper.
4. Close the lid and cook the green beans on medium heat for 10 minutes more.

Nutritional info per serve: Calories 58, Fat 4.6, Fiber 1.9, Carbs 4.1, Protein 1

Onion Mushroom and Spinach

Prep time: 10 minutes
Cook time: 30 minutes
Servings: 4
Ingredients:
- 2 cups spinach, chopped
- 1 teaspoon ground black pepper
- 2 cups cremini mushrooms, sliced
- 2 spring onions, diced
- 1 tablespoon coconut oil
- 1 tablespoon apple cider vinegar

Method:
1. Preheat the coconut oil well and put the mushrooms in it.
2. Add ground black pepper, scallions, and carefully mix.
3. Roast the vegetables for 10 minutes.
4. Then add apple cider vinegar and spinach.
5. Close the lid and cook the meal on medium heat for 20 minutes more.

Nutritional info per serve: Calories 50, Fat 3.5, Fiber 1, Carbs 3.7, Protein 1.5

Herbed Spaghetti Squash

Prep time: 35 minutes
Cook time: 10 minutes
Servings: 4
Ingredients:

- 10 oz spaghetti squash, peeled, chopped
- 1 tablespoon coconut oil
- 1 tablespoon cream cheese
- ½ teaspoon ground coriander

Method:
1. Grease the baking tray with coconut oil.
2. Then mix ground coriander with spaghetti squash and put in the tray.
3. Add cream cheese and bake the meal at 360F for 35 minutes.

Nutritional info per serve: Calories 60, Fat 4.7, Fiber 0, Carbs 5, Protein 0.6

Bacon Okra

Prep time: 10 minutes
Cook time: 15 minutes
Servings: 6
Ingredients:
- 1 tomato, chopped
- 1 teaspoon ground black pepper
- 2 scallions, chopped
- 4 cups okra, chopped
- 1 tablespoon coconut oil
- 1 teaspoon ground paprika
- 2 oz bacon, chopped

Method:
1. Put the bacon in the skillet and roast it for 1 minute.
2. Then stir it and add scallions, coconut oil, okra, and ground paprika.
3. Add tomato and carefully mix the mixture.
4. Close the lid and cook the meal on medium heat for 10 minutes. Stir it from time to time to avoid burning.

Nutritional info per serve: Calories 108, Fat 6.5, Fiber 2.7, Carbs 7.7, Protein 5.2

Cauliflower Tortillas

Prep time: 10 minutes
Cook time: 5 minutes
Servings: 6
Ingredients:
- 1 cup cauliflower, shredded
- 1 tablespoon almond flour
- 1 egg, beaten
- 1 oz Parmesan, grated

Method:
1. In the mixing bowl, mix cauliflower with almond flour, egg, and Parmesan.
2. Knead the soft dough and make 6 tortillas.
3. Put them in the lined with the baking paper tray and bake at 360F for 5 minutes.

Nutritional info per serve: Calories 37, Fat 2.3, Fiber 0.6, Carbs 1.4, Protein 3

Onion Edamame

Prep time: 10 minutes
Cook time: 12 minutes
Servings: 4
Ingredients:
- 1 cup edamame beans, soaked, cooked
- 1 teaspoon onion powder
- 1 tablespoon coconut oil

- 1 teaspoon dried oregano

Method:
1. Melt the coconut oil in the skillet.
2. Add edamame beans and sprinkle them with dried oregano and onion powder.
3. Roast the beans for 10 minutes on medium heat.

Nutritional info per serve: Calories 80, Fat 5.5, Fiber 2.2, Carbs 4.5, Protein 4.4

Coriander Eggplant Slices

Prep time: 10 minutes
Cook time: 10 minutes
Servings: 4
Ingredients:
- 1 large eggplant, trimmed, sliced
- 1 tablespoon ground coriander
- 1 teaspoon salt
- 1 tablespoon avocado oil

Method:
1. Sprinkle the eggplant slices with ground coriander and salt. Carefully mix and leave for 10 minutes.
2. Then preheat the avocado oil in the skillet.
3. Add eggplant slices and roast them for 1 minute per side.

Nutritional info per serve: Calories 33, Fat 0.7, Fiber 4.2, Carbs 6.9, Protein 1.2

Chili Collard Greens

Prep time: 10 minutes
Cook time: 15 minutes
Servings: 5
Ingredients:
- 8 oz collard greens, chopped
- 1 teaspoon chili powder
- 1 cup of water
- 1 spring onion, diced
- 1 tablespoon coconut oil

Method:
1. Melt the coconut oil in the saucepan.
2. Then add collard greens and sprinkle them with chili powder and diced spring onion.
3. Roast the vegetables for 4 minutes.
4. Add water and close the lid.
5. Cook the collard greens on medium heat for 10 minutes.

Nutritional info per serve: Calories 46, Fat 3.2, Fiber 2.2, Carbs 4.8, Protein 1.3

Paprika Cauliflower Rice

Prep time: 10 minutes
Cook time: 10 minutes
Servings: 4
Ingredients:
- 2 cups cauliflower, shredded
- 1 tablespoon butter
- 1 teaspoon garlic powder
- 1 teaspoon ground paprika
- ¼ cup beef broth

1. Bring the beef broth to boil.
2. Add shredded cauliflower, butter, garlic powder, and ground paprika.
3. Carefully mix the mixture and cook it on low heat for 10 minutes. Stir it from time to time to avoid burning.

Nutritional info per serve: Calories 44, Fat 3.1, Fiber 1.5, Carbs 3.5, Protein 1.5

Mozzarella Eggplant

Prep time: 15 minutes
Cook time: 20 minutes
Servings: 4
Ingredients:
- 1 eggplant, sliced
- 1 teaspoon salt
- 3 oz Mozzarella, sliced
- 1 tablespoon coconut oil

Method:
1. Grease the baking tray with coconut oil.
2. Then sprinkle the eggplants with salt and mix. Leave the vegetables for 10 minutes.
3. Then put eggplants in the tray in one layer and top with Mozzarella.
4. Bake the meal at 360F for 20 minutes.

Nutritional info per serve: Calories 118, Fat 7.4, Fiber 4, Carbs 7.5, Protein 7.1

Provolone Kale

Prep time: 10 minutes
Cook time: 10 minutes
Servings: 3
Ingredients:
- 3 cups kale, chopped
- 1 oz bacon, chopped, cooked
- 2 oz Provolone cheese, grated
- ½ cup coconut cream
- 1 teaspoon ground turmeric

Method:
1. Mix chopped kale with bacon, coconut cream, ground turmeric, and Provolone cheese.
2. Put the mixture in the tray and gently flatten.
3. Cook it at 360F for 10 minutes.

Nutritional info per serve: Calories 245, Fat 18.6, Fiber 2, Carbs 10.2, Protein 11.3

Coconut Broccoli

Prep time: 10 minutes
Cook time: 10 minutes
Servings: 4
Ingredients:
- 1 cup broccoli, chopped
- ½ cup coconut cream
- 1 teaspoon garlic, diced
- 1 tablespoon fresh parsley, chopped
- 1 teaspoon ground nutmeg

Method:
1. Put water in a saucepan, add the salt, and bring to a boil over medium-high heat.
2. Place broccoli florets in a steamer basket, place into saucepan, cover, and steam for 8 minutes. Drain and transfer to a bowl.
3. Heat a pan with the coconut butter over medium heat, add the lemon juice, lemon zest, and almonds, stir, and take off the heat.

4. Add the broccoli, toss to coat, divide between plates, and serve.
Nutritional info per serve: Calories 81, Fat 7.4, Fiber 1.4, Carbs 3.7, Protein 1.4

Lemon Spinach

Prep time: 5 minutes
Cook time: 10 minutes
Servings: 4
Ingredients:
- 2 cups spinach, chopped
- 1 tablespoon coconut oil
- ¼ cup of water
- 1 tablespoon lemon juice
- 1 teaspoon lemon zest, grated

Method:
1. Pour coconut cream in the skillet and bring it to boil.
2. Add chopped spinach and sprinkle it with turmeric and ground black pepper. Mix up well.
3. Close the lid and saute spinach for 5 minutes over the medium heat.
4. Then open the lid and stir the spinach well. Add almond flakes and grated Parmesan.
5. Mix up the spinach until all cheese is melted.
6. Then close the lid and leave the spinach rest for 5 minutes.

Nutritional info per serve: Calories 34, Fat 3.5, Fiber 0.4, Carbs 0.7, Protein 0.5

Cheesy Broccoli

Prep time: 10 minutes
Cook time: 22 minutes
Servings: 4
Ingredients:
- 5 tablespoons coconut oil
- 1 garlic clove, diced
- 1-pound broccoli florets
- 1 oz Cheddar cheese, shredded

Method:
1. Put water in a saucepan, add salt, bring to a boil over medium-high heat, add broccoli, cook for 5 minutes, and drain.
2. Heat a pan with oil over medium-high heat, add garlic, stir, and cook for 2 minutes. Add broccoli, stir, and cook for 15 minutes.
3. Take off heat, sprinkle Parmesan cheese, divide between plates, and serve.

Nutritional info per serve: Calories 215, Fat 19.7, Fiber 3, Carbs 7.9, Protein 5

Baked Parmesan Broccoli

Prep time: 10 minutes
Cook time: 15 minutes
Servings: 7
Ingredients:
- 2-pound broccoli florets
- 2 oz Parmesan, grated
- ½ teaspoon ground paprika
- 1 tablespoon sesame oil
- 1 tablespoon coconut flour

Method:
1. Pour water in the saucepan and bring it to boil.
2. Then toss broccoli florets in the hot water and boil them for 3 minutes over the high heat.
3. Drain the water and chill broccoli florets little. Meanwhile, line the tray with baking paper. Preheat the oven to 365F.
4. Place the broccoli florets in the tray and sprinkle over with the paprika and chili flakes.
5. Cook the vegetables in the oven for 5 minutes.
6. Then sprinkle broccoli with grated cheese and cook for 5 minutes more.
7. When the broccoli florets start to have light brown edges, the meal is cooked.

Nutritional info per serve: Calories 96, Fat 4.4, Fiber 4.1, Carbs 10.1, Protein 6.5

Tender Onions

Prep time: 10 minutes
Cook time: 20 minutes
Servings: 4
Ingredients:
- 1 tablespoon coconut oil
- 2 spring onions, sliced
- ¼ cup chicken broth
- 1 teaspoon ground black pepper

Direction:
1. Melt the coconut oil in the saucepan.
2. Add spring onion and sprinkle it with ground black pepper.
3. Add chicken broth and boil the onions on low heat for 20 minutes or until the onion is tender.

Nutritional info per serve: Calories 55, Fat 3.6, Fiber 1.3, Carbs 5.5, Protein 1

Cauliflower Puree

Prep time: 10 minutes
Cook time: 15 minutes
Servings: 4
Ingredients:
- 10 oz cauliflower
- ¼ cup coconut cream
- ½ teaspoon dried cilantro
- 1 cup of water

Method:
1. Bring the water to boil and then add cauliflower.
2. Boil it for 15 minutes or until it is soft.
3. Then drain water and blend the cauliflower.
4. Add coconut cream and dried cilantro.
5. Carefully mix the puree.

Nutritional info per serve: Calories 52, Fat 3.7, Fiber 2.1, Carbs 4.6, Protein 1.7

Baked Zucchini

Prep time: 10 minutes
Cook time: 20 minutes
Servings: 6
Ingredients:
- 3 zucchinis, sliced
- 1 tablespoon sesame oil
- 1 teaspoon salt

- 1 oz Parmesan, grated

Method:
1. Sprinkle the baking tray with sesame oil.
2. Put the zucchini slices in the baking tray in one layer and sprinkle with salt and Parmesan.
3. Bake at 360F for 20 minutes.

Nutritional info per serve: Calories 51, Fat 3.5, Fiber 1.1, Carbs 3.5, Protein 2.7

Creamy Cabbage

Prep time: 10 minutes
Cook time: 35 minutes
Servings: 5
Ingredients:
- 3 cups white cabbage, shredded
- 1 cup coconut cream
- 1 teaspoon salt
- 1 teaspoon ground nutmeg
- 1 tablespoon coconut oil

Method:
1. Pour the coconut cream in the saucepan.
2. Add white cabbage, salt, ground nutmeg, and coconut oil. Carefully mix the mixture.
3. Cook it on medium heat for 35 minutes.

Nutritional info per serve: Calories 147, Fat 14.4, Fiber 2., Carbs 5.3, Protein 1.7

Garlic Swiss Chard

Prep time: 10 minutes
Cook time: 10 minutes
Servings: 2
Ingredients:
- 2 tablespoons coconut oil
- 1 oz bacon, chopped
- 7 oz Swiss chard, chopped
- ½ teaspoon garlic, minced

Method:
1. Melt the coconut oil in the saucepan.
2. Add bacon and roast it for 1 minute per side.
3. Add Swiss chard and garlic.
4. Carefully mix the meal and cook it for 3 minutes per side.

Nutritional info per serve: Calories 214, Fat 19.8, Fiber 1.7, Carbs 4.1, Protein 7.1

Cauliflower Mix

Prep time: 10 minutes
Cook time: 10 minutes
Servings: 4
Ingredients:
- 2 cups cauliflower, shredded
- 1 oz chives, chopped
- 2 oz provolone, grated
- ½ teaspoon salt
- 1 teaspoon chili pepper
- 1 teaspoon cream cheese
- 3 eggs, beaten

Method:
1. In the mixing bowl, mix cream cheese and eggs.
2. Add chili pepper, salt, and chives.
3. Then mix the shredded cauliflower with cheese and egg mixture.

4. Put it in the baking pan and cook at 360F for 10 minutes.

Nutritional info per serve: Calories 115, Fat 7.5, Fiber 1.5, Carbs 3.7, Protein 9.1

Prosciutto Salad

Prep time: 10 minutes
Cook time: 12 minutes
Servings: 4
Ingredients:
- 2 tablespoons coconut oil
- 1 pound white mushrooms, chopped
- 2 tablespoons avocado oil
- 2 oz prosciutto, sliced
- 1 tablespoon lemon juice
- ½ cup coconut cream

Method:
1. Melt the coconut oil in the pan.
2. Add mushrooms and coconut cream, and roast them for 5 minutes per side on medium heat.
3. Then transfer the mushrooms in the salad bowl.
4. Add all remaining ingredients and carefully mix.

Nutritional info per serve: Calories 183, Fat 16, Fiber 2.1, Carbs 6.1, Protein 7.3

Lime Cabbage Mix

Prep time: 10 minutes
Cook time: 5 minutes
Servings: 6
Ingredients:
- 3 tablespoons lime juice
- 1 tablespoon ground black pepper
- 1/3 cup water
- 2 cups white cabbage, shredded
- 1 tablespoon avocado oil

Method:
1. Bring water to boil and add cabbage. Boil it for 5 minutes on medium heat.
2. Then transfer the cabbage in the big bowl.
3. Add all remaining ingredients and carefully mix.

Nutritional info per serve: Calories 12, Fat 0.4, Fiber 1, Carbs 2.2, Protein 0.5

Nutmeg Mushroom Mix

Prep time: 10 minutes
Cook time: 30 minutes
Servings: 6
Ingredients:
- ½ pounds mushrooms, chopped
- 1 tablespoon avocado oil
- 1 teaspoon ground coriander
- 1 tomato, chopped
- 1 tablespoon coconut oil
- 1 teaspoon ground nutmeg

Method:
1. Melt the coconut oil in the skillet.
2. Add mushrooms and roast them for 10 minutes. Stir them from time to time.
3. After this, add avocado oil, ground coriander, and ground nutmeg.

4. Add tomato and close the lid.
5. Simmer the meal for 15 minutes on medium-low heat.
Nutritional info per serve: Calories 33, Fat 2.7, Fiber 0.6, Carbs 1.8, Protein 1.3

Keto Pesto
Prep time: 10 minutes
Servings: 6
Ingredients:
- 1 avocado, peeled
- 1 oz Parmesan, grated
- ½ teaspoon minced garlic
- 1 jalapeno, minced
- 1 oz fresh cilantro, chopped
- 3 tablespoons avocado oil

Method:
1. Put all ingredients in the blender and blend until smooth.
2. Transfer it in the glass can and store it in the fridge for up to 4 days.
Nutritional info per serve: Calories 106, Fat 9.9, Fiber 2.4, Carbs 3.4, Protein 2.3

Basil Tomato Mix
Prep time: 10 minutes
Cook time: 0 minutes
Servings: 5
Ingredients:
- 2 tomatoes, chopped
- 1 teaspoon dried basil
- 2 scallions, sliced
- 1 teaspoon salt
- 1 tablespoon avocado oil

Method:
1. Put the chopped tomatoes in the bowl in one layer.
2. Add scallions over tomatoes and sprinkle with salt, avocado oil, and dried basil.
Nutritional info per serve: Calories 21, Fat 0.5, Fiber 1.2, Carbs 4.1, Protein 0.7

Turmeric Eggplant
Prep time: 15 minutes
Cook time: 10 minutes
Servings: 5
Ingredients:
- 2 eggplants, trimmed
- 1 teaspoon ground turmeric
- 1 teaspoon salt
- 2 tablespoons sesame oil

Method:
1. Slice the eggplants and sprinkle them with salt and ground turmeric.
2. Then leave them for 10 minutes to rest.
3. After this, preheat the sesame oil in the skillet.
4. Put the sliced eggplants in the skillet in one layer and roast for 2 minutes per side on medium heat.
Nutritional info per serve: Calories 104, Fat 5.9, Fiber 7.8, Carbs 13.2, Protein 2.2

Cucumber Salad
Prep time: 10 minutes
Cook time: 0 minutes
Servings: 6
Ingredients:
- 2 cucumbers, sliced
- ¼ cup radish, sliced
- 2 tablespoons cream cheese
- 1 teaspoon ground black pepper

Method:
1. Mix cucumbers with radish in the salad bowl.
2. Add cream cheese and ground black pepper.
3. Carefully mix the salad.
Nutritional info per serve: Calories 28, Fat 1.3, Fiber 0.7, Carbs 4.1, Protein 1

Mozzarella Salad
Prep time: 10 minutes
Servings: 4
Ingredients:
- ½ teaspoon white pepper
- 8 oz Mozzarella, shredded
- 1 teaspoon dried dill
- 1 tablespoon avocado oil
- 1 tablespoon apple cider vinegar
- 1 cup radish, chopped

Method:
1. Mix all ingredients in the salad bowl and leave for 10 minutes in the fridge before serving.
Nutritional info per serve: Calories 171, Fat 10.5, Fiber 0.7, Carbs 3.5, Protein 16.3

Dill Tomatoes
Prep time: 5 minutes
Cook time: 0 minutes
Servings: 4
Ingredients:
- 2 tomatoes, sliced
- 1 tablespoon avocado oil
- 1 teaspoon dried dill
- 1 teaspoon apple cider vinegar

Method:
1. Put the tomatoes in the plate in one layer and sprinkle with avocado oil.
2. Then sprinkle them with dried dill and apple cider vinegar.
Nutritional info per serve: Calories 17, Fat 0.6, Fiber 0.9, Carbs 2.7, Protein 0.6

Cinnamon Rutabaga
Prep time: 10 minutes
Cook time: 15 minutes
Servings: 3
Ingredients:
- 8 oz rutabaga, peeled
- 1 tablespoon coconut oil
- 1 teaspoon ground cinnamon

Method:
1. Chop the rutabaga and mix it with ground cinnamon and coconut oil.

2. Bake the meal at 360F for 15 minutes or until rutabaga is tender.
Nutritional info per serve: Calories 68, Fat 4.7, Fiber 2.3, Carbs 6.8, Protein 0.9

Fennel Salad

Prep time: 10 minutes
Cook time: 0 minutes
Servings: 4
Ingredients:
- 8 oz fennel, chopped
- 1 oz fresh cilantro, chopped
- 1 tablespoon avocado oil
- 1 teaspoon lemon juice
- 1 teaspoon ground paprika
- 1 teaspoon dried oregano

Method:
1. Put all ingredients in the salad bowl.
2. Carefully mix the salad.

Nutritional info per serve: Calories 27, Fat 0.7, Fiber 2.5, Carbs 5.2, Protein 1

Artichoke Bake

Prep time: 15 minutes
Cook time: 20 minutes
Servings: 4
Ingredients:
- 2 artichokes, halved
- 1 teaspoon minced garlic
- 1 tablespoon coconut oil
- 1 tablespoon lemon juice

Method:
1. Mix coconut oil with minced garlic.
2. Rub the artichoke halves with coconut oil mixture.
3. Then sprinkle them with lemon juice and bake at 365F for 20 minutes.

Nutritional info per serve: Calories 69, Fat 3.6, Fiber 4.4, Carbs 8.8, Protein 2.7

Avocado Mix

Prep time: 10 minutes
Cook time: 10 minutes
Servings: 4
Ingredients:
- 1 eggplant, chopped
- 1 tablespoon coconut oil
- 1 teaspoon salt
- 1 tablespoon lemon juice
- 1 teaspoon dried parsley
- ½ avocado, peeled, chopped
- 1 teaspoon avocado oil

Method:
1. Sprinkle the eggplant with salt and put it in the skillet.
2. Add avocado oil and roast it for 10 minutes or until the eggplant is soft.
3. Cool it to the room temperature and transfer it in the bowl.
4. Add all remaining ingredients and carefully mix.

Nutritional info per serve: Calories 121, Fat 9.7, Fiber 5.8, Carbs 9, Protein 1.6

Lemon Zucchini

Prep time: 10 minutes
Cook time: 5 minutes
Servings: 5
Ingredients:
- 2 zucchinis, chopped
- 1 teaspoon ground paprika
- 1 tablespoon lemon juice
- ¼ teaspoon ground nutmeg
- 1 tablespoon coconut oil

Method:
1. Melt the coconut oil in the skillet.
2. Add chopped zucchini and cook it for 2 minutes on medium heat.
3. Then carefully mix the vegetables and sprinkle them with ground paprika, lemon juice, and ground nutmeg.
4. Carefully mix and cook the meal on medium heat for 1 minute more.

Nutritional info per serve: Calories 39, Fat 3, Fiber 1.1, Carbs 3, Protein 1

Baked Eggplant

Prep time: 2 hours and 10 minutes
Cook time: 30 minutes
Servings: 5
Ingredients:
- 1 teaspoon Italian seasonings
- 1 tablespoon butter, softened
- 3 eggplants, roughly chopped
- ¼ cup of water

Method:
1. Mix eggplants with Italian seasonings and put them in the tray.
2. Add water and butter.
3. Bake the vegetables at 360F for 30 minutes.

Nutritional info per serve: Calories 105, Fat 3.2, Fiber 11.6, Carbs 19.4, Protein 3.2

Cream Cauliflower Mix

Prep time: 10 minutes
Cook time: 30 minutes
Servings: 4
Ingredients:
- 1 cup cauliflower florets
- ½ cup coconut cream
- 1 oz Cheddar cheese, shredded
- 1 tablespoon coconut oil
- 1 teaspoon dried basil

Method:
1. Grease the baking pan with coconut oil.
2. Then mix cauliflower florets with coconut cream, cheese, and dried basil.
3. Put the mixture in the baking pan, flatten it gently and cook at 360F for 30 minutes.

Nutritional info per serve: Calories 133, Fat 12.9, Fiber 1.3, Carbs 3.1, Protein 3

Endive Salad

Prep time: 5 minutes
Cook time: 0 minutes
Servings: 4
Ingredients:

- 4 endives, sliced (1-pound)
- 1 cup arugula, chopped
- 1 cup lettuce, chopped
- 1 tablespoon avocado oil
- 1 tablespoon apple cider vinegar

Method:
1. Put all ingredients in the salad bowl.
2. Carefully mix the salad.

Nutritional info per serve: Calories 30, Fat 0.8, Fiber 4.3, Carbs 5.1, Protein 1.8

Cilantro Turnip Bake

Prep time: 15 minutes
Cook time: 30 minutes
Servings: 3
Ingredients:
- 1 cup turnip, peeled, chopped
- 1/3 cup Cheddar cheese, shredded
- 1 tablespoon dried cilantro
- 1 teaspoon dried oregano
- 1 teaspoon coconut oil

Method:
1. Grease the baking ramekins with coconut oil.
2. Then mix turnip with dried cilantro and dried oregano.
3. Put the vegetables in the ramekins and top with Cheddar cheese.
4. Bake the meal at 360F for 30 minutes.

Nutritional info per serve: Calories 77, Fat 5.8, Fiber 1, Carbs 3.3, Protein 3.6

Radish Salad

Prep time: 10 minutes
Cook time: 0 minutes
Servings: 6
Ingredients:
- 1 teaspoon Italian seasonings
- 1 tablespoon avocado oil
- 1 teaspoon apple cider vinegar
- 4 cups radish, sliced
- 1 teaspoon salt

Method:
1. Mix all ingredients in the salad bowl and leave the salad for 10 minutes in the fridge before serving.

Nutritional info per serve: Calories 18, Fat 0.6, Fiber 1.3, Carbs 2.9, Protein 0.6

Curry Tofu

Prep time: 15 minutes
Cook time: 5 minutes
Servings: 2
Ingredients:
- 7 oz firm tofu
- 1 teaspoon curry powder
- ½ cup of coconut milk
- 1 teaspoon butter

Method:
1. In the mixing bowl, mix the curry powder and coconut milk.
2. Cut the tofu into cubes and put them in the curry mixture. Leave it for 10 minutes to marinate.
3. Then melt the butter in the skillet.
4. Add tofu and cook it for 2 minutes per side on medium heat.

Nutritional info per serve: Calories 228, Fat 20.5, Fiber 2.5, Carbs 5.6, Protein 9.7

Mint Sauce

Prep time: 0 minutes
Cook time: 10 minutes
Servings: 5
Ingredients:
- 1 teaspoon dried mint
- 1 oz Parmesan, grated
- 1/3 cup coconut cream
- 1 teaspoon butter

Method:
1. Melt the butter in the saucepan.
2. Add mint and coconut cream.
3. Bring the liquid to boil and add Parmesan.
4. Simmer it until the cheese is melted.

Nutritional info per serve: Calories 62, Fat 5.8, Fiber 0.4, Carbs 1.1, Protein 2.2

Baked Radishes

Prep time: 10 minutes
Cook time: 25 minutes
Servings: 3
Ingredients:
- 1 cup radish, trimmed, halved
- ½ teaspoon cayenne pepper
- ¼ teaspoon chili pepper
- 1 tablespoon coconut oil
- 1 teaspoon dried rosemary

Method:
1. Mix the radish with coconut oil, dried rosemary, chili pepper, and cayenne pepper.
2. Put the vegetables in the tray and bake at 360F for 25 minutes.

Nutritional info per serve: Calories 48, Fat 4.7, Fiber 0.9, Carbs 1.8, Protein 0.3

Jalapeno Sauce

Prep time: 7 minutes
Cook time: 10 minutes
Servings: 3
Ingredients:
- 1 tablespoon coconut shred
- 1 jalapeno, minced
- 1 teaspoon mustard seeds
- 1/3 cup coconut cream
- 1 teaspoon coconut oil
- ½ teaspoon curry powder

Method:
1. Melt the coconut oil in the saucepan.
2. Add mustard seeds and roast them for 3 minutes on medium heat. Stir them from time to time to avoid burning.
3. Then add jalapeno, coconut shred, coconut cream, and curry powder.
4. Carefully mix the sauce and simmer it for 5 minutes on low heat.

Nutritional info per serve: Calories 99, Fat 9.9, Fiber 1.3, Carbs 3, Protein 1

Rosemary Zucchini Mix

Prep time: 10 minutes
Cook time: 7 minutes
Servings: 4
Ingredients:
- 3 oz white mushrooms, chopped
- 1 teaspoon dried rosemary
- 1 teaspoon ground nutmeg
- ½ cup of water
- 2 tablespoon coconut oil, melted
- 1 zucchini, chopped

Method:
1. Put all ingredients in the saucepan and gently mix.
2. Close the lid and simmer the meal on medium heat for 3 minutes.

Nutritional info per serve: Calories 75, Fat 7.2, Fiber 1, Carbs 2.8, Protein 1.3

Masala Fennel

Prep time: 10 minutes
Cook time: 20 minutes
Servings: 4
Ingredients:
- 1 teaspoon garam masala
- 7 oz fennel bulb, chopped
- 1 tablespoon coconut oil

Method:
1. Sprinkle the fennel bulb with garam masala and carefully mix.
2. Then mix the vegetables with coconut oil and put in the tray.
3. Bake the fennel at 360F for 20 minutes or until it is tender.

Nutritional info per serve: Calories 45, Fat 3.5, Fiber 1.5, Carbs 3.6, Protein 0.6

Cardamom Eggplant

Prep time: 15 minutes
Cook time: 30 minutes
Servings: 4
Ingredients:
- 2 eggplants, chopped
- 1 teaspoon avocado oil
- 1 teaspoon apple cider vinegar
- 1 teaspoon ground cardamom
- 1 teaspoon salt

Method:
1. Sprinkle the eggplants with salt, ground cardamom, and apple cider vinegar. Leave them for 10 minutes.
2. Then transfer them in the baking tray, flatten the vegetables well and sprinkle with avocado oil.
3. Bake the eggplants for 30 minutes at 360F.

Nutritional info per serve: Calories 72, Fat 0.7, Fiber 9.9, Carbs 16.5, Protein 2.8

Dill Bell Peppers

Prep time: 10 minutes
Cook time: 10 minutes
Servings: 4
Ingredients:
- 1 tablespoon coconut oil
- 1 cup bell pepper, chopped
- 1 teaspoon dried dill

Method:
1. Melt the coconut oil in the skillet and preheat well.
2. Add bell pepper and dried dill.
3. Roast the bell pepper for 6 minutes (3 minutes per side).

Nutritional info per serve: Calories 39, Fat 3.5, Fiber 0.4, Carbs 2.4, Protein 0.4

Clove Carrots

Prep time: 10 minutes
Cook time: 15 minutes
Servings: 4
Ingredients:
- 2 carrots, sliced
- 1 tablespoon coconut oil
- 1 teaspoon ground clove
- ½ cup of water

Method:
1. Bring water to boil and add the carrot.
2. Boil it for 10 minutes.
3. Then preheat the coconut oil and put the boiled carrot in it.
4. Add ground clove and cook the carrots for 2-3 minutes. Carefully mix the vegetables.

Nutritional info per serve: Calories 44, Fat 3.5, Fiber 0.9, Carbs 3.3, Protein 0.3

Red Chard Stew

Prep time: 8 minutes
Cook time: 50 minutes
Servings: 4
Ingredients:
- 2 tablespoons coconut oil
- 1 tablespoon lemon juice
- 1 teaspoon ground black pepper
- 8 oz red chard, chopped
- ½ cup beef broth

Method:
1. Put all ingredients in the pot and carefully mix.
2. Then put the pot on the oven and bake at 355F for 50 minutes.

Nutritional info per serve: Calories 77, Fat 7.1, Fiber 1.4, Carbs 2.9, Protein 1.8

Bacon and Oregano Broccoli

Prep time: 10 minutes
Cook time: 30 minutes
Servings: 4
Ingredients:
- 2 cups broccoli, chopped
- 1/3 cup coconut cream
- 5 oz provolone cheese, shredded
- 1 tablespoon coconut oil
- ½ teaspoon ground black pepper
- ½ teaspoon salt
- 1 teaspoon oregano
- 3 oz bacon, chopped
- ¾ cup of water

Method:
1. Put the bacon in the saucepan and roast for 1 minute per side.
2. Then add coconut oil, broccoli, ground black pepper, and oregano.
3. Roast the vegetables for 10 minutes on medium heat, stir them from time to time.
4. Then add all remaining ingredients and close the lid.
5. Cook the broccoli on medium-low heat for 15 minutes.

Nutritional info per serve: Calories 332, Fat 26.7, Fiber 1.9, Carbs 5.6, Protein 18.7

Apple Cider Vinegar Kale

Prep time: 10 minutes
Cook time: 5 minutes
Servings: 4
Ingredients:
- 1 cup of water
- 1 tablespoon apple cider vinegar
- 1 pecan, chopped
- 1 teaspoon garlic powder
- 2 cups kale, chopped
- 1 teaspoon avocado oil

Method:
1. Bring the water to boil and add kale.
2. Boil it for 5 minutes.
3. Then remove it from the water and mix with all remaining ingredients. Carefully mix the kale.

Nutritional info per serve: Calories 46, Fat 2.7, Fiber 1, Carbs 4.6, Protein 1.5

Cheesy Cauliflower Florets

Prep time: 10 minutes
Cook time: 30 minutes
Servings: 3
Ingredients:
- 8 oz cauliflower florets
- 1 tablespoon coconut flour
- 2 oz Parmesan, grated
- 1 tablespoon avocado oil

Method:
1. Line the baking tray with baking paper and put the cauliflower florets inside. Flatten them well.
2. Then sprinkle the vegetables with avocado oil, coconut flour, and Parmesan.
3. Bake the meal at 360F for 30 minutes.

Nutritional info per serve: Calories 98, Fat 5.2, Fiber 3.2, Carbs 6.6, Protein 8.2

Cabbage and Arugula Salad

Prep time: 10 minutes
Cook time: 0 minutes
Servings: 4
Ingredients:
- 1 cup white cabbage, shredded
- 2 tablespoons coconut cream
- ½ teaspoon minced garlic
- 1 cup arugula, chopped
- 1 oz Parmesan, grated

Method:
1. Put all ingredients in the salad bowl.
2. Carefully mix the salad.

Nutritional info per serve: Calories 46, Fat 3.4, Fiber 0.7, Carbs 2, Protein 2.8

Cheddar Kale

Prep time: 10 minutes
Cook time: 10 minutes
Servings: 4
Ingredients:
- 2 oz pork rinds, chopped
- 2 cups kale, chopped
- 1 tablespoon dried dill
- 1 tablespoon avocado oil
- 1 teaspoon coconut oil
- 1 teaspoon dried oregano
- 2 oz Cheddar cheese, shredded

Method:
1. In the mixing bowl, mix pork rinds with kale, dried dill, avocado oil, coconut oil, and dried oregano.
2. Put the mixture in the lined with the baking paper tray and flatten well.
3. Then top it with Cheddar cheese.
4. Bake the kale at 360F for 10 minutes.

Nutritional info per serve: Calories 172, Fat 11.4, Fiber 0.9, Carbs 4.6, Protein 13.9

Pepper Cabbage

Prep time: 10 minutes
Cook time: 20 minutes
Servings: 4
Ingredients:
- 2 cups white cabbage, shredded
- 1 teaspoon ground black pepper
- 3 tablespoons coconut oil
- ½ teaspoon ground paprika

Method:
1. Mix white cabbage with ground paprika and ground black pepper.
2. Then melt the coconut oil in the saucepan and preheat well.
3. Add cabbage and cook it for 20 minutes on the medium heat. Stir it from time to time.

Nutritional info per serve: Calories 99, Fat 10.3, Fiber 1.1, Carbs 2.5, Protein 0.6

Zucchini Sticks

Prep time: 10 minutes
Cook time: 20 minutes
Servings: 4
Ingredients:
- 2 zucchini, cut into sticks
- 1 oz Parmesan, grated
- ½ teaspoon ground black pepper
- 1 teaspoon sesame oil

Method:
1. Line the baking tray with baking paper.
2. Then put the zucchini sticks inside in one layer.
3. Sprinkle them with sesame oil, ground black pepper, and Parmesan.
4. Bake the vegetables at 360F for 20 minutes or until Parmesan is light brown.

Nutritional info per serve: Calories 49, Fat 2.8, Fiber 1.2, Carbs 3.7, Protein 3.5

Scallions Green Beans

Prep time: 10 minutes
Cook time: 25 minutes
Servings: 4
Ingredients:
- 6 oz green beans, trimmed, chopped
- 1 oz scallions, chopped
- 1 teaspoon white pepper
- 1 teaspoon ground paprika
- 1 tablespoon coconut oil
- ¼ cup beef broth

Method:
1. Preheat the coconut oil in the saucepan.
2. Add green beans and roast them for 10 minutes.
3. Stir the bean carefully and add all remaining ingredients.
4. Close the lid and simmer the meal for 15 minutes on medium heat.

Nutritional info per serve: Calories 50, Fat 3.6, Fiber 2, Carbs 4.3, Protein 1.3

Lemon Cauliflower Shred

Prep time: 10 minutes
Cook time: 15 minutes
Servings: 6
Ingredients:
- 2 cups cauliflower, shredded
- 2 tablespoons lemon juice
- 1 tablespoon coconut oil
- 1 teaspoon ground clove

Method:
1. Preheat the coconut oil in the saucepan.
2. Add cauliflower and ground clove.
3. Carefully mix the cauliflower and cook it for 10 minutes on medium heat.
4. Add lemon juice and mix the meal before serving.

Nutritional info per serve: Calories 30, Fat 2.4, Fiber 1, Carbs 2.1, Protein 0.7

Cajun Zucchini

Prep time: 10 minutes
Cook time: 5 minutes
Servings: 4
Ingredients:
- 2 zucchinis, chopped
- 1 teaspoon Cajun seasonings
- 2 tablespoons coconut oil

Method:
1. Sprinkle zucchini with Cajun seasonings.
2. Preheat the coconut oil in the skillet well and add zucchini.
3. Roast the vegetables for 2 minutes per side.

Nutritional info per serve: Calories 74, Fat 7, Fiber 1.1, Carbs 3.3, Protein 1.2

Onion Spinach

Prep time: 10 minutes
Cook time: 10 minutes
Servings: 6
Ingredients:
- 1 cup spinach, steamed, chopped
- 2 spring onions, diced
- 1 tablespoon avocado oil
- 1 teaspoon sesame seeds

Method:
1. Preheat the skillet well.
2. Add spinach and spring onion.
3. Roast the ingredients for 10 minutes over the medium heat.
4. Then sprinkle the meal with sesame seeds and mix it well.

Nutritional info per serve: Calories 14, Fat 0.6, Fiber 0.7, Carbs 2.1, Protein 0.5

Oregano Olives

Prep time: 3 hours
Cook time: 0 minutes
Servings: 6
Ingredients:
- 6 Kalamata olives pitted
- 1 teaspoon dried oregano
- 1 teaspoon avocado oil
- 1 teaspoon apple cider vinegar

Method:
1. Put the Kalamata olives in the bowl.
2. Add all remaining ingredients and mix well.
3. Marinate the meal in the fridge for 3 hours.

Nutritional info per serve: Calories 7, Fat 0.6, Fiber 0.3, Carbs 0.8, Protein 0.1

Zucchini Cakes

Prep time: 1 minute
Cook time: 10 minutes
Servings: 6
Ingredients:
- 3 zucchinis, grated
- 1/3 cup coconut flour
- 1 egg, beaten
- 1 teaspoon garlic powder
- 1 teaspoon avocado oil

Method:
1. In the mixing bowl, mix zucchini with coconut flour, egg, and garlic powder.
2. Then preheat the avocado oil well.
3. Make the small cakes from the zucchini mixture with the help of the spoon and put in the hot avocado oil.
4. Roast the zucchini cakes for 3 minutes per side over the medium heat.

Nutritional info per serve: Calories 32, Fat 1.1, Fiber 1.4, Carbs 4.2, Protein 2.3

Cajun Zucchini Noodles

Prep time: 5 minutes
Cook time: 5 minutes
Servings: 6
Ingredients:
- 2 zucchinis, spiralized
- 1 teaspoon Cajun seasonings
- 1 teaspoon butter
- 2 tablespoons coconut milk

Method:
1. Melt the butter in the saucepan.
2. Add coconut milk and bring the mixture to boil.
3. Add spiralized zucchini and Cajun seasonings.
4. Carefully mix the meal and cook it for 2 minutes on medium heat.

Nutritional info per serve: Calories 28, Fat 1.9, Fiber 0.8, Carbs 2.5, Protein 0.9

Broccoli Puree

Prep time: 10 minutes
Cook time: 10 minutes
Servings: 6
Ingredients:
- 2 cups broccoli florets
- 1 cup of water
- 1 tablespoon butter
- 1 teaspoon salt
- 1/3 cup coconut cream

Method:
1. Bring the water to boil and add broccoli.
2. Boil the vegetables for 10 minutes. Then drain water and transfer the broccoli in the blender.
3. Add all remaining ingredients and blend until you get a smooth puree.

Nutritional info per serve: Calories 58, Fat 5.2, Fiber 1.1, Carbs 2.8, Protein 1.2

Dijon Brussel Sprouts

Prep time: 10 minutes
Cook time: 15 minutes
Servings: 4
Ingredients:
- 1 pound Brussels sprouts, trimmed and halved
- 1 cup of water
- 1 tablespoon Dijon mustard
- 1 teaspoon avocado oil
- 1 teaspoon ground paprika

Method:
1. Bring the water to boil and add Brussel sprouts, Boil them for 10 minutes.
2. Then drain water and transfer the Brussel sprouts in the well-preheated skillet.
3. Add avocado oil, Dijon mustard, and ground paprika.
4. Carefully mix the vegetables and cook them on medium heat for 5 minutes.

Nutritional info per serve: Calories 55, Fat 0.8, Fiber 4.6, Carbs 10.9, Protein 4.1

Ricotta Cabbage

Prep time: 15 minutes
Servings: 2
Ingredients:
- 1 cup white cabbage, shredded
- 1 tablespoon ricotta cheese
- 1 tablespoon coconut cream
- ½ teaspoon ground paprika

Method:
1. Put all ingredients in the mixing bowl and carefully mix.
2. Transfer the mixture in the serving bowl and leave in the fridge for 10-15 minutes before serving.

Nutritional info per serve: Calories 38, Fat 2.5, Fiber 1.3, Carbs 3.2, Protein 1.6

Monterey Jack Cheese Sauce

Prep time: 5 minutes
Cook time: 5 minutes
Servings: 8
Ingredients:
- 1 teaspoon butter
- 1 tablespoon ricotta cheese
- ½ cup coconut cream
- 1 cup Monterey Jack cheese, shredded
- 1 teaspoon garlic powder

Method:
1. Bring the coconut cream to boil.
2. Add ricotta cheese, butter, and garlic powder.
3. Simmer the mixture for 1 minute and add Monterey Jack cheese. Stir ti well until cheese is dissolved.

Nutritional info per serve: Calories 95, Fat 8.5, Fiber 0.4, Carbs 1.3, Protein 4.1

Dill Pickled Zucchini

Prep time: 15 minutes
Cook time: 10 minutes
Servings: 3
Ingredients:
- 1 cup zucchini, chopped
- ¼ cup of water
- 1 teaspoon dried dill
- 1 tablespoon apple cider vinegar
- ½ teaspoon ground black pepper

Method:
1. Bring the water to boil and add zucchini. Remove the mixture from the heat.
2. Add all remaining ingredients and leave the zucchini in the liquid for 10-15 minutes.

Nutritional info per serve: Calories 9, Fat 0.1, Fiber 0.5, Carbs 1.7, Protein 0.6

Parsley Kohlrabi

Prep time: 8 minutes
Cook time: 15 minutes
Servings: 4
Ingredients:
- 2 cups kohlrabi, chopped
- ½ teaspoon white pepper
- 1 tablespoon fresh parsley, chopped
- 1 tablespoon coconut oil
- ½ teaspoon minced garlic
- ¼ cup chicken broth

Method:
1. Melt the coconut oil in the saucepan. Add kohlrabi and roast it for 2-3 minutes.
2. Then add white pepper, parsley, minced garlic, and chicken broth. Carefully mix the meal and

cook it on medium heat for 10 minutes. Stir it from time to time.
Nutritional info per serve: Calories 51, Fat 3.6, Fiber 2.5, Carbs 4.6, Protein 1.5

Cheddar Jalapenos

Prep time: 5 minutes
Cook time: 15 minutes
Servings: 4
Ingredients:
- 4 jalapenos
- 1 teaspoon coconut oil
- 1 oz Cheddar cheese, shredded
- ½ teaspoon ricotta cheese
- ½ teaspoon dried cilantro

Method:
1. Trim the jalapenos and remove seeds. Slice them.
2. Then melt the coconut oil in the saucepan and add sliced jalapenos.
3. Add all cheese and dried cilantro.
4. Mix the mixture well and close the lid. Cook the meal on medium-low heat for 10 minutes. Stir it from time to time.

Nutritional info per serve: Calories 43, Fat 3.6, Fiber 0.4, Carbs 1, Protein 2

Garlic Turnips Sticks

Prep time: 10 minutes
Cook time: 15 minutes
Servings: 4
Ingredients:
- 1-pound turnips, peeled and cut into sticks
- 1 tablespoon coconut oil
- 1 teaspoon garlic powder
- 1 oz Cheddar cheese, shredded

Method:
1. Grease the baking tray with coconut oil and put the turnip sticks inside. Flatten them in one layer and sprinkle with garlic powder and cheddar cheese.
2. Bake the meal at 360F doe 15 minutes.

Nutritional info per serve: Calories 93, Fat 5.8, Fiber 1.9, Carbs 8, Protein 2.8

Cilantro Jalapenos

Prep time: 10 minutes
Cook time: 15 minutes
Servings: 6
Ingredients:
- 6 jalapeno peppers
- 2 tablespoons lemon juice
- 3 tablespoons water
- 1 teaspoon dried cilantro
- ½ teaspoon onion powder
- 1 teaspoon coconut oil

Method:
1. Put all ingredients in the saucepan and carefully mix.
2. Simmer the meal on low heat for 15 minutes. Stir the meal from time to time.

Nutritional info per serve: Calories 14, Fat 1, Fiber 0.6, Carbs 1.3, Protein 0.3

Butter Cauliflower Puree

Prep time: 10 minutes
Cook time: 10 minutes
Servings: 6
Ingredients:
- 3 cups cauliflower, chopped
- 1 cup chicken broth
- 1 tablespoon butter
- 1 teaspoon salt

Method:
1. Bring the chicken broth to boil and add cauliflower. Boil it for 10 minutes. Then drain the chicken broth and transfer the cauliflower in the food processor.
2. Add butter, salt, and ¼ cup of chicken broth. Blend the mixture until you get a smooth puree.

Nutritional info per serve: Calories 36, Fat 2.2, Fiber 1.3, Carbs 2.8, Protein 1.8

Coconut Bread

Prep time: 10 minutes
Cook time: 10 minutes
Servings: 2
Ingredients:
- 1 tablespoon coconut oil
- 1 tablespoon coconut flour
- ¾ teaspoon baking powder
- ¼ teaspoon apple cider vinegar
- 1 teaspoon psyllium husk powder

Method:
1. Mix all ingredients in the mixing bowl and knead the dough.
2. Transfer the dough in the non-stick baking pan and flatten it in the shape of the bread. Bake the bread at 350F for 10 minutes.

Nutritional info per serve: Calories 83, Fat 7.4, Fiber 2.7, Carbs 4.5, Protein 0.8

Zucchini and Pancetta Mix

Prep time: 10 minutes
Cook time: 10 minutes
Servings: 4
Ingredients:
- 1 cup zucchini, chopped
- 2 oz pancetta, chopped
- 2 spring onions, diced
- 1 jalapeno, chopped
- 1 teaspoon coconut oil

Method:
1. Preheat the coconut oil in the skillet well.
2. Add pancetta and roast it for 5 minutes. Stir it from time to time.
3. Add spring onion, jalapeno, and zucchini. Mix the mixture and cook it for 5-minute son medium heat.

Nutritional info per serve: Calories 103, Fat 7.2, Fiber 1, Carbs 3.9, Protein 5.9

Cabbage Stew

Prep time: 5 minutes
Cook time: 60 minutes
Servings: 4

Ingredients:
- 1 teaspoon keto tomato paste
- ¼ cup zucchini, chopped
- 1 cup white cabbage, shredded
- 1 tablespoon avocado oil
- 1 teaspoon dried cilantro
- 1 teaspoon ground black pepper
- ½ cup chicken broth

Method:
1. Put all ingredients in the saucepan and carefully mix.
2. Cook the stew on medium-low heat for 60 minutes.

Nutritional info per serve: Calories 17, Fat 0.7, Fiber 0.9, Carbs 2.2, Protein 1.1

Sausage Side Dish

Prep time: 10 minutes
Cook time: 20 minutes
Servings: 4
Ingredients:
- 4 ounces sausages, chopped
- 1 tablespoon coconut oil
- 1 teaspoon keto tomato paste
- ½ cup of water
- 1 teaspoon dried oregano

Method:
1. Bring the water to boil and add chopped sausages and coconut oil.
2. Then add keto tomato paste and dried oregano.
3. Simmer the meal on medium heat for 15 minutes.

Nutritional info per serve: Calories 128, Fat 11.5, Fiber 0.2, Carbs 0.5, Protein 5.6

Garlic Radicchio

Prep time: 10 minutes
Cook time: 5 minutes
Servings: 4
Ingredients:
- 8 oz radicchio
- 1 teaspoon avocado oil
- ½ teaspoon lemon juice
- ¼ cup coconut cream
- 1 teaspoon minced garlic
- 1 teaspoon dried parsley

Method:
1. Chop the radicchio roughly and mix with avocado oil.
2. Put it in the hot skillet and roast on high heat for 3 minutes.
3. Then stir the radicchio well and add all remaining ingredients.
4. Carefully mix the meal.

Nutritional info per serve: Calories 50, Fat 3.9, Fiber 0.9, Carbs 3.7, Protein 1.2

Parsley Pilaf

Prep time: 10 minutes
Cook time: 20 minutes
Servings: 4
Ingredients:
- 2 tablespoons coconut oil
- 1 pecan, chopped
- 1 cup cremini mushrooms, chopped
- 1 teaspoon flax seeds
- Salt and ground black pepper, to taste
- 1 tablespoon fresh parsley
- ½ cup cauliflower, shredded
- ½ cup chicken broth

Method:
1. Heat a pan with the butter over medium heat, add almonds and mushrooms, stir, and cook for 4 minutes.
2. Add hemp seeds and stir. Add salt, pepper, parsley, garlic powder, stock, stir, reduce the heat, cover the pan, and simmer until stock is absorbed.
3. Divide between plates and serve.

Nutritional info per serve: Calories 196, Fat 17.4, Fiber 1.5, Carbs 3.3, Protein 8.2

Walnut Salad

Prep time: 5 minutes
Servings: 2
Ingredients:
- 1 cup lettuce
- 2 tablespoons walnuts, chopped
- 1 tablespoon sesame oil
- ½ teaspoon sesame seeds
- 1 teaspoon apple cider vinegar
- ½ teaspoon lime zest, grated
- 1 tomato, chopped

Method:
1. Put all ingredients in the salad bowl.
2. Carefully mix the salad.

Nutritional info per serve: Calories 123, Fat 11.9, Fiber 1.2, Carbs 3.1, Protein 2.4

Zucchini Noodle Salad

Prep time: 5 minutes
Cook time: 0 minutes
Servings: 4
Ingredients:
- 1 zucchini, spiralized
- 1 tablespoon scallions, chopped
- 1 teaspoon avocado oil
- 1 teaspoon chili flakes
- 1 cup lettuce, chopped
- 1 teaspoon lemon juice

Method:
1. Put all ingredients in the salad bowl.
2. Carefully mix the salad with the help of two spoons.

Nutritional info per serve: Calories 12, Fat 0.3, Fiber 0.7, Carbs 2.3, Protein 0.7

Taco Jicama

Prep time: 10 minutes
Cook time: 15 minutes
Servings: 4
Ingredients:
- 1 cup jicama, cut into strips
- 1 teaspoon taco seasonings
- 1 teaspoon coconut oil

Method:

1. Grease the baking tray with coconut oil and put jicama sticks inside in one layer/
2. Sprinkle the jicama sticks with taco seasonings and bake them at 350F for 15 minutes.
Nutritional info per serve: Calories 24, Fat 1.2, Fiber 1.5, Carbs 3.2, Protein 0.2

Broccoli and Spinach Bowl

Prep time: 10 minutes
Cook time: 15 minutes
Servings: 4
Ingredients:
- 1 cup broccoli, chopped
- 2 tablespoons avocado oil
- 1 teaspoon chili powder
- 1 cup spinach, chopped
- ½ cup beef broth

Method:
1. Bring the beef broth to boil and add broccoli.
2. Boil it for 10 minutes.
3. Then transfer the broccoli in the saucepan and add avocado oil.
4. Add chili powder and spinach. Mix the meal and cook it on medium heat for 5 minutes. Stir it from time to time to avoid burning.

Nutritional info per serve: Calories 26, Fat 1.3, Fiber 1.3, Carbs 2.6, Protein 1.6

Sriracha Slaw

Prep time: 10 minutes
Cook time: 20 minutes
Servings: 4
Ingredients:
- 1 cup white cabbage, shredded
- 2 tablespoons sriracha
- 1 tablespoon coconut oil
- ¼ cup of water
- 1 teaspoon salt
- 1 teaspoon ground paprika

Method:
1. Mix cabbage with salt and leave for 10 minutes.
2. Then melt the coconut oil in the saucepan and add cabbage. Roast it for 10 minutes. Stir it from time to time.
3. After this, add all remaining ingredients and cook the meal on medium heat for 10 minutes.

Nutritional info per serve: Calories 39, Fat 3.5, Fiber 0.6, Carbs 2.1, Protein 0.3

Cauliflower Polenta

Prep time: 10 minutes
Cook time: 15 minutes
Servings: 2
Ingredients:
- 1 cup cauliflower, shredded
- 1 pecan, chopped
- 1 tablespoon coconut oil
- 1 teaspoon nutritional yeast
- 1 teaspoon dried oregano
- ¼ cup beef broth

Method:

1. Bring the beef broth to boil.
2. Add coconut oil, oregano, and shredded cauliflower. Carefully mix the mixture.
3. Add pecan and nutritional yeast.
4. Remove the meal from the heat and mix it well.

Nutritional info per serve: Calories 133, Fat 12.2, Fiber 2.7, Carbs 5, Protein 3.2

Mushroom Pan

Prep time: 10 minutes
Cook time: 20 minutes
Servings: 6
Ingredients:
- 10 oz white mushrooms, chopped
- 2 scallions, sliced
- 1 tablespoon coconut oil
- 1 teaspoon ground black pepper
- 1 tablespoon cream cheese

Method:
1. Melt the coconut oil in the saucepan and add white mushrooms and scallions.
2. Roast the vegetables for 15 minutes. Stir them from time to time.
3. Add ground black pepper and cream cheese. Carefully mix the meal and cook it for 5 minutes more.

Nutritional info per serve: Calories 44, Fat 3, Fiber 1, Carbs 3.5, Protein 1.9

Cheese and Peppers Bowl

Prep time: 10 minutes
Cook time: 20 minutes
Servings: 8
Ingredients:
- 1 cup bell peppers, chopped
- ½ cup Cheddar cheese, shredded
- 1 teaspoon taco seasonings
- 2 tablespoons sesame oil

Method:
1. Mix bell peppers with sesame oil and put in the baking tray. Flatten the vegetables and sprinkle with taco seasonings and Cheddar cheese.
2. Bake the bell peppers for 20 minutes at 360F.

Nutritional info per serve: Calories 66, Fat 5.8, Fiber 0.2, Carbs 1.6, Protein 2

Lime Salad

Prep time: 7 minutes
Servings: 5
Ingredients:
- 2 cups lettuce, chopped
- 1 cup arugula, chopped
- 1 pecan, chopped
- 1 teaspoon coconut cream
- 1 tablespoon lime juice
- ½ teaspoon lime zest, grated

Method:
1. Put all ingredients in the salad bowl.
2. Carefully mix the lime salad.

Nutritional info per serve: Calories 26, Fat 2.3, Fiber 0.5, Carbs 1.3, Protein 0.5

Nutmeg Mushrooms

Prep time: 10 minutes
Cook time: 20 minutes
Servings: 4
Ingredients:
- 4 tablespoons coconut oil
- 16 oz baby mushrooms
- 1 teaspoon ground nutmeg
- 1 teaspoon garlic powder
- ¼ cup beef broth

Method:
1. Melt the coconut oil in the saucepan.
2. Add baby mushrooms and roast them for 10 minutes.
3. Stir the mushrooms and sprinkle with ground nutmeg and garlic powder.
4. Add beef broth and cook the mushrooms on medium heat for 10 minutes more.

Nutritional info per serve: Calories 149, Fat 14.2, Fiber 1.3, Carbs 4.6, Protein 4

Sweet Cranberry Sauce

Prep time: 5 minutes
Servings: 6
Ingredients:
- 1 cup cranberries
- 1 teaspoon lemon zest, grated
- 1 tablespoon Erythritol
- 2 tablespoons water

Method:
1. Mash the cranberries and put them in the saucepan.
2. Add lemon zest, Erythritol, and water.

Nutritional info per serve: Calories 10, Fat 0, Fiber 0.7, Carbs 1.7, Protein 0

Cumin Green Beans

Prep time: 10 minutes
Cook time: 10 minutes
Serving: 8
Ingredients:
- 1 teaspoon apple cider vinegar
- 2 cups green beans, chopped
- ½ cup of water
- 1 teaspoon ground cumin
- 1 teaspoon avocado oil

Method:
1. Mix green beans with water and avocado oil and bring the vegetables to boil.
2. Add ground cumin and cook the meal for 5 minutes.
3. Add apple cider vinegar and transfer in the serving bowls.

Nutritional info per serve: Calories 10, Fat 0.2, Fiber 1, Carbs 2.1, Protein 0.6

Cauliflower Tots

Prep time: 10 minutes
Cook time: 10 minutes
Servings: 8
Ingredients:
- 2 cups cauliflower, shredded
- 1 egg, beaten
- ¼ cup Cheddar cheese, shredded
- 3 tablespoons coconut flour
- 1 teaspoon sesame oil

Method:
1. In the mixing bowl, mix egg, cheddar cheese, and coconut flour.
2. Make the small tots.
3. Preheat the sesame oil in the skillet. Add cauliflower tots and roast them for 2-3 minutes per side until they are light brown.

Nutritional info per serve: Calories 45, Fat 2.7, Fiber 1.6, Carbs 2.9, Protein 2.5

Eggplant Sauce

Prep time: 10 minutes
Cook time: 15 minutes
Servings: 4
Ingredients:
- 1 eggplant, diced
- 3 scallions, diced
- 1 tablespoon avocado oil
- ½ teaspoon minced garlic
- 2 tablespoons coconut aminos
- 1 teaspoon coconut oil
- ¼ cup of water

Method:
1. Mix all ingredients in the saucepan and close the lid.
2. Simmer the sauce for 15 minutes.
3. Cool the cooked meal till the room temperature.

Nutritional info per serve: Calories 57, Fat 1.8, Fiber 4.5, Carbs 9.8, Protein 1.3

Chili Zucchini Rounds

Prep time: 10 minutes
Cook time: 15 minutes
Servings: 3
Ingredients:
- 1 large zucchini, sliced
- 1 teaspoon chili powder
- 1 oz Parmesan, grated
- 1 teaspoon butter, melted

Method:
1. Mix sliced zucchini with chili powder and butter and put in the lined with baking paper tray.
2. Top the zucchini with Parmesan and bake at 360F for 15 minutes.

Nutritional info per serve: Calories 62, Fat 3.6, Fiber 1.5, Carbs 4.4, Protein 4.5

Cheese Ramekins

Prep time: 10 minutes
Cook time: 15 minutes
Servings: 8
Ingredients:
- 1 teaspoon coconut oil, softened
- ½ cup Cheddar cheese, shredded
- 2 eggs, beaten
- 3 tablespoons cream cheese
- 1 teaspoon dried dill

Method:

1. Grease the ramekins with coconut oil.
2. Then mix Cheddar cheese with eggs, cream cheese, and dried dill.
3. Put the mixture in the ramekins and bake at 360F for 15 minutes.
Nutritional info per serve: Calories 63, Fat 5.3, Fiber 0, Carbs 0.3, Protein 3.5

Harissa Turnip

Prep time: 10 minutes
Cook time: 8 minutes
Servings: 4
Ingredients:
- 9 oz turnip, peeled, chopped
- 1 tablespoon lemon juice
- 2 tablespoons coconut oil
- 1 teaspoon harissa

Method:
1. Melt the coconut oil in the saucepan.
2. Add turnip and roast it for 2 minutes per side, Add harissa and lemon juice.
3. Carefully mix the meal and cook it for 1 minute more.
Nutritional info per serve: Calories 82, Fat 7.1, Fiber 1.2, Carbs 4.7, Protein 0.7

Sweet Cauliflower Salad

Prep time: 10 minutes
Cook time: 0 minutes
Servings: 6
Ingredients:
- 3 cup cauliflower, boiled, chopped
- 1 teaspoon Erythritol
- 1 egg, hard-boiled, chopped
- 1 tablespoon cream cheese
- 1 tablespoon coconut cream
- 1 teaspoon coconut aminos
- 1 teaspoon onion powder

Method:
1. Mix all ingredients in the salad bowl and carefully mix.
Nutritional info per serve: Calories 37, Fat 2, Fiber 1.3, Carbs 3.4, Protein 2.1

Marinated Garlic

Prep time: 15 minutes
Cook time: 0 minutes
Servings: 3
Ingredients:
- 3 big garlic cloves, peeled
- 1 teaspoon avocado oil
- 1 teaspoon coconut aminos
- ½ teaspoon dried cilantro

Method:
1. Mix garlic with avocado oil, coconut aminos, and dried cilantro.
2. Carefully mix the mixture and leave it for 10 minutes to marinate.
Nutritional info per serve: Calories 8, Fat 0.2, Fiber 0.1, Carbs 1.4, Protein 0.2

Spicy Risotto

Prep time: 10 minutes
Cook time: 20 minutes
Servings: 4
Ingredients:
- 2 cups cauliflower, shredded
- ½ cup beef broth
- 1 teaspoon ground black pepper
- ¼ teaspoon ginger powder
- 1 teaspoon chili flakes
- 1 teaspoon coconut oil
- 4 oz white mushrooms, chopped

Method:
1. Put mushrooms in the saucepan and add coconut oil.
2. Roast them for 10 minutes and carefully mix.
3. Add beef broth, cauliflower, ground black pepper, ginger powder, and chili flakes. Mix the mixture.
4. Cook the risotto for 10 minutes more.
Nutritional info per serve: Calories 35, Fat 1.5, Fiber 1.7, Carbs 4.1, Protein 2.6

Baked Okra

Prep time: 10 minutes
Cook time: 15 minutes
Servings: 4
Ingredients:
- 1 ½ cup okra, roughly chopped
- 1 tablespoon coconut oil
- ½ teaspoon chili pepper
- ½ teaspoon salt

Method:
1. Grease the baking tray with coconut oil.
2. Add okra, chili pepper, and salt.
3. Mix the mixture and bake it at 365F for 15 minutes or until okra is light brown.
Nutritional info per serve: Calories 45, Fat 3.5, Fiber 1.2, Carbs 2.9, Protein 0.7

KETOGENIC SNACKS AND APPETIZERS RECIPES

Egg Balls

Prep time: 20 minutes
Cook time: 0 minutes
Servings: 4
Ingredients:
- 4 eggs, hard-boiled, chopped
- 1 teaspoon apple cider vinegar
- ¼ teaspoon minced garlic
- 1 teaspoon ricotta cheese
- 1 oz scallions, chopped

Method:
1. Mix all ingredients in the mixing bowl.
2. Make the small balls.

Nutritional info per serve: Calories 68, Fat 4.5, Fiber 0.2, Carbs 1, Protein 5.8

Pork Kebabs

Prep time: 15 minutes
Cook time: 8 minutes
Servings: 4
Ingredients:
- 1 cup ground pork
- ½ zucchini, grated
- 1 teaspoon chili powder
- ½ teaspoon dried basil

Method:
5. In the mixing bowl, mix ground pork with grated zucchini, chili powder, and dried dill.
6. Then make the kebabs using the wooden skewers and put them in the preheated to 400F grill.
7. Bake the kebabs for 4 minutes per side.

Nutritional info per serve: Calories 68, Fat 4.5, Fiber 0.2, Carbs 1, Protein 5.8

Chorizo Dip

Prep time: 10 minutes
Cook time: 10 minutes
Servings: 4
Ingredients:
- 1 teaspoon coconut oil
- ½ cup coconut cream
- 2 oz Cheddar cheese, shredded
- 12 oz chorizo, chopped
- ¼ cup green onions, chopped

Method:
1. Put the chorizo in the hot skillet and roast for 2 minutes per side.
2. Add coconut oil, coconut cream, and mix carefully. Cook the mixture for 10 minutes. Stir it from time to time.
3. Then add cheese and green onions. Carefully mix the dip and cook it until the cheese is melted.

Nutritional info per serve: Calories 528, Fat 45.5, Fiber 0.8, Carbs 3.9, Protein 24.8

Chili Biscuits

Prep time: 15 minutes
Cook time: 15 minutes
Servings: 8
Ingredients:
- 1 cup almond flour
- 1 teaspoon chili powder
- 1 teaspoon smoked paprika
- 3 teaspoons coconut oil
- 1 tablespoon sesame oil

Method:
1. Brush the baking pan with sesame oil.
2. Then mix all remaining ingredients in the mixing bowl and knead the dough.
3. Make the small biscuits and put them in the baking pan.
4. Bake the meal ta 360F for 15 minutes.

Nutritional info per serve: Calories 51, Fat 5.2, Fiber 0.6, Carbs 1.1, Protein 0.8

Cauliflower Sauce

Prep time: 10 minutes
Cook time: 10 minutes
Servings: 6
Ingredients:
- 2 cups cauliflower, shredded
- 2 tablespoons ricotta cheese
- 1 garlic clove, diced
- ½ teaspoon ground coriander
- ½ cup of coconut milk
- 1 teaspoon butter

Method:
1. Put all ingredients in the saucepan and bring to boil. Simmer it for 5 minutes on low heat.
2. Then remove it from the heat and cool to the room temperature.

Nutritional info per serve: Calories 68, Fat 5.8, Fiber 1.3, Carbs 3.3, Protein 1.8

Jalapeno Stuffed Eggs

Prep time: 10 minutes
Cook time: 0 minutes
Servings: 4
Ingredients:
- 4 eggs, hard-boiled, peeled
- 2 jalapenos, diced
- ½ tablespoon ricotta cheese
- ¼ teaspoon chili flakes

Method:
1. In the mixing bowl mix jalapenos with ricotta cheese, and chili flakes.
2. Then cut the eggs into halves and remove the egg yolks.
3. Add the egg yolks in the jalapeno mixture.
4. Fill the egg white halves with a jalapeno mixture.

Nutritional info per serve: Calories 68, Fat 4.6, Fiber 0.2, Carbs 0.9, Protein 5.9

Cilantro Crackers

Prep time: 10 minutes
Cook time: 10 minutes
Servings: 6
Ingredients:
- ½ teaspoon baking powder

- ¼ teaspoon ground black pepper
- 1¼ cups coconut flour
- ¼ teaspoon dried cilantro
- 1 teaspoon pesto sauce
- 2 tablespoon coconut oil

Method:
1. In the mixing bowl mix all ingredients and knead the dough.
2. Then roll it up and cut into small pieces (crackers).
3. Bake the crackers at 360F for 10 minutes or until they are crunchy.

Nutritional info per serve: Calories 143, Fat 8.2, Fiber 8.4, Carbs 13.7, Protein 3.4

Oregano Mushroom Caps

Prep time: 15 minutes
Cook time: 25 minutes
Servings: 8
Ingredients:
- 2 cups mushroom caps
- 1 teaspoon dried oregano
- ½ cup ground beef
- ½ teaspoon chili powder
- 1 tablespoon coconut oil

Method:
1. Melt the coconut oil and mix it with dried oregano, ground beef, and chili powder.
2. Then fill the mushroom caps with ground beef mixture and put in the tray.
3. Bake the mushroom caps for 25 minutes at 360F.

Nutritional info per serve: Calories 36, Fat 2.8, Fiber 0.3, Carbs 0.8, Protein 2.2

Herbed Muffins

Prep time: 10 minutes
Cook time: 14 minutes
Servings: 6
Ingredients:
- 3 tablespoons butter
- 1 tablespoon flax seeds
- 1 cup almond flour
- 1 tablespoon Erythritol
- ½ teaspoon baking powder
- 1 egg, beaten

Method:
1. In the mixing bowl, mix butter with flax seeds, almond flour, and baking powder. Add egg.
2. Stir the mixture until you get a smooth batter.
3. Then pour it in the silicone muffin molds (fill ½ part of every muffin mold) and bake at 360F for 14 minutes.

Nutritional info per serve: Calories 95, Fat 9.2, Fiber 0.8, Carbs 1.6, Protein 2.2

Spinach Dip

Prep time: 5 minutes
Cook time: 10 minutes
Servings: 6
Ingredients:
- 1 ½ cup spinach, chopped

- 2 tablespoons cream cheese
- 1 tablespoon coconut oil
- ¼ cup Cheddar cheese, grated
- ¼ cup heavy cream
- ½ teaspoon chili powder

Method:
1. Put all ingredients in the saucepan and carefully mix.
2. Then cook the mixture on low heat for 10 minutes or until it starts to boil.
3. Blend the mixture with the help of the immersion blender and simmer for 2-3 minutes more.

Nutritional info per serve: Calories 70, Fat 6.9, Fiber 0.3, Carbs 0.7, Protein 1.8

Seeds Chips

Prep time: 10 minutes
Cook time: 6 minutes
Servings: 6
Ingredients:
- 2 tablespoons flax seeds
- 1 egg, beaten
- 2 tablespoons almond flour
- ¼ teaspoon dried oregano
- Cooking spray

Method:
1. Spray the baking tray with cooking spray.
2. Then mix flax seeds with egg, almond flour, and dried oregano.
3. Roll up the mixture and cut it into small pieces (chips).
4. Put the chips in the prepared baking tray and cook at 360F for 5-6 minutes or until chips are crunchy.

Nutritional info per serve: Calories 36, Fat 2.6, Fiber 0.9, Carbs 1.3, Protein 1.9

Crab Dip

Prep time: 10 minutes
Cook time: 0 minutes
Servings: 6
Ingredients:
- 10 oz crab meat, canned
- 1 teaspoon garlic powder
- 1 tablespoon cream cheese
- ¼ cup Cheddar cheese, shredded
- ½ teaspoon ground paprika
- 1 teaspoon butter

Method:
1. Put all ingredients in the mixing bowl.
2. Carefully mix the mixture until smooth. The dip is cooked.

Nutritional info per serve: Calories 75, Fat 3.6, Fiber 0.1, Carbs 1.4, Protein 7.3

Pork Rinds Balls

Prep time: 10 minutes
Cook time: 0 minutes
Servings: 3
Ingredients:
- 4 oz pork rinds
- 2 tablespoons ricotta cheese
- ½ carrot, grated

- ½ teaspoon chili powder
- 1 egg, hard-boiled, chopped

Method:
1. In the mixing bowl, mix pork rinds with ricotta cheese, grated carrot, chili powder, and chopped eggs.
2. Make the small balls with the help of the ice cream scooper.

Nutritional info per serve: Calories 257, Fat 15.8, Fiber 0.4, Carbs 1.9, Protein 27.5

Paprika Wings

Prep time: 10 minutes
Cook time: 30 minutes
Servings: 4
Ingredients:
- 4 chicken wings, skinless
- 1 teaspoon avocado oil
- 1 teaspoon ground paprika
- 1 teaspoon salt

Method:
1. Put the chicken wings in the baking tray and sprinkle them with avocado oil, ground paprika, and salt.
2. Bake the chicken wings at 360F for 30 minutes.

Nutritional info per serve: Calories 31, Fat 0.9, Fiber 0.3, Carbs 0.4, Protein 5

Pepperoni Balls

Prep time: 15 minutes
Cook time: 0 minutes
Servings: 6
Ingredients:
- 14 pepperoni slices, chopped
- 4 oz ricotta cheese
- 2 tablespoons fresh parsley, chopped

Method:
1. Mix pepperoni slices with ricotta cheese and fresh parsley.
2. Make the medium size balls and refrigerate them for 10-15 minutes before serving.

Nutritional info per serve: Calories 90, Fat 7.1, Fiber 0, Carbs 1.1, Protein 5.1

Cheese Plate

Prep time: 10 minutes
Servings: 4
Ingredients:
- 1 oz Provolone cheese, chopped
- 1 oz Cheddar cheese, chopped
- 1 oz Swiss cheese, chopped
- 1 teaspoon olive oil
- 1 kalamata olive, sliced

Method:
1. Put all types of cheese on the plate one-by-one.
2. Then sprinkle the cheese with olive oil and slices olives.

Nutritional info per serve: Calories 92, Fat 7.5, Fiber 0, Carbs 0.7, Protein 5.5

Pork Muffins

Prep time: 10 minutes
Cook time: 18 minutes
Servings: 5
Ingredients:
- 2 tablespoons almond flour
- 1 cup ground pork
- 1 teaspoon minced garlic
- ¼ teaspoon dried basil
- 1 egg, beaten
- Cooking spray

Method:
1. Spray the muffin molds with cooking spray from inside. Preheat the oven to 360F.
2. Then mix ground pork with minced garlic, dried basil, and egg.
3. Put the mixture in the muffin molds and bake at 360F for 18 minutes.

Nutritional info per serve: Calories 263, Fat 19.5, Fiber 1.2, Carbs 2.7, Protein 19.6

Cheddar Peppers

Prep time: 15 minutes
Cook time: 30 minutes
Servings: 8
Ingredients:
- 4 bell peppers
- ¼ cup Cheddar cheese, shredded
- ½ cup ground chicken
- 1 egg, beaten
- 1 teaspoon avocado oil
- 1 teaspoon taco seasoning
- 1 tablespoon fresh cilantro, chopped

Method:
1. In the mixing bowl, mix ground chicken with Cheddar cheese, egg, cilantro, and Taco seasonings.
2. Then trim the bell peppers and remove the seeds.
3. Fill the peppers with ground chicken mixture and put in the baking tray.
4. Sprinkle the bell peppers with avocado oil and bake at 365F for 30 minutes.

Nutritional info per serve: Calories 60, Fat 2.6, Fiber 0.8, Carbs 4.9, Protein 4.7

Cream Cheese Dip

Prep time: 10 minutes
Cook time: 0 minutes
Servings: 4
Ingredients:
- 4 oz cream cheese
- ½ cup Cheddar cheese, shredded
- ¼ cup cream
- 1 teaspoon taco seasonings
- 1 teaspoon butter

Method:
1. Put all ingredients in the food processor and blend the mixture until smooth.
2. Transfer it in the serving bowl.

Nutritional info per serve: Calories 179, Fat 16.4, Fiber 0, Carbs 2.4, Protein 5.8

Chicken Caps

Prep time: 10 minutes
Cook time: 30 minutes
Servings: 4
Ingredients:
- ½ cup ground chicken
- ½ cup mushroom caps
- 1 teaspoon butter
- 1 teaspoon chili flakes

Method:
1. In the mixing bowl, mix ground chicken with butter and chili flakes.
2. Fill the mushroom caps with ground chicken mixture and put it in the baking tray.
3. Bake the chicken caps at 360F for 30 minutes.

Nutritional info per serve: Calories 44, Fat 2.3, Fiber 0.1, Carbs 0.3, Protein 5.4

Chorizo Muffins

Prep time: 10 minutes
Cook time: 15 minutes
Servings: 8
Ingredients:
- 2 tablespoons butter
- 1 egg, beaten
- ½ cup coconut flour
- 2 oz chorizo, chopped, cooked
- 1 teaspoon dried basil
- Cooking spray

Method:
1. Spray the muffin molds with cooking spray.
2. Then mix butter with egg, coconut flour, chorizo, and dried basil.
3. Transfer the muffin mixture in the muffin molds, flatten gently, and bake at 360F for 15 minutes.

Nutritional info per serve: Calories 69, Fat 6.3, Fiber 0.3, Carbs 0.7, Protein 2.6

Bacon Wraps

Prep time: 10 minutes
Cook time: 20 minutes
Servings: 2
Ingredients:
- 2 jalapeno peppers
- 2 bacon slices
- ¼ teaspoon onion powder

Method:
1. Sprinkle the bacon slices with onion powder.
2. Then wrap the jalapeno peppers in the bacon slices and transfer in the baking tray.
3. Cook the meal at 360F for 10 minutes. Then flip it on another side and cook for 10 minutes more.

Nutritional info per serve: Calories 110, Fat 8.2, Fiber 0.6, Carbs 1.6, Protein 7.3

Fried Halloumi

Prep time: 10 minutes
Cook time: 5 minutes
Servings: 4
Ingredients:
- 6 oz halloumi, roughly chopped
- ½ teaspoon avocado oil
- ¼ teaspoon dried thyme

Method:
1. Preheat the avocado oil well.
2. Add roughly chopped halloumi and sprinkle it with dried thyme.
3. Roast the cheese for 2 minutes per side.

Nutritional info per serve: Calories 138, Fat 10.7, Fiber 0.1, Carbs 1.6, Protein 9.1

Bacon Eggs

Prep time: 15 minutes
Cook time: 4 minutes
Servings: 4
Ingredients:
- 2 eggs, hard-boiled
- 4 bacon slices
- 1 teaspoon smoked paprika

Method:
1. Roast the bacon in the skillet for 2 minutes per side.
2. Then chop the bacon.
3. Peel the eggs and cut them into halves.
4. Top the egg halves with chopped bacon and smoked paprika.

Nutritional info per serve: Calories 136, Fat 10.2, Fiber 0.2, Carbs 0.7, Protein 9.9

Energy Bars

Prep time: 10 minutes
Cook time: 20 minutes
Servings: 8
Ingredients:
- ½ cup flaxseed
- 2 pecans, chopped
- ½ cup coconut flour
- 3 tablespoons coconut oil
- 1 tablespoon Erythritol
- 1 teaspoon xanthan gum
- 1 tablespoon butter, softened
- 1 teaspoon vanilla extract

Method:
1. Line the baking tray with baking paper.
2. Then mix all ingredients from the list above in the mixing bowl.
3. Transfer it in the baking tray and flatten well.
4. Cut the mixture into bars and bake at 360F for 20 minutes.
5. Cook the cooked energy bars well.

Nutritional info per serve: Calories 155, Fat 12.2, Fiber 6, Carbs 7.8, Protein 2.7

Turmeric Eggs

Prep time: 15 minutes
Cook time: 0 minutes
Servings: 4
Ingredients:
- 4 eggs, hard-boiled, peeled, halved
- 1 oz pancetta, chopped, roasted
- 1 teaspoon ground turmeric
- 1 teaspoon mustard

- 1 teaspoon heavy cream

Method:
1. Mix pancetta with ground turmeric, mustard, and heavy cream.
2. Then add egg yolks and stir the mixture until smooth.
3. Fill the egg white halves with turmeric mixture.

Nutritional info per serve: Calories 111, Fat 8.1, Fiber 0.2, Carbs 1.1, Protein 8.5

Chia Crackers

Prep time: 10 minutes
Cook time: 20 minutes
Servings: 8
Ingredients:
- 4 tablespoons chia seeds
- 2 tablespoons flax seeds
- ½ teaspoon garlic powder
- ½ teaspoon dried cilantro
- 1 egg, beaten
- 1 teaspoon coconut oil

Method:
1. Put all ingredients in the mixing bowl and carefully mix.
2. Line the baking tray with baking paper.
3. Put the chia mixture in the baking tray and flatten ell.
4. Cut the mixture into squares and bake at 355F for 20 minutes.

Nutritional info per serve: Calories 57, Fat 3.9, Fiber 2.9, Carbs 3.7, Protein 2.2

Parmesan Chips

Prep time: 15 minutes
Cook time: 5 minutes
Servings: 4
Ingredients:
- 2 oz Parmesan, grated
- 1 tablespoon almond flour
- ¼ teaspoon avocado oil

Method:
1. Brush the baking tray with avocado oil.
2. Then mix Parmesan with almond flour.
3. Make the small rounds from the cheese mixture in the tray (chips shape) and bake at 360fF for 5 minutes.
4. Cool the chips.

Nutritional info per serve: Calories 86, Fat 6.6, Fiber 0.8, Carbs 2.2, Protein 6.1

Thyme Cupcakes

Prep time: 10 minutes
Cook time: 13 minutes
Servings: 6
Ingredients:
- 5 tablespoons coconut oil
- 1 tablespoon psyllium husk
- ½ cup coconut flour
- 1 teaspoon dried thyme
- 1 teaspoon garlic, minced
- 2 oz Feta cheese, crumbled

Method:
1. In the mixing bowl, mix up coconut oil, psyllium husk, coconut flour, dried thyme, garlic, and crumbled feta.
2. When the mixture is smooth, transfer it in the muffin molds and flatten well.
3. Bake the meal at 360F for 13 minutes.

Nutritional info per serve: Calories 143, Fat 13.5, Fiber 5.2, Carbs 7, Protein 1.6

Ham Bites

Prep time: 10 minutes
Servings: 4
Ingredients:
- ¼ cucumber, cubed
- 2 oz ham, sliced
- 2 oz Cheddar cheese, cubed

Method:
1. String the cucumber cubes and cheese cubes into the toothpicks.
2. Then fol the ham and add it to the cheese and cucumber cubes.

Nutritional info per serve: Calories 83, Fat 5.9, Fiber 0.3, Carbs 1.4, Protein 6

Garlic and Avocado Spread

Prep time: 10 minutes
Cook time: 0 minutes
Servings: 4
Ingredients:
- 1 avocado, pitted, peeled
- 2 tablespoons fresh parsley, chopped
- 4 tablespoons cream cheese
- 1 teaspoon minced garlic

Method:
1. Put the avocado in the blender and blend until smooth.
2. Add parsley, cream cheese, and minced garlic.
3. Pulse the mixture for 10 seconds more.

Nutritional info per serve: Calories 139, Fat 13.3, Fiber 3.4, Carbs 4.9, Protein 1.8

Chorizo Tacos

Prep time: 10 minutes
Cook time: 15 minutes
Servings: 4
Ingredients:
- 4 spinach leaves
- 2 oz chorizo, chopped
- ½ teaspoon chili flakes
- ½ teaspoon dried thyme
- 1 teaspoon coconut oil
- 1 tablespoon fresh cilantro, chopped
- 1 tablespoon lemon juice

Method:
1. Put the chorizo in the skillet and roast it for 10 minutes. Stir it from time to time.
2. Then add chili flakes, dried thyme, coconut oil, and lemon juice. Roast the ingredients for 5 minutes more.
3. After this, fill the leaves in the chorizo mixture and sprinkle with fresh cilantro.

Nutritional info per serve: Calories 78, Fat 6.6, Fiber 0.3, Carbs 0.8, Protein 3.8

Shrimp Bites

Prep time: 10 minutes
Cook time: 10 minutes
Servings: 4
Ingredients:
- 1 tablespoon coconut oil
- 6 oz shrimps, peeled, boiled, chopped
- 1 tablespoon coconut flour
- 1 egg, beaten
- ½ teaspoon dried oregano

Method:
1. Mix shrimps with coconut flour, egg, and dried oregano.
2. Then melt the coconut oil in the skillet.
3. Make the small bites from the shrimp mixture with the help of the spoon and put them in the hot coconut oil.
4. Roast the meal for 3 minutes per side.

Nutritional info per serve: Calories 104, Fat 5.5, Fiber 0.7, Carbs 1.9, Protein 11.3

Roasted Cauliflower Florets

Prep time: 10 minutes
Cook time: 15 minutes
Servings: 4
Ingredients:
- 1 cup cauliflower florets, boiled
- 3 eggs, beaten
- 1 tablespoon coconut flour
- 1 teaspoon onion powder
- ½ teaspoon salt
- 1 tablespoon coconut oil

Method:
1. Grease the baking tray with coconut oil.
2. Then put the cauliflower florets in the tray in one layer.
3. Sprinkle them with coconut flour, onion powder, and salt.
4. After this, sprinkle the cauliflower with eggs and bake at 360F for 10-15 minutes or until the cauliflower is light brown.

Nutritional info per serve: Calories 92, Fat 7, Fiber 1.3, Carbs 3.1, Protein 5

Zucchini Rolls

Prep time: 20 minutes
Servings: 4
Ingredients:
- 1 large zucchini
- 2 scallions, julienned
- ¼ cup white cabbage, shredded
- 1 teaspoon ricotta cheese
- ¼ teaspoon garlic powder
- ½ teaspoon dried parsley

Method:
1. Slice the zucchini lengthwise.
2. Then mix scallions with shredded cabbage, ricotta cheese, garlic powder, and dried parsley.
3. Make the layer from the zucchini on the baking paper and put the cabbage mixture on it. Spread it well.
4. Roll the zucchini and press gently.
5. Slice the meal into servings.

Nutritional info per serve: Calories 19, Fat 0.3, Fiber 1.2, Carbs 3.8, Protein 1.3

Broccoli Biscuits

Prep time: 10 minutes
Cook time: 20 minutes
Servings: 5
Ingredients:
- 2 cups broccoli, shredded
- 1½ cup almond flour
- 1 teaspoon cayenne powder
- 1 egg, beaten
- ½ cup Cheddar cheese, shredded

Method:
1. Put all ingredients in the mixing bowl and mix well.
2. Then make the small balls and put them in the non-stick baking tray.
3. Bake the biscuits for 20 minutes at 360F and then cool to the room temperature.

Nutritional info per serve: Calories 248, Fat 20.2, Fiber 4.4, Carbs 9.4, Protein 11.6

Turmeric Sausages

Prep time: 15 minutes
Cook time: 10 minutes
Servings: 4
Ingredients:
- 2 tablespoons coconut oil
- 2 tablespoons coconut cream
- 1 cup coconut flour
- 4 sausages
- 1 egg, beaten

Method:
1. Melt the coconut oil in the skillet.
2. Meanwhile, mix the egg with coconut cream.
3. Dip the sausages in the egg mixture and then coat into coconut flour.
4. Repeat the same steps one more time and transfer the sausages in the hot coconut oil.
5. Roast the sausages on medium heat for 4 minutes per side.

Nutritional info per serve: Calories 256, Fat 17.4, Fiber 10.2, Carbs 16.5, Protein 18.1

Kalamata Snack

Prep time: 10 minutes
Cook time: 0 minutes
Servings: 4
Ingredients:
- 4 kalamata olives
- 5 oz goat cheese, crumbled
- 1 teaspoon fresh cilantro, chopped
- 2 tablespoons sesame oil

Method:
1. Put Kalamata olives on the plate and top them with the crumbled goat cheese.

2. Then sprinkle the meal with cilantro and sesame oil.
Nutritional info per serve: Calories 225, Fat 19.9, Fiber 0.1, Carbs 1.1, Protein 10.9

Peppers Nachos

Prep time: 10 minutes
Cook time: 20 minutes
Servings: 6
Ingredients:
- ½ cup bell peppers, chopped
- ¼ teaspoon minced garlic
- ½ teaspoon smoked paprika
- ½ cup ground beef
- 1 teaspoon coconut oil
- ¼ cup Cheddar cheese, shredded
- 1 tablespoon coconut cream

Method:
1. Put the ground beef in the saucepan and roast it for 5 minutes. Carefully mix it.
2. Then add minced garlic, smoked paprika, coconut oil, and coconut cream.
3. Add bell peppers and carefully mix the mixture. Cook it for 10 minutes.
4. Then stir the mixture and top it with Cheddar cheese. Cook the meal for 5 minutes more.
Nutritional info per serve: Calories 52, Fat 4, Fiber 0.3, Carbs 1.1, Protein 3.1

Mozzarella Bites

Prep time: 15 minutes
Servings: 4
Ingredients:
- 4 mozzarella balls
- 4 cherry tomatoes
- ½ teaspoon avocado oil
- ¼ teaspoon Italian seasonings

Method:
1. String the cherry tomatoes and mozzarella into the toothpicks one by one.
2. Then sprinkle the meal with avocado oil and Italian seasonings.
Nutritional info per serve: Calories 114, Fat 6.4, Fiber 1.5, Carbs 4.8, Protein 6.1

Almond Bars

Prep time: 10 minutes
Cook time: 10 minutes
Servings: 4
Ingredients:
- 2 tablespoons coconut shred
- 2 tablespoons almond butter
- 1 tablespoon Erythritol
- 1 tablespoon almonds, chopped
- 1 tablespoon coconut flakes

Method:
1. Put all ingredients in the mixing bowl and knead the dough.
2. Then line the baking tray with baking paper and put the dough inside.
3. Roll it up and cut into bars.
4. Bake the almond bars for 10 minutes at 360F.

Nutritional info per serve: Calories 87, Fat 8.2, Fiber 1.6, Carbs 3, Protein 2.1

Almond Zucchini

Prep time: 10 minutes
Cook time: 10 minutes
Servings: 4
Ingredients:
- 1 large zucchini, trimmed
- 2 tablespoons almond flour
- ¼ teaspoon ground black pepper
- ¼ teaspoon dried oregano
- 2 tablespoons coconut oil

Method:
1. Slice the zucchini and sprinkle it with ground black pepper, dried oregano, and almond flour.
2. Melt the coconut oil in the skillet and add sliced zucchini. Put them in one layer.
3. Roast the zucchini for 2 minutes per side.
Nutritional info per serve: Calories 152, Fat 14, Fiber 2.5, Carbs 5.9, Protein 4

Coated Zucchinis

Prep time: 10 minutes
Cook time: 8 minutes
Servings: 4
Ingredients:
- 4 Cheddar cheese slices
- 1 zucchini, sliced
- ¼ teaspoon ground nutmeg

Method:
1. Sprinkle the zucchini with ground nutmeg and coat into cheese slices.
2. Bake the zucchini at 360F for 8 minutes.
Nutritional info per serve: Calories 121, Fat 9.4, Fiber 0.6, Carbs 2.1, Protein 7.6

Bacon Peppers

Prep time: 15 minutes
Cook time: 15 minutes
Servings: 8
Ingredients:
- 8 mini peppers, trimmed
- 8 bacon slices
- ½ teaspoon ground black pepper
- ½ teaspoon avocado oil

Method:
1. Wrap the mini peppers into the bacon slices and sprinkle with ground black pepper and avocado oil.
2. Put the prepared peppers into the tray and bake them at 365F for 15 minutes.
Nutritional info per serve: Calories 108, Fat 8.1, Fiber 0.4, Carbs 1.2, Protein 7.2

Zucchini Chips

Prep time: 10 minutes
Cook time: 60 minutes
Servings: 8
Ingredients:
- 3 zucchinis, sliced thin
- ½ teaspoon avocado oil

Method:
1. Line the baking tray with baking paper and put the zucchini inside in one layer.
2. Sprinkle the zucchini with avocado oil and bake them at 350F for 60 minutes.
Nutritional info per serve: Calories 12, Fat 0.2, Fiber 0.8, Carbs 2.5, Protein 0.9

Ham Bites

Prep time: 10 minutes
Servings: 4
Ingredients:
- 4 ham slices
- 4 pickled cucumbers

Method:
1. Fold the ham slices and string into the toothpicks.
2. Then string the pickled cucumbers over the ham.
Nutritional info per serve: Calories 91, Fat 2.7, Fiber 1.9, Carbs 12, Protein 6.6

Zucchini Sauce

Prep time: 10 minutes
Cook time: 12 minutes
Servings: 5
Ingredients:
- 2 cups zucchini, diced
- 2 tablespoons coconut oil
- ½ teaspoon chili powder
- 1 teaspoon keto tomato paste
- 1 tablespoon lemon juice

Method:
1. Melt the coconut oil in the saucepan and add zucchini, chili powder, and lemon juice.
2. Cook the mixture for 10 minutes on medium heat. Stir it from time to time.
3. Then add keto tomato paste, carefully mix, and cook for 2 minutes more.
Nutritional info per serve: Calories 57, Fat 5.6, Fiber 0.6, Carbs 1.9, Protein 0.7

Cayenne Shrimp

Prep time: 10 minutes
Cook time: 10 minutes
Servings: 6
Ingredients:
- 1-pound shrimps, peeled
- 1 teaspoon cayenne pepper
- 1 teaspoon lime juice

Method:
1. Sprinkle the shrimps with cayenne pepper and put in the tray on layer. Bake the shrimps for 10 minutes at 360F.
2. Then sprinkle the cooked shrimps with lemon juice.
Nutritional info per serve: Calories 91, Fat 1.3, Fiber 0.1, Carbs 1.3, Protein 17.3

Celery Boats

Prep time: 10 minutes
Cook time: 0 minutes
Servings: 8
Ingredients:
- 1 cup ground chicken, roasted
- 1 oz Parmesan, grated
- 2 tablespoons cream cheese
- 8 celery stalks

Method:
1. Mix the ground chicken with grated Parmesan and cream cheese.
2. Then fill the celery stalks with the chicken mixture.
Nutritional info per serve: Calories 56, Fat 3, Fiber 0.3, Carbs 0.7, Protein 6.5

Fish Pancakes

Prep time: 10 minutes
Cook time: 10 minutes
Servings: 4
Ingredients:
- ½ cup coconut flour
- 3 tablespoons coconut milk
- ½ teaspoon coconut oil
- 4 oz salmon, canned, shredded
- 1 tablespoon ricotta cheese

Method:
1. Melt the coconut oil in the skillet well.
2. Meanwhile, mix all remaining ingredients in the mixing bowl and stir until smooth.
3. Pour the small amount of the salmon mixture in the hot oil and flatten it in the shape of the pancake.
4. Roast the pancakes for 4 minutes per side on medium-low heat.
Nutritional info per serve: Calories 134, Fat 6.8, Fiber 6.3, Carbs 10.8, Protein 8.2

Jerky

Prep time: 8 hours
Cook time: 4 hours
Servings: 8
Ingredients:
- ½ cup coconut aminos
- ½ teaspoon cayenne pepper
- 1 teaspoon apple cider vinegar
- ½ teaspoon chili powder
- 1-pound beef round, sliced

Method:
1. Sprinkle the sliced beef with chili powder, apple cider vinegar, cayenne pepper, and coconut aminos.
2. Leave the mixture overnight to marinate.
3. Then transfer it in the baking tray in one layer and bake at 350F for 4 hours.
Nutritional info per serve: Calories 62, Fat 2.1, Fiber 0.1, Carbs 4.2, Protein 9.1

Paprika Beef Jerky

Prep time: 60 minutes
Cook time: 3 hours
Servings: 10
Ingredients:
- 1-pound beef round, sliced
- ½ teaspoon salt
- 1 tablespoon smoked paprika

- 3 tablespoons apple cider vinegar
- 3 tablespoons coconut aminos

Method:
1. In the mixing bowl, mix salt with smoked paprika, apple cider vinegar, and coconut aminos.
2. Put the sliced beef inside and marinate it for 1 hour.
3. Then transfer it in the baking tray in one layer and bake at 355F for 3 hours.

Nutritional info per serve: Calories 44, Fat 1.7, Fiber 0.3, Carbs 2.1, Protein 7.4

Crab Spread

Prep time: 10 minutes
Cook time: 0 minutes
Servings: 8
Ingredients:
- 10 oz crab meat, chopped, canned
- 3 tablespoons cream cheese
- 1 teaspoon chives, chopped
- ½ teaspoon ground paprika

Method:
1. Put all ingredients in the food processor and blend until smooth.
2. Transfer the cooked spread in the serving bowl.

Nutritional info per serve: Calories 45, Fat 2, Fiber 0.1, Carbs 0.8, Protein 4.7

Spinach Wraps

Prep time: 15 minutes
Cook time: 10 minutes
Servings: 6
Ingredients:
- 8 oz chicken fillet
- 1 cup spinach leaves
- 1 tablespoon ricotta cheese
- ½ teaspoon salt
- 1 teaspoon avocado oil
- 1 teaspoon chili powder

Method:
1. Slice the chicken fillet and sprinkle with chili powder and salt.
2. Then preheat the avocado oil and put the chicken in it.
3. Roast the chicken for 4 minutes per side.
4. After this, spread the spinach leaves with ricotta cheese and top with cooked chicken.
5. For the spinach leaves into wraps.

Nutritional info per serve: Calories 79, Fat 3.2, Fiber 0.3, Carbs 0.6, Protein 11.4

Nutmeg Balls

Prep time: 10 minutes
Cook time: 13 minutes
Servings: 10
Ingredients:
- 2 tablespoons coconut oil
- 1 egg, beaten
- 1 cup coconut flour
- 1 cup spinach, chopped
- 6 oz goat cheese, crumbled
- 1 teaspoon ground nutmeg

Method:
1. Put all ingredients in the mixing bowl and carefully mix.
2. Make the medium-size balls from the mixture and put them in the lined with baking paper tray.
3. Bake the nutmeg balls for 13 minutes at 360F.

Nutritional info per serve: Calories 156, Fat 10.9, Fiber 4.1, Carbs 7, Protein 7.4

Kale Chips

Prep time: 10 minutes
Cook time: 7 minutes
Servings: 5
Ingredients:
- 3 cups Kale, roughly chopped
- 1 teaspoon nutritional yeast
- 1 tablespoon avocado oil

Method:
1. Line the baking tray with baking paper.
2. Put the kale into the tray and flatten it in one layer.
3. Then sprinkle it with avocado oil and nutritional yeast and bake at 350F for 7 minutes.

Nutritional info per serve: Calories 26, Fat 0.4, Fiber 0.9, Carbs 4.7, Protein 1.5

Parsley Dip

Prep time: 10 minutes
Cook time: 7 minutes
Servings: 6
Ingredients:
- 1 cup Cheddar cheese, shredded
- ½ cup of coconut milk
- 1 teaspoon cayenne pepper
- 1/3 cup fresh parsley, chopped

Method:
1. Put all ingredients in the saucepan and bring to boil.
2. Then blend the mixture until smooth with the help of the immersion blender and remove from the heat.

Nutritional info per serve: Calories 124, Fat 11.1, Fiber 0.6, Carbs 1.7, Protein 5.3

Cucumber Bites

Prep time: 10 minutes
Servings: 3
Ingredients:
- 1 cucumber, roughly sliced
- 1 tablespoon cream cheese
- ¼ teaspoon minced garlic
- ¼ teaspoon chili flakes

Method:
1. Mix cream cheese with minced garlic and chili flakes.
2. Then spread the cucumbers with cream cheese mixture.

Nutritional info per serve: Calories 27, Fat 1.3, Fiber 0.5, Carbs 3.8, Protein 0.9

Mushrooms with Shrimps

Prep time: 10 minutes
Cook time: 11 minutes
Servings: 5
Ingredients:
- 5 Portobello mushroom caps
- 7 oz shrimps, peeled, chopped
- 1 teaspoon avocado oil
- ¼ teaspoon dried thyme

Method:
1. Preheat the avocado oil in the skillet.
2. Add mushrooms and roast them for 2 minutes per side.
3. Then top the mushrooms with shrimps and dried thyme.
4. Cook the meal for 7 minutes more.

Nutritional info per serve: Calories 56, Fat 0.9, Fiber 0.5, Carbs 2.1, Protein 9.8

Basil Bites

Prep time: 5 minutes
Servings: 4
Ingredients:
- 1 big tomato
- 4 basil leaves
- ½ teaspoon avocado oil

Method:
1. Slice the tomato into 4 slices.
2. Then top every tomato slice with a basil leaf and sprinkle with avocado oil.

Nutritional info per serve: Calories 9, Fat 0.2, Fiber 0.6, Carbs 1.8, Protein 0.4

Cheese Cubes

Prep time: 5 minutes
Cook time: 0 minutes
Servings: 8
Ingredients:
- 7 oz Cheddar cheese, cubed
- ½ teaspoon ground paprika
- ¼ teaspoon lemon juice

Method:
1. Put the cheese cubes on the plate and sprinkle with ground paprika and lemon juice.

Nutritional info per serve: Calories 100, Fat 8.2, Fiber 0.1, Carbs 0.4, Protein 6.2

Chili Caps

Prep time: 10 minutes
Cook time: 10 minutes
Servings: 4
Ingredients:
- 4 mushroom caps
- 1 oz Parmesan, grated
- ½ teaspoon chili powder

Method:
1. Put the mushroom caps in the baking tray in one layer and top with chili powder and parmesan.
2. Bake the mushrooms at 360F for 10 minutes.

Nutritional info per serve: Calories 28, Fat 1.6, Fiber 0.3, Carbs 1, Protein 2.9

Turkey Meatballs

Prep time: 10 minutes
Cook time: 15 minutes
Servings: 4
Ingredients:
- 4 oz ground turkey
- 1 teaspoon minced garlic
- ½ teaspoon ground black pepper
- 1 teaspoon dried cilantro

Method:
1. Mix ground turkey with minced garlic, ground black pepper, and dried cilantro.
2. Then make the small meatballs and bake them at 360F for 15 minutes.

Nutritional info per serve: Calories 57, Fat 3.1, Fiber 0.1, Carbs 0.4, Protein 7.8

Escargot Ramekins

Prep time: 10 minutes
Cook time: 10 minutes
Servings: 4
Ingredients:
- 1 cup Escargot snails, boiled
- 4 oz provolone cheese, shredded
- 1 teaspoon coconut oil
- ¼ cup mushrooms, chopped

Method:
1. Roast the mushrooms with coconut oil in the skillet for 10 minutes. Stir them from time to time.
2. Then mix mushrooms with provolone cheese and fill the snails.

Nutritional info per serve: Calories 135, Fat 9, Fiber 0.5, Carbs 1.3, Protein 12.4

Italian Style Wings

Prep time: 10 minutes
Cook time: 30 minutes
Servings: 6
Ingredients:
- 6 chicken wings
- 1 tablespoon Italian seasoning
- 1 tablespoon avocado oil
- ½ teaspoon ground black pepper

Method:
1. Put the chicken wings in the baking tray in one layer and sprinkle with Italian seasonings, avocado oil, and ground black pepper.
2. Bake the chicken wings for 30 minutes at 360F.

Nutritional info per serve: Calories 169, Fat 11.7, Fiber 0.3, Carbs 5.9, Protein 9.8

Thyme Halloumi

Prep time: 10 minutes
Cook time: 3 minutes
Servings: 4
Ingredients:
- 8 oz Halloumi cheese
- 1 tablespoon dried thyme
- 1 tablespoon avocado oil

Method:
1. Preheat the grill to 400F.
2. Then chop the cheese roughly and sprinkle with avocado oil.

3. Put the cheese in the grill and sprinkle with thyme. Roast it for 1 minute per side.
Nutritional info per serve: Calories 213, Fat 17.4, Fiber 0.4, Carbs 2.1, Protein 12.3

Italian Sticks

Prep time: 15 minutes
Cook time: 20 minutes
Servings: 4
Ingredients:
- 1 egg, beaten
- 1 oz Parmesan, grated
- 1 large zucchini

Method:
1. Cut the zucchini into sticks and dip into the egg.
2. Then coat every zucchini stick in the cheese and transfer in the baking tray.
3. Flatten the zucchini sticks in one layer and bake at 360F for 20 minutes.
Nutritional info per serve: Calories 51, Fat 2.8, Fiber 0.9, Carbs 3, Protein 4.6

Crispy Bites

Prep time: 5 minutes
Cook time: 5 minutes
Servings: 4
Ingredients:
- 3 oz Parmesan, grated
- ½ teaspoon dried basil

Method:
1. Preheat the non-stick skillet well.
2. Make the small rounds from Parmesan in the skillet and top them with basil.
3. Roast the cheese for 1-2 minutes or until it is light brown.
4. Cool the cheese.
Nutritional info per serve: Calories 68, Fat 4.6, Fiber 0, Carbs 0.8, Protein 6.8

Cauliflower Florets in Cheese

Prep time: 10 minutes
Cook time: 25 minutes
Servings: 8
Ingredients:
- 1 cup cauliflower, cut into florets
- 2 eggs, beaten
- 2 oz Parmesan, grated

Method:
1. Dip the cauliflower florets in the eggs and coat into the parmesan.
2. Put them in the baking tray in one layer and bake for 25 minutes at 365F.
Nutritional info per serve: Calories 42, Fat 2.6, Fiber 0.3, Carbs 1, Protein 3.9

Eggplant Chips

Prep time: 15 minutes
Cook time: 12 minutes
Servings: 4
Ingredients:
- 1 large eggplant, thinly sliced
- 1 teaspoon avocado oil
- 1 teaspoon salt

Method:
1. Sprinkle the sliced eggplant with salt and leave for 10 minutes.
2. Then drain the eggplant juice.
3. Preheat the avocado oil in the skillet well.
4. Put the sliced eggplants in the skillet in one layer and roast them for 3 minutes per side.
Nutritional info per serve: Calories 30, Fat 0.4, Fiber 4.1, Carbs 6.8, Protein 1.1

Chocolate Bacon

Prep time: 10 minutes
Cook time: 3 minutes
Servings: 4
Ingredients:
- 4 bacon slices, cooked
- 1 oz dark chocolate

Method:
1. Freeze the cooked bacon slices.
2. Meanwhile, melt the chocolate well.
3. Sprinkle the frozen bacon with chocolate.
Nutritional info per serve: Calories 141, Fat 10, Fiber 0.2, Carbs 4.5, Protein 7.6

Carrot Chips

Prep time: 10 minutes
Cook time: 40 minutes
Servings: 2
Ingredients:
- 1 carrot, thinly sliced
- 1 teaspoon avocado oil

Method:
1. Line the baking tray with baking paper and put the carrot slices inside in one layer.
2. Then sprinkle the carrot with avocado oil and bake at 355F for 40 minutes or until the carrot is crunchy.
Nutritional info per serve: Calories 16, Fat 0.3, Fiber 0.9, Carbs 3.1, Protein 0.3

Asparagus Chips

Prep time: 10 minutes
Cook time: 75 minutes
Servings: 5
Ingredients:
- 8 oz asparagus, thinly sliced
- ¼ teaspoon dried rosemary

Method:
1. Sprinkle the asparagus with dried rosemary and put in the baking tray in one layer.
2. Bake the asparagus chips at 350F for 75 minutes.
Nutritional info per serve: Calories 20, Fat 0.1, Fiber 0.9, Carbs 4.6, Protein 0.8

Sweet Bacon

Prep time: 5 minutes
Cook time: 5 minutes
Servings: 5
Ingredients:
- 5 bacon slices
- 1 teaspoon Erythritol

Method:
1. Put the bacon slices in the hot skillet and roast for 2 minutes.
2. Then flip the bacon on another side and sprinkle with Erythritol.
3. Cook the bacon for 2 minutes more.
Nutritional info per serve: Calories 103, Fat 7.9, Fiber 0, Carbs 0.3, Protein 7

Chicken Wraps
Prep time: 20 minutes
Cook time: 40 minutes
Servings: 4
Ingredients:
- 8 oz chicken fillet
- ½ cup spinach, chopped
- 1 tablespoon cream cheese

Method:
1. Slice the chicken fillet into 4 fillets and top with spinach and cream cheese.
2. For the chicken fillets and secure with toothpicks.
3. Then wrap the chicken in the foil and bake at 360F for 40 minutes.
Nutritional info per serve: Calories 117, Fat 5.1, Fiber 0.1, Carbs 0.2, Protein 16.7

Garlic Rinds
Prep time: 5 minutes
Cook time: 3 minutes
Servings: 4
Ingredients:
- 6 oz pork rinds
- 1 teaspoon garlic powder
- ½ teaspoon ground paprika

Method:
1. Mix pork rinds with garlic powder and ground paprika and roast in the well-preheated oven for 3 minutes.
Nutritional info per serve: Calories 246, Fat 15.2, Fiber 0.2, Carbs 0.7, Protein 27.5

Marinara Bites
Prep time: 10 minutes
Cook time: 10 minutes
Servings: 4
Ingredients:
- ¼ cup marinara sauce
- 5 oz Halloumi, cubed
- 1 teaspoon coconut oil

Method:
1. Melt the coconut oil in the skillet and add cubed Halloumi.
2. Sprinkle it with marinara sauce and roast for 3 minutes per side.
Nutritional info per serve: Calories 103, Fat 7.6, Fiber 0.4, Carbs 2.9, Protein 6

Pepper Cucumbers
Prep time: 10 minutes
Servings: 2
Ingredients:
- 1 cucumber
- 1 teaspoon fresh dill, chopped
- 1 bell pepper, diced

Method:
1. Remove the flesh from the cucumber to get the holes in cucumbers.
2. Then fill the hole with bell pepper and fresh dill.
3. Cut the cucumber into halves.
Nutritional info per serve: Calories 43, Fat 0.3, Fiber 1.6, Carbs 10.2, Protein 1.7

Jalapeño Bites
Prep time: 15 minutes
Cook time: 0 minutes
Servings: 4
Ingredients:
- 4 jalapenos
- 3 oz ground chicken, cooked
- 1 teaspoon ricotta cheese
- 1 teaspoon chives, chopped

Method:
1. In the mixing bowl, mix ground chicken with ricotta cheese, and chives.
2. Trim the jalapenos and remove the seeds.
3. Fill the jalapenos with ground chicken mixture.
Nutritional info per serve: Calories 46, Fat 1.8, Fiber 0.4, Carbs 0.9, Protein 6.5

Baked Coconut Eggs
Prep time: 10 minutes
Cook time: 12 minutes
Servings: 5
Ingredients:
- 1 egg, beaten
- 1 scallion, sliced
- 2 tablespoons coconut flour

Method:
1. Line the baking tray with baking paper.
2. Then crack the eggs on the baking papper.
3. Sprinkle them with coconut flour and scallions.
4. Bake the eggs for 12 minutes at 360F.
Nutritional info per serve: Calories 37, Fat 1.3, Fiber 1.6, Carbs 4.5, Protein 1.8

Stuffed Cucumber
Prep time: 10 minutes
Cook time: 0 minutes
Servings: 4
Ingredients:
- 1 cucumber
- 4 oz tuna, canned, shredded
- 1 tablespoon coconut cream
- ¼ teaspoon salt

Method:
1. Cut the cucumber into halves and them into 4 pieces.
2. Remove the flesh from the cucumbers to get the cucumber boats.
3. Then mix shredded tuna with coconut cream and salt.
4. Fill the cucumbers with tuna mixture.

Nutritional info per serve: Calories 73, Fat 3.3, Fiber 0.5, Carbs 2.9, Protein 8.1

Seaweed Chips

Prep time: 10 minutes
Cook time: 3 minutes
Servings: 4
Ingredients:
- 4 nori sheets
- 1 teaspoon nutritional yeast
- 1 tablespoon water

Method:
1. Cut the nori sheets into the chips and sprinkle with water and nutritional yeast.
2. Then put the nori chips in the baking tray in one layer and cook for 3 minutes at 355F.

Nutritional info per serve: Calories 13, Fat 0.1, Fiber 1.2, Carbs 0.4, Protein 1.4

Eggs Salad

Prep time: 10 minutes
Cook time: 0 minutes
Servings: 4
Ingredients:
- 2 eggs, hard-boiled, peeled, chopped
- 1 tablespoon heavy cream
- 1 tablespoon coconut cream
- 1 kalamata olive, chopped

Method:
1. Put all ingredients in the salad bowl.
2. Carefully mix the salad.

Nutritional info per serve: Calories 54, Fat 4.6, Fiber 0.1, Carbs 0.6, Protein 3

Berry Cubes

Prep time: 15 minutes
Cook time: 10 minutes
Servings: 4
Ingredients:
- 1 tablespoon Erythritol
- 1 oz strawberries
- 1 cup of water
- 1 tablespoon agar

Method:
1. Mash the strawberries and mix them with water and agar.
2. Ring the liquid to boil, add Erythritol, and carefully mix.
3. Then pour the hot liquid into ice cubes and refrigerate.

Nutritional info per serve: Calories 3, Fat 0, Fiber 0.2, Carbs 0.6, Protein 0.1

Peppers Kebabs

Prep time: 10 minutes
Cook time: 20 minutes
Servings: 6
Ingredients:
- 1 cup ground beef
- 1 cup bell pepper, diced
- 1 teaspoon minced garlic
- 1 teaspoon onion powder
- 1 teaspoon ground black pepper
- 1 teaspoon dried oregano

Method:
1. In the mixing bowl, mix ground beef with bell pepper, minced garlic, onion powder, ground black pepper, and dried oregano.
2. Then make the kebabs with the help of the wooden sticks.
3. Put the kebabs in the baking tray and bake for 20 minutes at 365F (for 10 minutes per side).

Nutritional info per serve: Calories 43, Fat 2.1, Fiber 0.5, Carbs 2.4, Protein 3.8

Pumpkin Bowls

Prep time: 5 minutes
Cook time: 0 minutes
Servings: 4
Ingredients:
- 2 tablespoons pumpkin seeds
- 1 tablespoon sunflower seeds
- 1 tablespoon chia seeds
- 1 teaspoon ground cinnamon
- ½ teaspoon salt

Method:
1. Put pumpkin seeds, sunflower seeds, and chia seeds in the serving bowl.
2. Sprinkle the seeds with ground cinnamon and salt and carefully mix.

Nutritional info per serve: Calories 63, Fat 4.5, Fiber 3, Carbs 4.4, Protein 2.4

Zucchini Rolls

Prep time: 15 minutes
Cook time: 0 minutes
Servings: 4
Ingredients:
- 1 zucchini, trimmed
- 1 tablespoon goat cheese
- 2 tablespoons heavy cream
- 1 oz scallions, chopped
- 1 kalamata olive, diced

Method:
1. Slice the zucchini lengthwise and put on the baking paper in one layer.
2. Then mix goat cheese with heavy cream, scallions, and olive.
3. Spread the mixture over the zucchini and roll the zucchini.
4. Cut the big roll into small rolls.

Nutritional info per serve: Calories 69, Fat 5.5, Fiber 0.8, Carbs 2.6, Protein 3

Egg Sandwich

Prep time: 10 minutes
Cook time: 0
Servings: 4
Ingredients:
- 4 eggs, boiled
- 4 ham slices
- 1 oz Parmesan, sliced
- 8 lettuce leaves

Method:
1. Slice the eggs into halves and put 2 egg halves on 4 lettuce leaves.

2. Add ham and Parmesan.
3. Cover the cheese with remaining lettuce leaves.
Nutritional info per serve: Calories 133, Fat 8.3, Fiber 0.4, Carbs 2, Protein 12.5

Basil Crackers

Prep time: 10 minutes
Cook time: 7 hours
Servings: 6
Ingredients:
- 2 nori sheets
- 4 tablespoons water
- ½ teaspoon dried basil

Method:
1. Cut the nori sheets into crackers' shape and sprinkle with water and dried basil.
2. Bake the cracker at 350F for 7 minutes or until the nori is dried.
Nutritional info per serve: Calories 3, Fat 0, Fiber 0.3, Carbs 0, Protein 0.3

Monterey Jack Cheese Rolls

Prep time: 10 minutes
Cook time: 15 minutes
Servings: 4
Ingredients:
- 4 mini sausages
- 4 Monterey Jack cheese slices
- 1 teaspoon coconut oil
- ½ teaspoon smoked paprika

Method:
1. Melt the coconut oil in the skillet.
2. Then sprinkle the mini sausages with smoked paprika and wrap it into cheese.
3. Put the sausages in the skillet in one layer and bake at 360F for 15 minutes.
Nutritional info per serve: Calories 333, Fat 29.2, Fiber 0.1, Carbs 2, Protein 15.1

Ham Terrine

Prep time: 15 minutes
Cook time: 30 minutes
Servings: 10
Ingredients:
- ¼ cup coconut cream
- 1 cup Cheddar cheese, shredded
- 1 cup ground chicken
- 1 teaspoon dried parsley
- 1 teaspoon dried dill
- 1 teaspoon dried basil

Method:
1. Mix the ground chicken with dried parsley, dill, basil.
2. Put it in the baking mold and flatten well.
3. Top the ground chicken with cheese and coconut cream.
4. Bake the terrine for 30 minutes at 360F.
Nutritional info per serve: Calories 86, Fat 6.2, Fiber 0.1, Carbs 0.5, Protein 7

Chocolate Pecans

Prep time: 5 minutes
Cook time: 1 minute
Servings: 4
Ingredients:
- 4 pecans
- 1 oz Dark chocolate
- 1 teaspoon coconut oil

Method:
1. Melt the chocolate with coconut oil in the microwave oven.
2. Then dip every pecan in the chocolate mixture and refrigerate until the chocolate is solid.
Nutritional info per serve: Calories 145, Fat 13.2, Fiber 1.7, Carbs 6.2, Protein 2

Jalapeno Salad

Prep time: 10 minutes
Cook time: 0 minutes
Servings: 4
Ingredients:
- ½ avocado, pitted, peeled, chopped
- 1 jalapeno, chopped
- 1 scallion, diced
- 1 teaspoon avocado oil
- ½ teaspoon sesame seeds

Method:
1. Put jalapeno in the salad bowl.
2. Add scallion, avocado oil, and sesame seeds.
3. Carefully mix the salad and top it with avocado.
Nutritional info per serve: Calories 68, Fat 6.3, Fiber 2, Carbs 3.1, Protein 0.7

Rosemary Tomatoes

Prep time: 5 minutes
Cook time: 0 minutes
Servings: 4
Ingredients:
- 4 cherry tomatoes
- ½ teaspoon dried rosemary
- ½ teaspoon avocado oil

Method:
1. Cut the cherry tomatoes into halves and sprinkle with rosemary and avocado oil.
Nutritional info per serve: Calories 23, Fat 0.3, Fiber 1.6, Carbs 4.9, Protein 1.1

Egg Halves

Prep time: 5 minutes
Cook time: 1 minute
Servings: 2
Ingredients:
- 1 oz Cheddar cheese, shredded
- 2 eggs, hard-boiled, peeled, halved

Method:
1. Top the egg halves with cheese and microwave for 1 minute.
Nutritional info per serve: Calories 120, Fat 9.1, Fiber 0, Carbs 0.5, Protein 9.1

Celery Skewers

Prep time: 10 minutes
Servings: 4
Ingredients:

- 2 celery stalks
- ½ carrot, roughly chopped
- 4 cherry tomatoes

Method:
1. String the carrot and cherry tomatoes into the wooden skewers.
2. Then cut the celery stalk roughly and string it in the skewers too.

Nutritional info per serve: Calories 27, Fat 0.3, Fiber 1.8, Carbs 5.8, Protein 1.2

Lemon Chips

Prep time: 10 minutes
Cook time: 10 minutes
Servings: 4
Ingredients:
- 1 cup coconut flour
- ¼ teaspoon ground paprika
- 1 teaspoons lemon zest, grated
- 1 teaspoon lemon juice
- 1 egg, beaten
- 1 tablespoon coconut oil

Method:
1. Put all ingredients in the mixing bowl and knead the dough.
2. Then roll it up and cut into small squares.
3. Bake the dough squares in the baking tray for 10 minutes at 360F or until the chips squares are light brown.

Nutritional info per serve: Calories 166, Fat 8.5, Fiber 10.1, Carbs 16.3, Protein 5.4

Scallions Sandwich

Prep time: 10 minutes
Cook time: 2 minutes
Servings: 4
Ingredients:
- 1 eggplant
- 2 oz scallions, chopped
- 1 teaspoon avocado oil
- ½ teaspoon salt
- 2 tablespoons ricotta cheese
- ¼ teaspoon minced garlic

Method:
1. Slice the eggplant lengthwise and rub with salt. Sprinkle the vegetables with avocado oil.
2. Then grill the eggplants at 400F for 1 minute per side.
3. After this, rub the eggplant slices with minced garlic and spread with ricotta cheese.
4. Sprinkle the sandwiches with scallions.

Nutritional info per serve: Calories 46, Fat 1, Fiber 4.5, Carbs 8.3, Protein 2.3

Artichoke Dip

Prep time: 10 minutes
Cook time: 10 minutes
Servings: 5
Ingredients:
- ½ cup coconut cream
- 4 artichoke hearts, canned, chopped
- 1 cup Cheddar cheese, shredded
- 1 tablespoon dried cilantro
- 1 teaspoon dried parsley

Method:
1. Put all ingredients in the saucepan and bring to boil.
2. Then remove it from the heat, carefully mix, and cool until warm.

Nutritional info per serve: Calories 207, Fat 13.4, Fiber 7.6, Carbs 15.3, Protein 10.4

Coffee Cubes

Prep time: 10 minutes
Cook time: 60 minutes
Servings: 1
Ingredients:
- ½ teaspoon instant coffee
- 6 tablespoons water
- 4 tablespoons coconut cream

Method:
1. Bring the water to boil.
2. Add coconut cream and instant coffee.
3. Then pour the liquid in the ice cubes molds and freeze for 1 hour.

Nutritional info per serve: Calories 138, Fat 14.3, Fiber 1.3, Carbs 3.3, Protein 1.4

KETOGENIC FISH AND SEAFOOD RECIPES

Tuna Pie

Prep time: 10 minutes
Cook time: 30 minutes
Servings: 6
Ingredients:
- 3 spring onions, chopped
- 1 cup coconut flour
- ¼ cup of coconut oil
- 1 egg, beaten
- 1 teaspoon baking powder
- 9 oz tuna, canned, shredded

Method:
1. In the mixing bowl mix baking powder with coconut oil, and coconut flour. Knead the dough and put it in the non-stick baking pan. Flatten the dough in the shape of the pie crust.
2. Then mix shredded tuna with chopped spring onion and egg.
3. Put the fish mixture over the pie crust and flatten well.
4. Bake the pie at 360F for 30 minutes.

Nutritional info per serve: Calories 186, Fat 13.6, Fiber 1.2, Carbs 3.8, Protein 12.7

Wrapped Scallops

Prep time: 10 minutes
Cook time: 6 minutes
Servings: 4
Ingredients:
- 1-pound scallops
- 5 oz bacon, sliced
- 1 teaspoon ground coriander
- ½ teaspoon avocado oil

Method:
1. Sprinkle the scallops with ground coriander and wrap in the bacon. Secure scallops with the help of the toothpicks if needed.
2. Preheat the avocado oil well and put the scallops in it.
3. Roast them for 3 minutes per side.

Nutritional info per serve: Calories 292, Fat 15.7, Fiber 0, Carbs 3.2, Protein 32.2

Lime Haddock

Prep time: 10 minutes
Cook time: 25 minutes
Servings: 4
Ingredients:
- 1-pound haddock
- 1 tablespoon avocado oil
- 1 teaspoon ground black pepper
- ½ teaspoon salt
- 1 lime

Method:
1. Sprinkle the haddock with avocado oil, ground black pepper, and salt and put in the lined with a baking paper baking tray.
2. Cut the lime into halves and squeeze over the fish.
3. Then sprinkle the fish with avocado oil and bake in the preheated to 360F oven for 25 minutes.

Nutritional info per serve: Calories 138, Fat 1.5, Fiber 0.8, Carbs 2.3, Protein 27.7

Salmon Boats

Prep time: 10 minutes
Servings: 6
Ingredients:
- 6 celery stalks
- 8 oz salmon, canned
- 1 teaspoon scallions, chopped
- 1 tablespoon ricotta cheese

Method:
1. Shred the salmon and mix it with scallions and ricotta cheese.
2. Then fill the celery with salmon mixture.

Nutritional info per serve: Calories 56, Fat 2.6, Fiber 0.3, Carbs 0.7, Protein 7.8

Cheddar Tilapia

Prep time: 10 minutes
Cook time: 30 minutes
Servings: 4
Ingredients:
- 4 tilapia fillets, boneless
- ½ cup Cheddar cheese, shredded
- 1 teaspoon lemon juice
- 1 teaspoon dried thyme
- 1 teaspoon salt

Method:
1. Rub the tilapia fillets with dried thyme and salt.
2. Put them in the casserole mold.
3. After this, sprinkle the fish with lemon juice and shredded cheese.
4. Bake the tilapia for 30 minutes at 355F.

Nutritional info per serve: Calories 151, Fat 5.7, Fiber 0.1, Carbs 0.4, Protein 24.6

Salmon Kababs

Prep time: 15 minutes
Cook time: 5 minutes
Servings: 4
Ingredients:
- 1-pound salmon fillet
- 1 tablespoon marinara sauce
- 1 teaspoon avocado oil
- ¼ teaspoon ground cumin

Method:
1. Cut the salmon fillet into the medium cubes and mix with marinara sauce, avocado oil, and ground cumin.
2. String the fish cubes in the skewers and grill t 400F for 2 minutes per side.

Nutritional info per serve: Calories 155, Fat 7.3, Fiber 0.2, Carbs 0.7, Protein 22.1

Soft Trout

Prep time: 10 minutes
Cook time: 25 minutes

Servings: 1
Ingredients:
- 3 oz trout fillet
- 2 tablespoons coconut oil
- ¼ cup coconut cream
- 1 teaspoon ground black pepper

Method:
1. Sprinkle the trout fillet with coconut oil, coconut cream, and ground black pepper.
2. Then put the fish and remaining mixture in the skillet and bake at 360F for 25 minutes.

Nutritional info per serve: Calories 539, Fat 48.8, Fiber 1.9, Carbs 4.7, Protein 24.3

Cod in Sauce

Prep time: 5 minutes
Cook time: 20 minutes
Servings: 2
Ingredients:
- 1-pound cod fillet
- 1 teaspoon keto tomato paste
- ½ cup coconut cream
- 1 teaspoon curry paste

Method:
1. Mix coconut cream with curry paste, and keto tomato paste and bring to boil.
2. Add cod and simmer the fish on medium heat for 15 minutes.

Nutritional info per serve: Calories 339, Fat 17.8, Fiber 1.4, Carbs 4.5, Protein 42.1

Lime Trout

Prep time: 10 minutes
Cook time: 30 minutes
Servings: 4
Ingredients:
- 4 trout fillets
- 1 lime
- 1 teaspoon dried thyme
- 1 teaspoon avocado oil

Method:
1. Slice the lime.
2. Put the trout fillets in the baking pan in one layer and sprinkle with avocado oil and dried thyme.
3. Then top it with sliced lime and bake at 360F for 30 minutes.

Nutritional info per serve: Calories 125, Fat 5.5, Fiber 0.6, Carbs 2, Protein 16.7

Cod with Chives

Prep time: 10 minutes
Cook time: 25 minutes
Servings: 4
Ingredients:
- 4 cod fillets
- ½ lemon
- 1 rosemary, fresh
- 1 oz chives, chopped
- ½ cup coconut cream
- ½ teaspoon salt

Method:
1. Rub the cod fillets with rosemary, chives, and salt, and transfer in the baking pan.
2. Squeeze the lemon over the fish and add all remaining ingredients.
3. Cook the cod in the oven at 360F for 25 minutes.

Nutritional info per serve: Calories 164, Fat 8.3, Fiber 1.2, Carbs 2.8, Protein 21

Spicy Salmon

Prep time: 10 minutes
Cook time: 12 minutes
Servings: 4
Ingredients:
- 2 tablespoons coconut oil, softened
- 1¼ pound salmon fillet
- 1 teaspoon chili powder

Method:
1. Sprinkle the salmon fillet with chili powder.
2. Then melt the coconut oil in the skillet and add salmon fillet.
3. Roast the salmon over the medium heat for 5 minutes per side.

Nutritional info per serve: Calories 473, Fat 26.2, Fiber 0.2, Carbs 0.4, Protein 60.6

Tilapia Bowl

Prep time: 10 minutes
Cook time: 10 minutes
Servings: 4
Ingredients:
- 9 oz tilapia fillet, chopped
- ½ cup white cabbage, shredded
- 1 teaspoon coconut oil
- 1 teaspoon chili powder
- ½ teaspoon cayenne pepper
- 1 cup coconut cream

Method:
1. Melt the coconut oil in the skillet.
2. Add tilapia and chili powder. Roast the fish for 2 minutes per side.
3. Then add cayenne pepper and cook the fish for 1 minute more.
4. Transfer the cooked tilapia in the bowl.
5. Add shredded cabbage and coconut cream.
6. Carefully mix the meal.

Nutritional info per serve: Calories 205, Fat 16.2, Fiber 1.8, Carbs 4.3, Protein 13.5

Salmon Meatballs

Prep time: 10 minutes
Cook time: 10 minutes
Servings: 4
Ingredients:
- 10 oz salmon, minced
- 1 teaspoon minced garlic
- 2 tablespoons coconut flour
- ½ teaspoon dried oregano
- ½ teaspoon dried cilantro
- 1 tablespoon coconut oil

Method:
1. In the mixing bowl, mix minced salmon, minced garlic, coconut flour, dried oregano, and cilantro.
2. Make the fish balls from the mixture.

3. Then preheat the coconut oil in the skillet well.
4. Add fish meatballs and roast them for 4 minutes per side over the low heat.
Nutritional info per serve: Calories 140, Fat 8.2, Fiber 1.6, Carbs 2.9, Protein 14.3

Cinnamon Hake

Prep time: 10 minutes
Cook time: 30 minutes
Servings: 4
Ingredients:
- 4 hake fillets
- 1 teaspoon salt
- ½ teaspoon ground cinnamon
- 1 tablespoon coconut oil, melted
- ½ teaspoon chili powder

Method:
1. Brush the baking pan with coconut oil and put the hake fillets inside one layer.
2. Sprinkle the fish with salt, ground cinnamon, and chili powder.
3. Bake the fish at 360F for 30 minutes.
Nutritional info per serve: Calories 145, Fat 4.7, Fiber 0.3, Carbs 1.7, Protein 25.5

Oregano Salmon

Prep time: 10 minutes
Cook time: 10 minutes
Servings: 3
Ingredients:
- 3 salmon fillets
- 1 teaspoon dried oregano
- 1 tablespoon avocado oil
- ½ teaspoon salt

Method:
1. Rub the salmon fillets with dried oregano and salt.
2. Then preheat the skillet well and add avocado oil.
3. Add the fish and roast it for 4 minutes per side over the medium heat.
Nutritional info per serve: Calories 243, Fat 11.6, Fiber 0.4, Carbs 0.6, Protein 34.7

Sage Cod Fillets

Prep time: 10 minutes
Cook time: 30 minutes
Servings: 2
Ingredients:
- 2 cod fillets
- 1 teaspoon dried sage
- 1 tablespoon coconut aminos
- 1 tablespoon avocado oil

Method:
1. Mix dried sage with coconut aminos and avocado oil.
2. Then mix fish with coconut aminos mixture and leave for 10 minutes to marinate.
3. Bake the cod at 360F for 30 minutes.
Nutritional info per serve: Calories 108, Fat 1.9, Fiber 0.4, Carbs 2.1, Protein 20.1

Herbed Oysters

Prep time: 5 minutes
Cook time: 10 minutes
Servings: 3
Ingredients:
- 6 oysters, shucked
- 1 teaspoon Italian seasonings
- 1 tablespoon dried cilantro
- 1 tablespoon coconut oil

Method:
1. Melt the coconut oil in the skillet and add oysters.
2. Sprinkle them with Italian seasonings and dried cilantro and roast for 7 minutes on medium heat. Stir them from time to time.
Nutritional info per serve: Calories 130, Fat 7.9, Fiber 0, Carbs 4.7, Protein 9.6

Cod Curry

Prep time: 10 minutes
Cook time: 25 minutes
Servings: 6
Ingredients:
- 1-pound cod fillet, chopped
- 1 tablespoon curry paste
- ½ teaspoon dried cilantro
- 1 teaspoon chili powder
- ½ bell pepper, diced
- 1 teaspoon coconut oil
- ½ cup coconut cream
- ½ teaspoon keto tomato paste

Method:
1. In the mixing bowl, mix keto tomato paste with coconut cream, chili powder, dried cilantro, and curry paste.
2. Then add cod and carefully mix the mixture. Add bell pepper and mix the mixture again.
3. Transfer it in the baking pan and bake at 360F for 25 minutes.
Nutritional info per serve: Calories 135, Fat 7.8, Fiber 0.7, Carbs 2.9, Protein 14.3

Parmesan Cod

Prep time: 10 minutes
Cook time: 30 minutes
Servings: 4
Ingredients:
- 2 oz Parmesan cheese, grated
- 1 teaspoon olive oil
- ½ teaspoon cayenne pepper
- 4 cod fillets

Method:
1. Brush the cod fillets with olive oil from each side and sprinkle with cayenne pepper.
2. Put the fish in the baking pan and top with grated cheese.
3. Cover the pan with foil and bake the cod for 30 minutes at 360F.
Nutritional info per serve: Calories 146, Fat 5.3, Fiber 0.1, Carbs 0.6, Protein 24.6

Roasted Sea Eel

Prep time: 10 minutes
Cook time: 15 minutes
Servings: 4
Ingredients:
- 10 oz sea eel
- 1 teaspoon cayenne pepper
- ½ teaspoon ground paprika
- ½ teaspoon chili flakes
- ½ teaspoon keto tomato paste
- 2 oz celery stalk, chopped
- 1 teaspoon coconut oil

Method:
1. Melt the coconut oil in the skillet.
2. Add sea eel and sprinkle it with cayenne pepper, ground paprika, chili flakes, and celery stalk.
3. Add keto tomato paste and carefully mix the mixture.
4. Cook it for 10 minutes on the medium-high heat or until the sea eel is tender.

Nutritional info per serve: Calories 182, Fat 11.9, Fiber 0.5, Carbs 1, Protein 17

Cilantro Salmon

Prep time: 10 minutes
Cook time: 8 minutes
Servings: 4
Ingredients:
- ½ teaspoon garlic powder
- 1-pound salmon fillet
- 1 tablespoon avocado oil
- 1 tablespoon dried cilantro

Method:
1. Sprinkle the salmon fillet with avocado oil, dried cilantro, and garlic powder.
2. Roast the fish in the well-preheater skillet for 4 minutes per side.

Nutritional info per serve: Calories 156, Fat 7.4, Fiber 0.2, Carbs 0.5, Protein 22.1

Italian Spices Seabass

Prep time: 10 minutes
Cook time: 40 minutes
Servings: 4
Ingredients:
- 1-pound seabass
- 2 tablespoons butter
- 1 tablespoon Italian seasonings

Method:
1. Rub the seabass with butter and Italian seasonings. Wrap it in the foil and put it in the baking tray.
2. Bake the fish at 360F for 40 minutes.

Nutritional info per serve: Calories 119, Fat 8.3, Fiber 0, Carbs 1.9, Protein 0.1

Mustard Cod

Prep time: 10 minutes
Cook time: 10 minutes
Servings: 4
Ingredients:
- 4 cod fillets
- 1 tablespoon mustard
- 1 tablespoon coconut cream
- 1 teaspoon avocado oil

Method:
1. Mix mustard with coconut cream.
2. Then mix cod fillets with mustard mixture and leave for 10 minutes to marinate.
3. Preheat the skillet well and put the avocado oil inside.
4. Add cod fillets and roast them for 5 minutes per side over the medium-low heat.

Nutritional info per serve: Calories 113, Fat 2.9, Fiber 0.5, Carbs 1.3, Protein 20.8

Shrimp Chowder

Prep time: 10 minutes
Cook time: 15 minutes
Servings: 5
Ingredients:
- 7 oz cod fillet, chopped
- 5 oz shrimps, peeled
- 1 oz pancetta, chopped
- 1 spring onion, diced
- ½ cup celery stalk
- ½ cup heavy cream
- 3 cups of water

Method:
1. Roast the pancetta in the saucepan for 2 minutes per side.
2. Then add all remaining ingredients and carefully mix.
3. Cook the chowder on medium-low heat for 10 minutes.

Nutritional info per serve: Calories 144, Fat 7.7, Fiber 0.4, Carbs 2.2, Protein 16.1

Onion Salmon

Prep time: 10 minutes
Cook time: 40 minutes
Servings: 4
Ingredients:
- 4 salmon fillets
- 1 tablespoon avocado oil
- 1 teaspoon ground coriander
- 1 teaspoon sweet paprika
- 2 scallions, diced
- 1 teaspoon onion powder

Method:
1. In the mixing bowl, mix salmon fillets with avocado oil, ground coriander, sweet paprika, and onion powder.
2. Put the mixture in the non-stick baking pan.
3. Then top the fish with scallions and cover the baking pan with foil.
4. Bake the salmon at 360F for 40 minutes.

Nutritional info per serve: Calories 249, Fat 11.5, Fiber 0.7, Carbs 2.3, Protein 34.9

Cheddar Pollock

Prep time: 10 minutes
Cook time: 25 minutes
Servings: 3
Ingredients:
- 11 oz pollock fillet
- ½ cup Cheddar cheese, shredded

- 1 teaspoon white pepper
- 1 tablespoon avocado oil
- ¼ cup heavy cream

Method:
1. Brush the baking pan with avocado oil from inside.
2. Then slice the Pollock fillet and sprinkle it with white pepper.
3. Put the fish in the baking pan and top it with heavy cream and Cheddar cheese.
4. Cover the baking pan with foil and bake it at 360F for 25 minutes.

Nutritional info per serve: Calories 211, Fat 11.5, Fiber 0.4, Carbs 1.2, Protein 25.5

Parsley Tuna Fritters

Prep time: 10 minutes
Cook time: 10 minutes
Servings: 8
Ingredients:
- 12 ounces canned tuna, drained well and flaked
- 2 tablespoons fresh parsley, chopped
- 1 egg, beaten
- 2 tablespoons coconut oil
- 2 tablespoons coconut flour
- ½ teaspoon ground cumin

Method:
1. In the mixing bowl, mix canned tuna with parsley, egg, coconut flour, and cumin.
2. Then make the small fritters from the tuna mixture.
3. After this, melt the coconut oil in the skillet.
4. Add the tuna fritters and roast them for 4 minutes per side.

Nutritional info per serve: Calories 132, Fat 7.9, Fiber 1.3, Carbs 2.2, Protein 12.5

Clam Stew

Prep time: 5 minutes
Cook time: 15 minutes
Servings: 3
Ingredients:
- 5 oz clams
- ½ cup heavy cream
- ½ teaspoon curry paste
- ½ cup bell pepper, chopped
- 1 teaspoon keto tomato paste
- 1 cup of water
- 8 oz shrimps, peeled

Method:
1. Put all ingredients in the saucepan and bring to boil.
2. Close the lid and simmer the stew for 5 minutes on the medium-low heat.

Nutritional info per serve: Calories 195, Fat 9.3, Fiber 0.5, Carbs 9, Protein 18.2

Sour Cod

Prep time: 15 minutes
Cook time: 10 minutes
Servings: 4
Ingredients:
- 1 pound cod, cut into medium-sized pieces
- ½ teaspoon chives, chopped
- 2 tablespoons coconut aminos
- 1 teaspoon dried dill
- ½ teaspoon lemon zest, grated
- 1 teaspoon avocado oil

Method:
1. Put the cod in the big bowl and sprinkle it with chives, coconut aminos, dried dill, and lemon zest.
2. Add avocado oil and carefully mix the fish. Leave it for 10 minutes to marinate.
3. Then preheat the skillet well, add fish and roast it for 5 minutes per side on medium heat.

Nutritional info per serve: Calories 129, Fat 1.1, Fiber 0.1, Carbs 1.8, Protein 26

Fennel Seabass

Prep time: 10 minutes
Cook time: 40 minutes
Servings: 4
Ingredients:
- 1-pound seabass
- 1 tablespoon fennel seeds
- 1 teaspoon avocado oil
- ½ teaspoon salt
- 1 teaspoon minced garlic

Method:
1. In the shallow bowl, mix fennel seeds with avocado oil, salt, and minced garlic.
2. Then carefully rub the seabass with fennel mixture and wrap in the foil.
3. Bake the seabass for 40 minutes at 360F.

Nutritional info per serve: Calories 65, Fat 1.9, Fiber 0.6, Carbs 2.6, Protein 0.3

Cheesy Tuna Bake

Prep time: 10 minutes
Cook time: 25 minutes
Servings: 6
Ingredients:
- 4 oz Provolone cheese, grated
- 12 oz tuna fillet
- 1 teaspoon butter
- 1 teaspoon dried cilantro
- ½ teaspoon ground black pepper
- 1 tablespoon heavy cream

Method:
1. Chop the tuna and sprinkle it with dried cilantro and ground black pepper.
2. Then grease the ramekins with butter and put the tuna inside.
3. Add heavy cream and Provolone cheese.
4. Bake the meal at 360F for 25 minutes or until you get the crunchy crust.

Nutritional info per serve: Calories 287, Fat 24.2, Fiber 0.1, Carbs 0.6, Protein 16.8

Parsley Sea Bass

Prep time: 10 minutes
Cook time: 30 minutes
Servings: 4
Ingredients:

- ¼ lime, sliced
- 1-pound sea bass fillet
- 1 tablespoon dried parsley
- 1 teaspoon avocado oil
- ¼ teaspoon salt

Method:
1. Brush the seabass fillet with avocado oil and put it in the casserole mold.
2. Top the fish with sliced lime and sprinkle with salt and dried parsley.
3. Bake the fish at 355F for 30 minutes.

Nutritional info per serve: Calories 144, Fat 3.1, Fiber 0.2, Carbs 0.6, Protein 26.9

Scallions Salmon Cakes

Prep time: 10 minutes
Cook time: 10 minutes
Servings: 4
Ingredients:
- 8 oz salmon, canned, shredded
- 2 tablespoons almond flour
- 2 oz scallions, chopped
- 1 teaspoon ground coriander
- ½ teaspoon salt
- 1 egg, beaten
- 1 tablespoon coconut oil

Method:
1. In the mixing bowl, mix shredded salmon with almond flour, scallions, ground salt, and egg.
2. Then melt the coconut oil in the skillet well.
3. Make the small cakes from the salmon mixture with the help of the spoon and transfer them in the skillet.
4. Roast the salmon cakes for 3 minutes per side or until they are light brown.

Nutritional info per serve: Calories 205, Fat 15, Fiber 1.9, Carbs 4.1, Protein 15.6

Tilapia with Olives

Prep time: 10 minutes
Cook time: 20 minutes
Servings: 2
Ingredients:
- 2 tilapia fillets
- 1 tablespoon avocado oil
- 2 kalamata olives, sliced
- 1 teaspoon apple cider vinegar
- 1 teaspoon ground turmeric

Method:
1. Rub the tilapia fillets with ground turmeric and sprinkle with apple cider vinegar.
2. Then brush the baking pan with avocado oil from inside and put the fish.
3. Top it with olives and bake at 360F for 20 minutes.

Nutritional info per serve: Calories 112, Fat 2.5, Fiber 0.7, Carbs 1.4, Protein 21.2

Cod Sticks

Prep time: 10 minutes
Cook time: 15 minutes
Servings: 6
Ingredients:
- 10 oz cod fillet
- ½ cup almond flour
- 2 eggs, beaten
- 1 teaspoon salt
- ½ teaspoon smoked paprika
- 3 oz Parmesan, grated
- 1 teaspoon butter

Method:
1. Cut the cod fillet into the sticks and sprinkle with salt and smoked paprika.
2. Then dip the fish sticks in the eggs and coat in the almond flour and Parmesan.
3. Grease the baking tray with butter and put the fish sticks inside.
4. Bake the meal at 360F for 10-15 minutes or until the cod sticks are crunchy.

Nutritional info per serve: Calories 124, Fat 6.7, Fiber 0.3, Carbs 1.2, Protein 15.4

Halibut and Spinach

Prep time: 10 minutes
Cook time: 15 minutes
Servings: 2
Ingredients:
- 1 yellow bell pepper, seeded and chopped
- 1 teaspoon apple cider vinegar
- 1 tablespoon avocado oil
- 2 halibut fillets
- 2 cups spinach, chopped
- 1 teaspoon ground paprika
- 1 teaspoon ground coriander

Method:
1. Preheat the skillet well.
2. Sprinkle the halibut fillets with ground paprika and ground coriander and put in the skillet. Roast the fish fillets for 2 minutes per side.
3. Then add bell pepper, apple cider vinegar, and spinach.
4. Cover the skillet with foil and bake at 360F for 10 minutes.

Nutritional info per serve: Calories 357, Fat 8, Fiber 2.2, Carbs 6.6, Protein 62.2

Coriander Cod

Prep time: 15 minutes
Cook time: 10 minutes
Servings: 2
Ingredients:
- 12 oz cod fillet
- 1 tablespoon coconut oil
- 1 tablespoon ground coriander
- 1 teaspoon dried dill
- 1 teaspoon coconut aminos

Method:
1. Sprinkle the cod fillet with ground coriander, dried dill, and coconut aminos.
2. Leave the fish for 10 minutes to marinate.
3. After this, melt the coconut oil in the skillet and add marinated fish.
4. Roast it for 5 minutes per side on the medium heat.

Nutritional info per serve: Calories 199, Fat 8.3, Fiber 0.1, Carbs 0.8, Protein 30.5

White Fish Stew

Prep time: 10 minutes
Cook time: 40 minutes
Servings: 4
Ingredients:
- 4 tilapia fillets
- ½ cup turnip, chopped
- 1 cup of water
- 1 teaspoon avocado oil
- 2 spring onions, diced
- 1 teaspoon ground black pepper
- ½ teaspoon salt
- 1 teaspoon keto tomato paste

Method:
1. Mix water with keto tomato paste in the saucepan.
2. Add fish, turnip, avocado oil, spring onion, ground black pepper, and salt.
3. Close the lid and cook the stew on low heat for 40 minutes.

Nutritional info per serve: Calories 113, Fat 1.3, Fiber 1.1, Carbs 4.3, Protein 21.6

Crab Fritters

Prep time: 10 minutes
Cook time: 12 minutes
Servings: 4
Ingredients:
- 4 tablespoons ricotta cheese
- 1 teaspoon garlic powder
- 8 oz crab meat, canned, shredded
- 2 oz provolone cheese, shredded
- 1 teaspoon dried dill

Method:
1. Line the baking tray with baking paper.
2. Then mix ricotta cheese, garlic powder, shredded crab meat, provolone cheese, and dried dill.
3. Make the fritters from the mixture and put them in the baking tray.
4. Bake the crab fritters in the preheated to 360F oven for 12 minutes.

Nutritional info per serve: Calories 125, Fat 6, Fiber 0.1, Carbs 2.8, Protein 12.7

Lime Shrimp

Prep time: 5 minutes
Cook time: 10 minutes
Servings: 4
Ingredients:
- 1-pound shrimps, peeled
- ½ lemon
- 1 tablespoon butter
- ½ teaspoon chili powder

Method:
1. Melt the butter in the saucepan and add shrimps.
2. Sprinkle the shrimps with chili powder and roast for 2 minutes per side.
3. Then squeeze the lemon juice over the shrimps and cook them for 5 minutes more.

Nutritional info per serve: Calories 163, Fat 4.9, Fiber 0.3, Carbs 2.6, Protein 26

Ginger Cod

Prep time: 10 minutes
Cook time: 30 minutes
Servings: 4
Ingredients:
- 4 cod fillets
- 1 teaspoon minced ginger
- 2 tablespoons butter
- 1 teaspoon ground black pepper
- 1 teaspoon ground turmeric

Method:
1. In the shallow bowl, mix minced ginger, butter, ground black pepper, and ground turmeric.
2. Rub the cod fillets with the ginger mixture and wrap in the foil.
3. Bake the fish for 30 minutes at 360F.

Nutritional info per serve: Calories 146, Fat 6.9, Fiber 0.3, Carbs 1, Protein 20.2

Tomato Sea Bass

Prep time: 10 minutes
Cook time: 35 minutes
Servings: 4
Ingredients:
- 2 sea bass fillets
- 1 tablespoon keto tomato paste
- 1 tablespoon butter, softened
- ½ teaspoon ground black pepper
- ½ teaspoon dried rosemary

Method:
1. Rub the seabass fillets with ground black pepper and dried rosemary.
2. Then sprinkle the fish with butter and keto tomato paste. Wrap the seabass in the foil.
3. Bake the fish at 360F for 35 minutes.

Nutritional info per serve: Calories 93, Fat 4.2, Fiber 0.3, Carbs 1, Protein 12.2

Scallions Salmon Spread

Prep time: 15 minutes
Cook time: 0 minutes
Servings: 6
Ingredients:
- 1-pound salmon, canned, shredded
- 1 oz scallions, diced
- 1 tablespoon butter, softened
- 1 tablespoon ricotta cheese
- ½ teaspoon minced garlic
- ¼ teaspoon lime zest, grated

Method:
1. Put all ingredients in the food processor and blend until smooth.
2. Then transfer it in the bowl and refrigerate for 10-15 minutes before serving.

Nutritional info per serve: Calories 122, Fat 6.8, Fiber 0.1, Carbs 0.6, Protein 15.1

Tomato and Thyme Shrimps

Prep time: 10 minutes
Cook time: 10 minutes
Servings: 4
Ingredients:
- 1-pound shrimps

- 1 teaspoon dried thyme
- 1 teaspoon coconut oil
- 1 teaspoon keto tomato paste
- ¼ cup of coconut milk

Method:
1. Melt the coconut oil in the saucepan and add shrimps.
2. Then sprinkle them with dried thyme, keto tomato paste, and coconut milk.
3. Stir the mixture until you get tomato color.
4. Cook the shrimps on medium heat for 5 minutes.

Nutritional info per serve: Calories 181, Fat 6.7, Fiber 0.5, Carbs 3, Protein 26.3

Chili Cod

Prep time: 10 minutes
Cook time: 6 minutes
Servings: 1
Ingredients:
- 1 cod fillet
- 1 teaspoon coconut oil, melted
- ½ teaspoon garlic powder
- ½ teaspoon chili powder
- ½ teaspoon coconut aminos

Method:
1. Rub the cod fillet with chili powder and garlic powder.
2. Then sprinkle it with coconut oil and coconut aminos.
3. Preheat the skillet well and put the fish inside.
4. Roast it for 3 minutes per side on high heat.

Nutritional info per serve: Calories 143, Fat 5.8, Fiber 0.6, Carbs 2.2, Protein 21.4

Shrimp Bowl

Prep time: 10 minutes
Cook time: 5 minutes
Servings: 4
Ingredients:
- ½ cup celery stalk, chopped
- 1 spring onion, sliced
- 1 tablespoon avocado oil
- 10 oz shrimps, peeled
- 1 teaspoon ground coriander
- 1 tablespoon coconut oil

Method:
1. Melt the coconut oil in the skillet.
2. Add shrimps and ground coriander. Roast the seafood for 5 minutes. Stir it from time to time.
3. Then transfer the shrimps in the bowl and add all remaining ingredients.
4. Carefully mix the meal.

Nutritional info per serve: Calories 123, Fat 5.1, Fiber 0.5, Carbs 2.3, Protein 16.4

Tender Catfish

Prep time: 10 minutes
Cook time: 10 minutes
Servings: 7
Ingredients:
- 1-pound catfish, chopped
- ½ cup coconut cream
- 1 teaspoon ground turmeric
- ½ teaspoon smoked paprika

Method:
1. Bring the coconut cream to boil.
2. Meanwhile, sprinkle the catfish with ground turmeric and smoked paprika.
3. Put the fish in the boiling coconut cream and cook for 10 minutes on medium heat.

Nutritional info per serve: Calories 189, Fat 12.8, Fiber 1, Carbs 6.4, Protein 12.2

Cayenne Mahi Mahi

Prep time: 10 minutes
Cook time: 8 minutes
Servings: 2
Ingredients:
- 2 mahi-mahi fillets
- 1 teaspoon cayenne pepper
- 1 tablespoon coconut oil
- 1 teaspoon salt

Method:
1. Melt the coconut oil in the skillet.
2. Then sprinkle the fish fillets with cayenne pepper and salt.
3. Roast the fish fillets in the hot coconut oil for 4 minutes per side.

Nutritional info per serve: Calories 150, Fat 7.9, Fiber 0.2, Carbs 0.5, Protein 19

Sweet Salmon Steaks

Prep time: 10 minutes
Cook time: 6 minutes
Servings: 4
Ingredients:
- 4 salmon fillets (steaks)
- ½ teaspoon Erythritol
- 1 tablespoon water
- 1 teaspoon ground black pepper
- 1 teaspoon smoked paprika
- ¼ cup coconut cream
- 1 teaspoon coconut oil

Method:
1. In the mixing bowl, mix Erythritol, ground black pepper, and smoked paprika.
2. Rub the salmon fillets with mixture and them put in the skillet.
3. Add coconut oil and coconut cream.
4. Roast the fish for 5 minutes per side on the medium heat.

Nutritional info per serve: Calories 283, Fat 15.8, Fiber 0.7, Carbs 1.5, Protein 35

Pepper Shrimp

Prep time: 10 minutes
Cook time: 5 minutes
Servings: 2
Ingredients:
- ½ pound shrimp, peeled and deveined
- 1 tablespoon lime juice
- 1 teaspoon ground black pepper
- 2 tablespoons avocado oil

Method:

1. Preheat the skillet well and add avocado oil.
2. Add shrimps and sprinkle them with ground black pepper.
3. Roast the shrimps for 2 minutes per side.
4. Sprinkle the cooked shrimps with lime juice.
Nutritional info per serve: Calories 156, Fat 3.7, Fiber 0.9, Carbs 3.2, Protein 26.1

Jalapeno Tilapia

Prep time: 10 minutes
Cook time: 20 minutes
Servings: 4
Ingredients:
- 2 jalapenos, chopped
- 1/3 avocado, pitted, sliced
- 1 tablespoon lime juice
- 4 tilapia fillets
- 1 tablespoon avocado oil

Method:
1. Brush the baking pan with avocado oil.
2. Then put the tilapia fillets inside.
3. Sprinkle them with lime juice and top with jalapeno peppers.
4. Bake the tilapia for 20 minutes at 360F.
5. Then top the cooked fish with avocado.
Nutritional info per serve: Calories 159, Fat 7.8, Fiber 1.3, Carbs 1.9, Protein 21.4

Shrimp and Turnip Stew

Prep time: 10 minutes
Cook time: 20 minutes
Servings: 6
Ingredients:
- 1-pound shrimps, peeled
- 1 cup turnip, chopped
- 2 cups of water
- ½ cup coconut cream
- 1 teaspoon keto tomato paste
- 1 teaspoon ground coriander

Method:
1. Bring the water to boil and add keto tomato paste, ground coriander, and chopped turnip.
2. Cook the mixture on medium heat for 10 minutes.
3. Then add shrimps and coconut cream.
4. Simmet the stew on medium heat for 10 minutes.
Nutritional info per serve: Calories 143, Fat 6.1, Fiber 0.9, Carbs 3.8, Protein 17.9

Parmesan Tilapia Bites

Prep time: 10 minutes
Cook time: 10 minutes
Servings: 4
Ingredients:
- 7 oz Parmesan, grated
- ½ cup coconut flour
- 8 oz tilapia, boiled
- 1 egg, beaten
- 1 teaspoon dried parsley

Method:
1. Mix parmesan with coconut flour, boiled tilapia, egg, and dried parsley.
2. Carefully mix the mixture and make the small bites.
3. Bake the meal at 360F for 10 minutes.
Nutritional info per serve: Calories 282, Fat 13.7, Fiber 6, Carbs 11.9, Protein 29.9

Mushroom Shrimps

Prep time: 10 minutes
Cook time: 25 minutes
Servings: 4
Ingredients:
- 1-pound shrimps, peeled
- ½ cup heavy cream
- ½ cup cremini mushrooms, chopped
- 1 tablespoon coconut oil
- 1 teaspoon ground black pepper
- ½ teaspoon dried rosemary
- ½ cup of water

Method:
1. Melt the coconut oil in the saucepan.
2. Add mushrooms and ground black pepper.
3. Roast the shrimps on medium heat for 10 minutes.
4. Then stir them well and add ground black pepper, dried rosemary, water, and heavy cream.
5. Add shrimps and carefully mix the mixture.
6. Cook it for 15 minutes on medium heat.
Nutritional info per serve: Calories 220, Fat 10.9, Fiber 0.3, Carbs 3, Protein 26.4

Creamy Cod

Prep time: 10 minutes
Cook time: 15 minutes
Servings: 4
Ingredients:
- ½ cup heavy cream
- 4 cod fillets
- 1 teaspoon dried rosemary
- 1 teaspoon avocado oil
- ½ teaspoon salt

Method:
1. Roast the cod fillets in avocado oil for 1 minute per side.
2. Then sprinkle the fish with dried rosemary, salt, and heavy cream.
3. Close the lid and cook the cod on medium heat for 10 minutes.
Nutritional info per serve: Calories 144, Fat 6.8, Fiber 0.2, Carbs 0.7, Protein 20.3

Shrimp Soup

Prep time: 10 minutes
Cook time: 15 minutes
Servings: 4
Ingredients:
- 1 oz chives, chopped
- 1½ tablespoons avocado oil
- ½ teaspoon minced ginger
- 4 cups chicken stock
- 1-pound shrimps, peeled
- 2 oz leek, chopped

Method:

1. Put all ingredients in the saucepan and bring to boil.
2. Simmer the soup for 10 minutes.
Nutritional info per serve: Calories 182, Fat 5, Fiber 1.3, Carbs 6, Protein 27.2

Garlic Catfish

Prep time: 10 minutes
Cook time: 15 minutes
Servings: 2
Ingredients:
- 8 oz catfish, fillet
- 1 teaspoon minced garlic
- 1 tablespoon coconut cream
- 1 teaspoon ground turmeric
- ½ teaspoon cayenne pepper
- 1 tablespoon butter

Method:
1. In the mixing bowl, mix minced garlic with coconut cream, ground turmeric, and cayenne pepper.
2. Pour the liquid in the saucepan, add butter and bring to boil.
3. Then add catfish and cook the meal for 10 minutes on medium heat.
Nutritional info per serve: Calories 335, Fat 22.9, Fiber 1.3, Carbs 11, Protein 21

Lime Mussels

Prep time: 10 minutes
Cook time: 10 minutes
Servings: 4
Ingredients:
- 2-pound mussels, debearded and scrubbed
- 2 tablespoons lime juice
- 3 tablespoons butter
- ½ cup of water

Method:
1. Bring the water to boil and add mussels.
2. Cook them for 7 minutes.
3. Then drain water and add butter and lime juice.
4. Carefully mix the mussels and cook them for 3 minutes more.
Nutritional info per serve: Calories 271, Fat 13.7, Fiber 0, Carbs 8.4, Protein 27.1

Salmon Kababs

Prep time: 10 minutes
Cook time: 6 minutes
Servings: 3
Ingredients:
- 11 oz salmon fillet
- 1 teaspoon keto tomato paste
- 1 teaspoon chili powder
- ½ teaspoon ground paprika
- 3 tablespoons avocado oil

Method:
1. In the mixing bowl, mix keto tomato paste with chili powder, ground paprika, and avocado oil.
2. Then cut the salmon into medium cubes.
3. Coat every salmon cube in the keto tomato paste mixture and string in the skewers.
4. Grill the fish kababs at 400F for 3 minutes per side.
Nutritional info per serve: Calories 161, Fat 8.4, Fiber 1.1, Carbs 1.8, Protein 20.6

Sriracha Calamari

Prep time: 10 minutes
Cook time: 10 minutes
Servings: 2
Ingredients:
- 1 squid, cut into medium rings
- 1 tablespoon sriracha
- 2 tablespoons avocado oil
- ½ teaspoon dried rosemary

Method:
1. Preheat the avocado oil well.
2. Then mix squid with sriracha and dried rosemary. Put it in the hot oil.
3. Roast the meal for 3 minutes per side on medium heat.
Nutritional info per serve: Calories 66, Fat 2.4, Fiber 0.7, Carbs 3.8, Protein 6.8

Curry Cod

Prep time: 15 minutes
Cook time: 16 minutes
Servings: 4
Ingredients:
- 1-pound cod fillet
- ¾ cup heavy cream
- ¾ teaspoon coriander
- 1 teaspoon salt
- ½ teaspoon curry powder
- 1 teaspoon garlic powder
- 1 tablespoon coconut oil
- 1 teaspoon dried parsley

Method:
1. Sprinkle the cod fillet with coriander, salt, curry powder, garlic powder, and dried parsley.
2. Then melt the coconut oil in the skillet and add cod fillets.
3. Roast them for 3 minutes per side.
4. Add heavy cream and close the lid.
5. Cook the cod on medium heat for 10 minutes.
Nutritional info per serve: Calories 274, Fat 19.5, Fiber 0.2, Carbs 0.7, Protein 20.4

Turmeric Calamari

Prep time: 10 minutes
Cook time: 15 minutes
Servings: 2
Ingredients:
- 8 ounces calamari, cut into medium rings
- 1 teaspoon ground turmeric
- 2 tablespoons coconut oil
- ¼ cup heavy cream
- ½ teaspoon salt

Method:
1. Melt the coconut oil in the saucepan and add calamari.
2. Roast them for 2 minutes per side.

3. Then add the ground turmeric, salt, and heavy cream.
4. Carefully mix the calamari and cook them for 10 minutes on medium-low heat.
Nutritional info per serve: Calories 277, Fat 20.8, Fiber 0.2, Carbs 4.6, Protein 18.1

Parsley Cod

Prep time: 10 minutes
Cook time: 25 minutes
Servings: 2
Ingredients:
- 10 oz cod fillet
- ¼ cup almond flour
- ¾ teaspoon salt
- 1 tablespoon olive oil
- 6 tablespoons water
- 1 tablespoon lemon juice
- 1 tablespoon dried parsley

Method:
1. Brush the baking pan with olive oil and put the cod fillets inside.
2. Sprinkle them with salt, water, lemon juice, and dried parsley.
3. Massage the fish and top with almond flour.
4. Cover the baking pan with foil and bake the fish for 25 minutes at 360F.

Nutritional info per serve: Calories 260, Fat 15, Fiber 1.6, Carbs 3.3, Protein 28.4

Lemon Octopus

Prep time: 10 minutes
Cook time: 6 minutes
Servings: 2
Ingredients:
- 10 oz octopus, rinsed
- 2 tablespoons lemon juice
- 1 teaspoon ground coriander
- ½ teaspoon salt
- 2 tablespoons butter

Method:
1. Melt the butter in the skillet.
2. Add octopus, lemon juice, ground coriander, and salt.
3. Cook the meal on medium heat for 6 minutes. Stir it from time to time.

Nutritional info per serve: Calories 338, Fat 14.6, Fiber 0.1, Carbs 6.6, Protein 42.5

Cod Packets

Prep time: 15 minutes
Cook time: 30 minutes
Servings: 4
Ingredients:
- 4 cod fillet
- 2 bell peppers
- 1 zucchini
- ½ teaspoon onion powder
- 4 tablespoons coconut oil
- 1 teaspoon ground coriander
- 1 teaspoon dried cilantro

Method:
1. Make 4 packets from the baking paper.
2. Then rub the cod fillets with onion powder, ground coriander, and dried cilantro.
3. Put the fish inside the packets.
4. Chop zucchini and bell peppers and add them in the fish packest.
5. Bake the meal at 360F for 30 minutes.

Nutritional info per serve: Calories 240, Fat 14.6, Fiber 1.4, Carbs 6.4, Protein 21.9

Clam Soup with Pancetta

Prep time: 10 minutes
Cook time: 15 minutes
Servings: 4
Ingredients:
- 2 oz pancetta, chopped
- 8 oz clams
- 4 cups chicken stock
- 1 teaspoon ground cumin
- ½ teaspoon salt

Method:
1. Roast pancetta in the saucepan for 3-4 minutes on medium heat.
2. Stir it well and add chicken stock, ground cumin, and salt. Bring the mixture to the boil and add clams.
3. Cook the soup on medium heat for 10 minutes.

Nutritional info per serve: Calories 116, Fat 6.7, Fiber 0.3, Carbs 7.4, Protein 6.4

Tuna Meatballs

Prep time: 15 minutes
Cook time: 10 minutes
Servings: 6
Ingredients:
- 10 oz tuna, canned, shredded
- 1 jalapeno, minced
- 1 tablespoon almond flour
- ½ teaspoon cayenne pepper
- 1 egg, beaten
- ½ teaspoon ground coriander
- 2 tablespoons coconut oil

Method:
1. In the mixing bowl, mix tuna with minced jalapeno, almond flour, cayenne pepper, egg, and ground coriander.
2. Make the tuna meatballs.
3. Then melt the coconut oil in the skillet, add tuna meatballs and roast them for 3 minutes per side on the medium heat.

Nutritional info per serve: Calories 146, Fat 9.7, Fiber 0.2, Carbs 0.5, Protein 13.8

Lemon Flounder

Prep time: 10 minutes
Cook time: 25 minutes
Servings: 4
Ingredients:
- 1-pound flounder fillet
- 2 tablespoons lemon juice
- 1 teaspoon smoked paprika
- ½ teaspoon lemon zest, grated

Method:

1. Put the flounder fillet in the lined with baking paper tray.
2. Sprinkle the fish with lemon juice, smoked paprika, and lemon zest.
3. Bake the fish at 360F for 25 minutes.
Nutritional info per serve: Calories 136, Fat 1.9, Fiber 0.3, Carbs 0.5, Protein 27.6

Creamy Halibut

Prep time: 10 minutes
Cook time: 20 minutes
Servings: 6
Ingredients:
- 6 halibut fillets
- ½ cup coconut cream
- 1 garlic clove, diced
- 1 teaspoon ground turmeric
- ½ teaspoon dried rosemary
- 1 teaspoon avocado oil

Method:
1. Preheat the skillet well and add avocado oil.
2. Add halibut fillets and roast them for 3 minutes per side.
3. Then sprinkle the fish with garlic, ground turmeric, and rosemary.
4. Add coconut cream and close the lid.
5. Cook the halibut on medium heat for 15 minutes.
Nutritional info per serve: Calories 367, Fat 11.6, Fiber 0.6, Carbs 1.6, Protein 61

Shrimp Salad

Prep time: 10 minutes
Cook time: 0 minutes
Servings: 4
Ingredients:
- 1 cup lettuce, chopped
- 1-pound shrimps, peeled, boiled
- 1 tablespoon avocado oil
- 1 teaspoon salt
- ½ teaspoon ground black pepper
- 1 tablespoon apple cider vinegar

Method:
1. Put all ingredients in the salad bowl and carefully mix.
Nutritional info per serve: Calories 143, Fat 2.4, Fiber 0.3, Carbs 2.5, Protein 26

Salmon Quesadillas

Prep time: 15 minutes
Cook time: 10 minutes
Servings: 4
Ingredients:
- ¾ cup coconut flour
- 1 tablespoon coconut oil
- 10 oz salmon, canned, shredded
- 1 teaspoon ricotta cheese
- ¼ teaspoon chili powder
- 4 oz Provolone, grated

Method:
1. In the mixing bowl, mix coconut flour with coconut oil and ricotta cheese.
2. Knead the dough and make 2 buns. Roll them up in the shape of flatbreads.
3. Preheat the skillet well and roast the flatbreads for 1 minute per side.
4. After this, mix chili powder with provolone cheese, and shredded salmon.
5. Put one cooked flatbread in the skillet and top it with salmon mixture, flatten it carefully, and cover with second flatbread.
6. Close the lid and cook the meal on medium heat for 5 minutes.
Nutritional info per serve: Calories 236, Fat 15.8, Fiber 1, Carbs 2.3, Protein 21.6

Garlic Oysters

Prep time: 10 minutes
Cook time: 5 minutes
Servings: 4
Ingredients:
- 12 oysters, shucked
- 1 teaspoon minced garlic
- ½ teaspoon ground ginger
- 1 tablespoon coconut oil
- ½ teaspoon chili powder

Method:
1. Melt the coconut oil in the skillet.
2. Add chili powder, ground ginger, and minced garlic. Bring the mixture to boil.
3. Add oysters, carefully mix the mixture, and transfer in the serving plates.
Nutritional info per serve: Calories 161, Fat 7.8, Fiber 0.2, Carbs 7.4, Protein 14.5

Onion Mahi Mahi

Prep time: 15 minutes
Cook time: 15 minutes
Servings: 4
Ingredients:
- 1-pound mahi-mahi, chopped
- 2 spring onion, diced
- 1 tablespoon avocado oil
- ½ teaspoon ground black pepper
- 1 teaspoon ground paprika
- ¼ cup of water

Method:
1. Melt the coconut oil in the skillet.
2. Add onion, ground black pepper, and ground paprika. Roast the onion for 3 minutes.
3. Stir it carefully and add mahi-mahi.
4. Then add water and cook the fish on medium heat for 10 minutes.
Nutritional info per serve: Calories 142, Fat 1.6, Fiber 1, Carbs 3.2, Protein 27.4

Spicy Salmon

Prep time: 10 minutes
Cook time: 15 minutes
Servings: 12
Ingredients:
- 1-pound salmon, fillet
- 8 oz shrimps, peeled
- 1 teaspoon dried oregano
- 1 teaspoon dried basil

- 1 teaspoon dried cilantro
- 1 teaspoon salt
- ¼ cup of water
- 1 tablespoon coconut oil

Method:
1. Sprinkle the salmon and shrimps with dried oregano, basil, cilantro, and salt.
2. Then melt coconut oil in the saucepan, add shrimps and salmon and roast the seafood for 5 minutes, stir it occasionally.
3. Then add water and close the lid. Cook the meal o medium heat for 10 minutes.

Nutritional info per serve: Calories 83, Fat 3.8, Fiber 0.1, Carbs 0.4, Protein 11.6

Cod Sticks

Prep time: 10 minutes
Cook time: 10 minutes
Servings: 6
Ingredients:
- ½ cup coconut flour
- 4 oz Provolone cheese, grated
- 1-pound cod fillet
- 1 egg, beaten
- 2 tablespoons coconut oil

Method:
1. Melt the coconut oil in the skillet.
2. Meanwhile, cut the cod fillet into the sticks. Dip every fish stick in the egg.
3. Then mix coconut flour with Provolone cheese. Coat the fish in the cheese mixture.
4. Put the fish sticks in the skillet and roast them for 2 minutes per side or until they are light brown.

Nutritional info per serve: Calories 217, Fat 12, Fiber 4, Carbs 7.1, Protein 20.6

Tuna Skewers

Prep time: 10 minutes
Cook time: 5 minutes
Servings: 4
Ingredients:
- 1-pound tuna fillet, roughly chopped
- 1 tablespoon lemon juice
- 1 teaspoon ground paprika
- 1 teaspoon onion powder
- 1 teaspoon olive oil

Method:
1. String the tuna fillet in the skewers and sprinkle with ground paprika, onion powder, and lemon juice.
2. Then sprinkle the fish with olive oil and grill at 400F for 2 minutes per side.

Nutritional info per serve: Calories 426, Fat 36.4, Fiber 0.3, Carbs 0.9, Protein 24

Turmeric Salmon Balls

Prep time: 15 minutes
Cook time: 0 minutes
Servings: 4
Ingredients:
- 8 oz salmon, canned, shredded
- 3 tablespoons ricotta cheese
- 1 teaspoon dried parsley
- ½ teaspoon ground turmeric
- ½ garlic clove, diced

Method:
1. In the mixing bowl mix shredded salmon, ricotta cheese, parsley, ground turmeric, and garlic clove.
2. When the mixture is homogenous, make the salmon balls with the help of the scooper.

Nutritional info per serve: Calories 93, Fat 4.5, Fiber 0.1, Carbs 0.9, Protein 12.4

Basil Shrimp

Prep time: 10 minutes
Cook time: 5 minutes
Servings: 4
Ingredients:
- 1-pound shrimp, peeled and deveined
- 1 teaspoon dried basil
- 1 teaspoon sriracha
- 2 tablespoons coconut oil

Method:
1. Melt the coconut oil in the skillet.
2. Add shrimps and sprinkle them with dried basil. Roast the shrimps for 2 minutes per side.
3. Add sriracha and carefully mix the meal.
4. Cook it for 1 minute more.

Nutritional info per serve: Calories 195, Fat 8.7, Fiber 0, Carbs 2, Protein 25.8

Cumin Seabass

Prep time: 10 minutes
Cook time: 25 minutes
Servings: 4
Ingredients:
- 4 seabass fillets
- 1 teaspoon ground cumin
- 1 teaspoon coconut aminos
- 1 tablespoon canola oil
- ¼ teaspoon ground nutmeg

Method:
1. Sprinkle the seabass fillet with ground cumin, coconut aminos, canola oil, and ground nutmeg.
2. Bake the seabass at 360F for 25 minutes.

Nutritional info per serve: Calories 270, Fat 17.8, Fiber 1, Carbs 0.6, Protein 26.2

Calamari Salad

Prep time: 30 minutes
Cook time: 4 minutes
Servings: 8
Ingredients:
- 1 jalapeno, chopped
- 2 cups arugula, chopped
- 10 oz calamari, sliced
- 1 tablespoon butter
- ½ teaspoon chili powder
- 1 teaspoon avocado oil
- 1 teaspoon lemon juice

Method:
1. Melt the butter in the skillet, Add calamari, and chili powder.

2. Roast the calamari for 2 minutes per side and transfer in the salad bowl.
3. Add arugula, and all remaining ingredients. Carefully mix the salad.
Nutritional info per serve: Calories 72, Fat 4, Fiber 0.2, Carbs 2.9, Protein 5.9

Paprika Cod
Prep time: 10 minutes
Cook time: 10 minutes
Servings: 4
Ingredients:
- 4 cod fillets
- 1 teaspoon ground paprika
- 1 teaspoon ground ginger
- 1 tablespoon canola oil
- ½ teaspoon dried rosemary

Method:
1. Preheat the canola oil well.
2. Then put the cod fillet in the hot oil. Sprinkle it with ground paprika, ground ginger, and dried rosemary.
3. Roast the fish on medium heat for 4 minutes per side.
Nutritional info per serve: Calories 125, Fat 4.6, Fiber 0.3, Carbs 0.7, Protein 20.1

Lettuce and Cod Salad
Prep time: 10 minutes
Cook time: 7 minutes
Servings: 8
Ingredients:
- 1 jalapeno pepper, sliced
- 1 bell pepper, chopped
- 2 cups lettuce, chopped
- 3 cod fillets
- 1 teaspoon ground black pepper
- 1 teaspoon salt
- 1 tablespoon avocado oil
- 1 teaspoon lemon juice
- 1 teaspoon olive oil

Method:
1. Preheat the olive oil in the skillet.
2. Then sprinkle the cod fillets with ground black pepper and salt and put in the hot skillet. Roast the fish for 3 minutes per side. Then chop it.
3. Add all remaining ingredients and carefully mix the salad.
Nutritional info per serve: Calories 49, Fat 1.3, Fiber 0.5, Carbs 1.9, Protein 7.8

Marjoram Seabass
Prep time: 10 minutes
Cook time: 30 minutes
Servings: 2
Ingredients:
- 10 oz seabass
- 1 teaspoon dried marjoram
- 1 tablespoon avocado oil
- ½ teaspoon salt

Method:
1. Sprinkle the seabass with dried marjoram, avocado oil, and salt.
2. Then wrap it in the foil and bake at 365F for 30 minutes.
Nutritional info per serve: Calories 300, Fat 18.3, Fiber 1.5, Carbs 0.6, Protein 32.3

Sardine Salad
Prep time: 10 minutes
Cook time: 0 minutes
Servings: 1
Ingredients:
- 5 oz canned sardines in oil
- 1 tablespoon lime juice
- ½ tablespoon mustard
- 1 cup lettuce, chopped
- 1 teaspoon avocado oil

Method:
1. Mix lime juice with mustard, and avocado oil.
2. Then mix sardines with lettuce and top with mustard mixture.
Nutritional info per serve: Calories 335, Fat 18.5, Fiber 1.4, Carbs 3.9, Protein 36.6

Garlic Mackerel
Prep time: 10 minutes
Cook time: 30 minutes
Servings: 2
Ingredients:
- 10 oz mackerel fillet
- 1 teaspoon minced garlic
- 1 teaspoon avocado oil
- ½ teaspoon dried parsley

Method:
1. Rub the mackerel with minced garlic and dried parsley.
2. Then sprinkle the fish with avocado oil and put it in the baking pan.
3. Bake the mackerel for 30 minutes at 360F.
Nutritional info per serve: Calories 377, Fat 25.6, Fiber 0.1, Carbs 0.6, Protein 33.9

Rosemary Clams
Prep time: 10 minutes
Cook time: 20 minutes
Servings: 4
Ingredients:
- 3 tablespoons coconut oil
- 12 oz clams
- 1 teaspoon dried rosemary
- ½ cup of water

Method:
1. Preheat the coconut oil in the saucepan.
2. Add clams and rosemary and roast them for 2 minutes per side.
3. Then add water and cook the clams for 15 minutes.
Nutritional info per serve: Calories 130, Fat 10.4, Fiber 0.5, Carbs 9.5, Protein 0.5

Coconut Tilapia
Prep time: 10 minutes
Cook time: 15 minutes
Servings: 4

Ingredients:
- 4 tilapia fillets
- 1 tablespoon coconut shred
- ½ cup of coconut milk
- 1 teaspoon ground black pepper
- 1 teaspoon butter
- ½ teaspoon chili powder

Method:
1. Sprinkle the tilapia with ground black pepper and chili powder.
2. Then melt the butter in the saucepan.
3. Add tilapia and cook it for 2 minutes per side.
4. Sprinkle the fish with coconut shred and coconut milk. Close the lid and cook it for 10 minutes on medium heat.

Nutritional info per serve: Calories 185, Fat 10.5, Fiber 1.2, Carbs 2.7, Protein 21.8

Vinegar Salmon

Prep time: 15 minutes
Cook time: 10 minutes
Servings: 2
Ingredients:
- 10 oz salmon fillet
- 2 tablespoons apple cider vinegar
- 1 teaspoon avocado oil
- ½ teaspoon ground nutmeg

Method:
1. Sprinkle the salmon fillet with ground nutmeg and apple cider vinegar. Marinate the fish for 10 minutes.
2. Then preheat the avocado oil well.
3. Add marinated salmon and roast it for 5 minutes per side on the medium heat.

Nutritional info per serve: Calories 197, Fat 9.3, Fiber 0.2, Carbs 0.5, Protein 27.6

Boiled Crab Legs

Prep time: 5 minutes
Cook time: 10 minutes
Servings: 4
Ingredients:
- 1-pound king crab legs
- 3 cups of water

Method:
1. Bring the water to boil and add crab legs.
2. Boil them for 5 minutes.
3. Cool the crab legs.

Nutritional info per serve: Calories 115, Fat 1.7, Fiber 0, Carbs 0, Protein 21.8

Salmon Sauce

Prep time: 10 minutes
Cook time: 15 minutes
Servings: 4
Ingredients:
- ¼ cup heavy cream
- ½ teaspoon onion powder
- 1 teaspoon coconut flour
- 1 teaspoon butter
- 12 oz salmon, canned, shredded
- 1 teaspoon fresh dill, chopped

Method:
1. Melt the butter in the saucepan and add heavy cream, onion powder, coconut flour, and dill.
2. Whisk the mixture until smooth and add shredded salmon.
3. Carefully mix the mixture and bring it to boil.
4. Cool the sauce.

Nutritional info per serve: Calories 151, Fat 9.1, Fiber 0.3, Carbs 1, Protein 16.8

Tuna Salad

Prep time: 10 minutes
Servings: 3
Ingredients:
- 1 cup lettuce, chopped
- 6 oz tuna, canned, shredded
- 1 tomato, chopped
- 2 tablespoons canola oil
- 1 garlic clove, diced

Method:
1. Put all ingredients in the salad bowl.
2. Carefully mix the salad.

Nutritional info per serve: Calories 196, Fat 14, Fiber 0.4, Carbs 1.7, Protein 15.4

Hot Salmon

Prep time: 10 minutes
Cook time: 7 minutes
Servings: 6
Ingredients:
- 2-pound salmon
- 2 tablespoons keto hot sauce
- 1 tablespoon coconut oil
- ½ teaspoon dried parsley

Method:
1. Melt the coconut oil in the skillet.
2. Add salmon and sprinkle it with dried parsley.
3. Roast the fish for 4 minutes per side.
4. Then add keto hot sauce and roast the fish for 2 minutes more.

Nutritional info per serve: Calories 220, Fat 11.6, Fiber 0, Carbs 0.1, Protein 29.4

Cod Casserole

Prep time: 15 minutes
Cook time: 50 minutes
Servings: 4
Ingredients:
- 1 cup cauliflower, chopped
- ½ cup coconut cream
- 2 oz Monterey Jack cheese, shredded
- 10 oz cod fillet, chopped
- 1 cup celery stalk, chopped
- 1 teaspoon butter

Method:
1. Grease the casserole mold with butter.
2. Then add cod fillet and celery stalk.
3. Then top the mixture with Monterey Jack cheese, coconut cream, and cauliflower.
4. Cover the casserole with foil and bake it for 50 minutes at 360F.

Nutritional info per serve: Calories 198, Fat 13.1, Fiber 1.7, Carbs 3.8, Protein 17.5

Clams and Bacon

Prep time: 10 minutes
Cook time: 15 minutes
Servings: 4
Ingredients:
- 2 pounds clams, scrubbed
- 2 oz bacon, chopped
- 1 cup of water
- 1 teaspoon dried thyme

Method:
1. Put the bacon in the saucepan and roast it for 2 minutes per side.
2. Then add dried thyme and water. Bring the mixture to boil.
3. Add clams and cook them for 10 minutes.

Nutritional info per serve: Calories 161, Fat 7, Fiber 0.1, Carbs 3.3, Protein 19.8

Taco Tilapia

Prep time: 10 minutes
Cook time: 8 minutes
Servings: 2
Ingredients:
- 2 tilapia fillets
- 1 teaspoon taco seasonings
- 1 tablespoon coconut oil

Method:
1. Melt the coconut oil in the skillet.
2. Meanwhile, sprinkle the tilapia fillets with taco seasonings.
3. Put the fish in the hot skillet and roast it for 3 minutes per side.

Nutritional info per serve: Calories 157, Fat 7.8, Fiber 0, Carbs 1, Protein 21

Pomegranate Scallops

Prep time: 5 minutes
Cook time: 10 minutes
Servings: 4
Ingredients:
- 1-pound scallops
- 1 tablespoon coconut oil
- 3 tablespoons pomegranate juice
- 1 teaspoon dried basil

Method:
1. Melt the coconut oil in the skillet.
2. Add scallops and sprinkle them with dried basil.
3. Roast the scallops for 2 minutes per side.
4. After this, add pomegranate juice and close the lid.
5. Cook the meal on medium heat for 3 minutes more.

Nutritional info per serve: Calories 130, Fat 4.3, Fiber 0, Carbs 2.8, Protein 19.1

Tarragon Seabass

Prep time: 10 minutes
Cook time: 20 minutes
Servings: 4
Ingredients:
- 1 teaspoon dried tarragon
- 3 tablespoons butter
- 12 oz seabass fillet

Method:
1. Rub the seabass fillet with dried tarragon and put it in the baking pan.
2. Top the fish with butter and bake at 360F for 20 minutes.

Nutritional info per serve: Calories 251, Fat 19.1, Fiber 0.7, Carbs 0.1, Protein 19.4

Spicy Marjoram Oysters

Prep time: 10 minutes
Cook time: 15 minutes
Servings: 6
Ingredients:
- 18 oysters, scrubbed
- 1 teaspoon dried marjoram
- 1 teaspoon chili flakes
- ½ teaspoon ground paprika
- ½ teaspoon ground turmeric
- 1 tablespoon avocado oil
- ½ cup of water

Method:
1. Mix oysters with dried marjoram, chili flakes, ground paprika, and turmeric.
2. Then put them in the saucepan, add avocado oil and roast them for 5 minutes.
3. Add water and close the lid.
4. Cook the oysters on medium heat for 10 minutes.

Nutritional info per serve: Calories 134, Fat 4.7, Fiber 0.3, Carbs 7.3, Protein 14.5

Pepper Tuna Cakes

Prep time: 15 minutes
Cook time: 6 minutes
Servings: 4
Ingredients:
- 10 oz tuna, canned, shredded
- ½ cup bell pepper, diced
- 1 teaspoon cayenne pepper
- 1 teaspoon lemon zest, grated
- 2 eggs, beaten
- 2 tablespoons butter

Method:
1. In the mixing bowl, mix tuna with bell pepper, cayenne pepper, lemon zest, and eggs.
2. Melt the butter in the skillet.
3. Then make the tuna cakes and put in the butter.
4. Roast the cakes for 3 minutes per side.

Nutritional info per serve: Calories 221, Fat 13.8, Fiber 0.4, Carbs 1.7, Protein 21.8

Almond Squid

Prep time: 10 minutes
Cook time: 6 minutes
Servings: 2
Ingredients:
- ½ teaspoon chili flakes
- ½ cup organic almond milk

- 1 teaspoon ground paprika
- 10 oz squid, sliced

Method:
1. Sprinkle the squid with ground paprika and chili flakes.
2. Then put the squid in the hot skillet and roast for 1 minute per side.
3. Add almond milk and cook the squid for 5 minutes on medium heat.

Nutritional info per serve: Calories 149, Fat 2.7, Fiber 0.4, Carbs 7, Protein 22.5

Dill Crab Cakes

Prep time: 15 minutes
Cook time: 6 minutes
Servings: 7
Ingredients:
- 12 oz crabmeat, chopped, cooked
- 1 teaspoon salt
- 1 tablespoon dill, chopped
- 2 eggs, beaten
- 1 tablespoon coconut oil
- ½ teaspoon white pepper

Method:
1. In the mixing bowl, mix crabmeat with salt, dill, eggs, and white pepper.
2. Melt the coconut oil in the skillet.
3. Make the small crab cakes from the mixture and put in the hot coconut oil.
4. Roast the crab cakes for 3 minutes per side.

Nutritional info per serve: Calories 82, Fat 3.4, Fiber 0.3, Carbs 7.7, Protein 5.4

Coated Shrimps

Prep time: 10 minutes
Cook time: 10 minutes
Servings: 2
Ingredients:
- 4 king shrimps, peeled
- 1 tablespoon coconut shred
- 1 egg, beaten
- 1 teaspoon avocado oil

Method:
1. Preheat the avocado oil well.
2. Then dip the shrimps in egg and coat into the coconut shred.
3. Put the shrimps in the avocado oil and roast for 5 minutes per side on medium heat.

Nutritional info per serve: Calories 180, Fat 7, Fiber 0.6, Carbs 1.3, Protein 26.8

Tomato Mackerel

Prep time: 10 minutes
Cook time: 15 minutes
Servings: 4
Ingredients:
- 4 mackerel fillets
- 1 tablespoon keto tomato paste
- 2 tablespoons coconut cream
- ½ teaspoon ground coriander

Method:
1. In the saucepan mix ground coriander, coconut cream, and keto tomato paste.
2. Then bring it to boil and add mackerel fillets.
3. Boil the fish on medium heat for 15 minutes.
4. Serve the mackerel with tomato sauce.

Nutritional info per serve: Calories 251, Fat 17.5, Fiber 0.3, Carbs 1.2, Protein 21.3

Stuffed Salmon with Spinach

Prep time: 20 minutes
Cook time: 30 minutes
Servings: 2
Ingredients:
- 8 oz salmon fillet
- 1 teaspoon avocado oil
- ½ cup fresh spinach, chopped
- 1 teaspoon minced garlic
- 1 tablespoon cream cheese
- ½ teaspoon ground black pepper

Method:
1. Cut the fillet into 2 servings and rub with minced garlic and ground black pepper.
2. Then mix spinach with cream cheese.
3. Put the spinach mixture on the salon and fold them. Secure the salmon fillets with the help of the toothpicks and brush with avocado oil.
4. Bake the meal at 360F for 30 minutes.

Nutritional info per serve: Calories 176, Fat 9.1, Fiber 0.4, Carbs 1.3, Protein 22.8

Halibut with Mushrooms

Prep time: 10 minutes
Cook time: 30 minutes
Servings: 5
Ingredients:
- 4 oz mushrooms, chopped
- ½ teaspoon dried sage
- 10 oz halibut fillet, chopped
- 1 teaspoon chili powder
- 2 tablespoons butter
- ½ cup of water

Method:
1. Melt the butter in the saucepan.
2. Add mushrooms, chili powder, and dried sage. Roast the vegetables for 15 minutes. Stir them from time to time.
3. Add chopped halibut and water.
4. Close the lid and cook the meal on medium heat for 15 minutes.

Nutritional info per serve: Calories 61, Fat 5.8, Fiber 0.4, Carbs 1.1, Protein 1.9

Mustard Tilapia

Prep time: 10 minutes
Cook time: 8 minutes
Servings: 1
Ingredients:
- 1 tilapia fillet
- 1 tablespoon mustard
- 1 teaspoon lemon juice
- 1 teaspoon olive oil

Method:

1. Mix mustard with lemon juice. Rub the fillet with mustard mixture.
2. Then preheat the olive oil in the skillet and put the fillet inside.
3. Roast the tilapia on medium heat for 4 minutes per side.
4. Sprinkle the cooked tilapia with lemon juice.
Nutritional info per serve: Calories 187, Fat 9, Fiber 1.7, Carbs 4, Protein 23.9

Salmon Burger

Prep time: 15 minutes
Cook time: 15 minutes
Servings: 4
Ingredients:
- 1-pound salmon fillet, minced
- 1 teaspoon chili powder
- ½ teaspoon garlic powder
- 2 tablespoons coconut flour

Method:
1. Line the baking tray with baking paper.
2. Mix the salmon with chili powder, garlic powder, and coconut flour.
3. Make the burgers from the salmon mixture and put it in the baking tray.
4. Bake the salmon burgers for 15 minutes at 365F.
Nutritional info per serve: Calories 168, Fat 7.5, Fiber 1.8, Carbs 3.1, Protein 22.6

Salmon and Radish Stew

Prep time: 10 minutes
Cook time: 15 minutes
Servings: 4
Ingredients:
- 1-pound salmon fillet, chopped
- 1 cup radish, chopped
- 1 cup of water
- 1 teaspoon ground coriander
- 1 teaspoon salt
- 1 teaspoon dried dill
- 1 teaspoon ground nutmeg
- 1 tablespoon coconut oil

Method:
1. Melt the coconut oil in the saucepan.
2. Add salmon and sprinkle it with ground coriander, salt, dried dill, and ground nutmeg. Roast the salmon for 2-3 minutes.
3. Add radish and water.
4. Simmer the stew on medium-low heat for 10 minutes.
Nutritional info per serve: Calories 187, Fat 10.6, Fiber 0.6, Carbs 1.4, Protein 22.3

Cardamom Shrimp

Prep time: 5 minutes
Cook time: 10 minutes
Servings: 7
Ingredients:
- 12 oz shrimps, peeled
- 1 teaspoon ground cardamom
- 2 tablespoons butter, softened
- 1 teaspoon dried thyme
- ½ water

Method:
1. Bring the water to boil and add shrimps.
2. Then add ground cardamom, butter, and dried thyme.
3. Simmer the shrimps on medium heat for 10 minutes.
Nutritional info per serve: Calories 88, Fat 4.1, Fiber 0.1, Carbs 1, Protein 11.1

Oregano and Basil Scallops

Prep time: 10 minutes
Cook time: 6 minutes
Servings: 2
Ingredients:
- 6 scallops
- 1 teaspoon dried basil
- 1 teaspoon dried oregano
- 2 tablespoons butter
- ½ teaspoon salt

Method:
1. Sprinkle the scallops with dried basil, oregano, and salt.
2. Then melt the butter in the skillet well.
3. Add scallops and roast them for 3 minutes per side.
Nutritional info per serve: Calories 183, Fat 12.3, Fiber 0.3, Carbs 2.6, Protein 15.3

Fennel Mussels

Prep time: 7 minutes
Cook time: 10 minutes
Servings: 5
Ingredients:
- 1-pound mussels
- 1 teaspoon fennel seeds
- 1 tablespoon avocado oil
- 1 teaspoon dried thyme
- ¼ cup coconut cream

Method:
1. Mix fennel seeds with avocado oil, and dried thyme.
2. Preheat the mixture well and add coconut cream. Bring the liquid to boil.
3. Add mussels and boil them for 5 minutes.
Nutritional info per serve: Calories 111, Fat 5.3, Fiber 0.6, Carbs 4.5, Protein 11.2

Cilantro Cod

Prep time: 10 minutes
Cook time: 6 minutes
Servings: 2
Ingredients:
- 2 medium cod fillets
- 1 tablespoon fresh cilantro, chopped
- 1 teaspoon salt
- 1 tablespoon avocado oil

Method:
1. Preheat the avocado oil in the skillet.
2. Put the cod fillets in the skillet and sprinkle with salt.
3. Roast the fish on medium heat for 3 minutes per side.

4. Sprinkle the cod with chopped cilantro.
Nutritional info per serve: Calories 99, Fat 1.9, Fiber 0.3, Carbs 0.4, Protein 20.1

Basil Clam Chowder

Prep time: 10 minutes
Cook time: 15 minutes
Servings: 8
Ingredients:
- 1 cup organic almond milk
- 1 teaspoon dried basil
- 1-pound clams
- 1 teaspoon chili flakes
- 4 oz leek, chopped
- 1 tablespoon coconut oil
- ½ cup celery stalk, chopped
- 5 cups of water

Method:
1. Put all ingredients in the saucepan and bring to boil.
2. Boil the chowder on medium heat for 5 minutes and remove from the heat.

Nutritional info per serve: Calories 121, Fat 9, Fiber 1.3, Carbs 10.1, Protein 1.3

Chili Mussel Stew

Prep time: 10 minutes
Cook time: 15 minutes
Servings: 6
Ingredients:
- 2 pounds mussels
- 1 teaspoon chili flakes
- 1 chili pepper, chopped
- 5 cups chicken stock
- 2 spring onions, diced
- 1 tablespoon avocado oil

Method:
1. Preheat the avocado oil in the saucepan.
2. Add chili pepper and spring onion. Roast the vegetables on medium heat for 5 minutes.
3. Stir the mixture and add chili flakes, chicken stock, and mussels.
4. Close the lid and cook the stew on medium heat for 10 minutes.

Nutritional info per serve: Calories 149, Fat 4.2, Fiber 0.5, Carbs 8.1, Protein 18.8

Oysters Stir-Fry

Prep time: 10 minutes
Cook time: 10 minutes
Servings: 2
Ingredients:
- 6 oysters
- 1 tablespoon coconut oil
- 1 teaspoon ground black pepper

Method:
1. Preheat the coconut oil well.
2. Add oysters and sprinkle then with ground black pepper.
3. Roast the oysters for 10 minutes. Stir them from time to time.

Nutritional info per serve: Calories 190, Fat 11.2, Fiber 0.3, Carbs 7.5, Protein 14.5

Sweet Swordfish

Prep time: 10 minutes
Cook time: 15 minutes
Servings: 2
Ingredients:
- 7 oz swordfish fillet
- 1 teaspoon Erythritol
- 1 teaspoon butter
- ½ teaspoon dried oregano

Method:
1. Rub the swordfish fillet with dried oregano and Erythritol.
2. Melt the coconut oil in the skillet, add fish and roast it on medium heat for 6 minutes per side.

Nutritional info per serve: Calories 172, Fat 7.1, Fiber 0.2, Carbs 2.2, Protein 25.3

Stuffed Calamari with Herbs

Prep time: 15 minutes
Cook time: 50 minutes
Servings: 4
Ingredients:
- 4 calamari tubes, trimmed
- ½ cup celery stalk, chopped
- 2 oz mushrooms, chopped
- 1 teaspoon coconut oil
- ½ teaspoon ground black pepper
- ½ cup of water

Method:
1. Melt the coconut oil in the skillet.
2. Add mushrooms and ground black pepper.
3. Roast the vegetables for 15 minutes and cool them.
4. After this, mix cooked mushrooms with a celery stalk and fill the calamari tubes.
5. Secure the calamari tubes and put them in the casserole mold.
6. Add water and bake the meal at 360F for 35 minutes.

Nutritional info per serve: Calories 65, Fat 2.2, Fiber 0.4, Carbs 1, Protein 10.6

Greek-Style Tuna

Prep time: 10 minutes
Cook time: 30 minutes
Servings: 4
Ingredients:
- 12 oz tuna fillet
- ½ cup Plain yogurt
- 1 teaspoon ground coriander
- 1 teaspoon garlic powder
- ½ teaspoon ground turmeric

Method:
1. Mix Plain yogurt with ground coriander, garlic powder, and ground turmeric.
2. Then put tuna fillet inside and marinate it for 10 minutes.
3. Then transfer the mixture in the casserole mold and cover it with foil.
4. Bake the tuna at 360F for 30 minutes.

Nutritional info per serve: Calories 334, Fat 26.8, Fiber 0.1, Carbs 2.9, Protein 19.7

Curry Crabs

Prep time: 20 minutes
Cook time: 15 minutes
Servings: 2
Ingredients:
- 6 oz crab meat
- 1 teaspoon curry paste
- ¼ cup coconut cream
- 1 teaspoon avocado oil
- ½ teaspoon dried dill

Method:
1. In the mixing bowl, mix curry paste with coconut cream, and dried ill.
2. Put the crab meat in the curry mixture and leave it for 10-15 minutes to marinate.
3. Then preheat the avocado oil well and add crab meat.
4. Roast the crab meat on high heat for 2 minutes per side.
5. Add remaining curry paste mixture and cook the meal on medium heat for 10 minutes.

Nutritional info per serve: Calories 165, Fat 10.4, Fiber 0.8, Carbs 4.2, Protein 11.5

Rosemary Swordfish

Prep time: 10 minutes
Cook time: 10 minutes
Servings: 4
Ingredients:
- 1-pound swordfish fillet
- 1 teaspoon dried rosemary
- 1 tablespoon avocado oil
- 1 teaspoon apple cider vinegar

Method:
1. Sprinkle the swordfish with apple cider vinegar, dried rosemary, and avocado oil.
2. Then preheat the skillet well.
3. Put the fish in the hot skillet and roast it on medium heat for 5 minutes per side.

Nutritional info per serve: Calories 182, Fat 6.3, Fiber 0.3, Carbs 0.4, Protein 28.8

KETOGENIC POULTRY RECIPES

Garlic Chicken

Prep time: 10 minutes
Cook time: 12 minutes
Servings: 2
Ingredients:
- ½ cup almond flour
- 1 egg, beaten
- 2 tablespoons minced garlic
- 2 chicken breasts, skinless, boneless, chopped
- 2 tablespoons coconut oil

Method:
1. Melt the coconut oil in the skillet.
2. Then mix chicken with minced garlic and egg.
3. After this, coat the chicken in the almond flour and put in the melted oil.
4. Roast the chicken for 5 minutes per side on the medium heat.

Nutritional info per serve: Calories 479, Fat 30.2, Fiber 0.9, Carbs 4.5, Protein 47

Chili Drumsticks

Prep time: 10 minutes
Cook time: 20 minutes
Servings: 4
Ingredients:
- 4 chicken drumsticks
- 1 teaspoon chili flakes
- 1 teaspoon salt
- 1 teaspoon dried sage
- 1 tablespoon avocado oil

Method:
1. In the shallow bowl, mix chili flakes, salt, and dried sage.
2. Then mix chicken drumsticks with spice mixture.
3. After this, preheat the skillet well.
4. Put the chicken drumsticks in the skillet and roast the meal for 10 minutes per side on the medium heat.

Nutritional info per serve: Calories 83, Fat 3.1, Fiber 0.2, Carbs 0.3, Protein 12.7

Sage Chicken Wings

Prep time: 10 minutes
Cook time: 30 minutes
Servings: 6
Ingredients:
- 1 teaspoon dried sage
- 1 teaspoon ground black pepper
- 6 chicken wings
- 1 tablespoon avocado oil

Method:
1. Mix the chicken wings with ground black pepper and dried sage.
2. Then sprinkle the chicken wings with avocado oil and transfer in the tray.
3. Bake the chicken wings for 30 minutes at 360F.

Nutritional info per serve: Calories 98, Fat 6.6, Fiber 0.3, Carbs 3.6, Protein 5.8

Oregano Chicken Wings

Prep time: 10 minutes
Cook time: 30 minutes
Servings: 2
Ingredients:
- 4 chicken wings
- 1 tablespoon dried oregano
- 2 tablespoons avocado oil
- 1 tablespoon lemon juice

Method:
1. Sprinkle the chicken wings with dried oregano, avocado oil, and lemon juice.
2. Then put them in the baking tray and bake at 365F for 30 minutes. Flip the chicken wings on another side after 15 minutes of cooking.

Nutritional info per serve: Calories 345, Fat 23.4, Fiber 1.9, Carbs 13.1, Protein 20

Chicken Meatballs

Prep time: 10 minutes
Cook time: 10 minutes
Servings: 3
Ingredients:
- 1 teaspoon dried oregano
- 1 teaspoon chili powder
- 1 teaspoon dried cilantro
- 1 cup ground chicken
- 1 teaspoon coconut oil

Method:
1. In the mixing bowl, mix ground chicken, dried cilantro, chili powder, and dried oregano.
2. Then make the small meatballs.
3. Melt the coconut oil in the skillet.
4. Then put the chicken meatballs in the hot coconut oil and roast them for 4 minutes per side.

Nutritional info per serve: Calories 106, Fat 5.2, Fiber 0.5, Carbs 0.8, Protein 13.7

Paprika Chicken Wings

Prep time: 10 minutes
Cook time: 10 minutes
Servings: 4
Ingredients:
- 10 oz chicken wings
- 1 tablespoon ground paprika
- 1 tablespoon avocado oil
- 1 teaspoon salt

Method:
1. Sprinkle the chicken wings with ground paprika and salt.
2. Then sprinkle the chicken ings with avocado oil and put in the hot skillet.
3. Roast the chicken wings for 4 minutes per side.

Nutritional info per serve: Calories 144, Fat 5.9, Fiber 0.8, Carbs 1.2, Protein 20.8

Lime Chicken Wings

Prep time: 10 minutes
Cook time: 10 minutes
Servings: 5
Ingredients:
- 5 chicken wings
- 1 teaspoon lime zest, grated
- 1 tablespoon avocado oil
- 3 tablespoons lime juice

Method:
1. Mix lime juice, avocado oil, and lime zest.
2. Then rub the chicken wings with avocado oil mixture.
3. Grill the chicken wings at 400F for 4 minutes.

Nutritional info per serve: Calories 99, Fat 6.7, Fiber 0.3, Carbs 3.8, Protein 5.8

Coconut Chicken

Prep time: 10 minutes
Cook time: 20 minutes
Servings: 6
Ingredients:
- 1-pound chicken breast, skinless, boneless, chopped
- ½ cup coconut cream
- 1 teaspoon dried oregano
- 1 teaspoon garlic powder
- ½ teaspoon ground paprika
- 1 tablespoon coconut oil

Method:
1. In the shallow bowl, mix ground paprika, garlic powder, and dried oregano.
2. Then mix the chicken breast with ground paprika mixture.
3. Then melt the coconut oil in the saucepan.
4. Add chicken and roast it for 4 minutes per side.
5. Add coconut cream and close the lid.
6. Cook the meal on medium heat for 10 minutes.

Nutritional info per serve: Calories 155, Fat 9, Fiber 0.7, Carbs 1.7, Protein 16.6

Onion Chicken

Prep time: 10 minutes
Cook time: 15 minutes
Servings: 4
Ingredients:
- 1-pound chicken fillet, sliced
- 2 spring onions, sliced
- 1 tablespoon coconut oil
- ½ teaspoon onion powder
- ½ teaspoon salt

Method:
1. Sprinkle the chicken fillet with spring onion powder and salt.
2. Then melt the coconut oil in the skillet.
3. Add onion and roast it for 5 minutes.
4. After this, stir the onion and add chicken fillet.
5. Roast the chicken with onion for 10 minutes on medium heat.

Nutritional info per serve: Calories 257, Fat 11.8, Fiber 0.6, Carbs 2.8, Protein 33.1

Almond Chicken

Prep time: 10 minutes
Cook time: 40 minutes
Servings: 4
Ingredients:
- 11 oz chicken fillet
- 2 eggs, beaten
- ½ cup almond flour
- Cooking spray

Method:
1. Cut the chicken into 4 servings.
2. Then dip it in the eggs and coat in the almond flour.
3. Spray the baking tray with cooking spray and put the chicken inside.
4. Bake the chicken for 40 minutes at 355F.

Nutritional info per serve: Calories 200, Fat 9.7, Fiber 0.4, Carbs 0.9, Protein 26.1

Garlic and Dill Chicken

Prep time: 10 minutes
Cook time: 45 minutes
Servings: 4
Ingredients:
- 2 tablespoons avocado oil
- 1 teaspoon minced garlic
- 1 teaspoon dried dill
- 1-pound chicken breast, skinless, boneless

Method:
1. Mix dill with avocado oil and dried dill.
2. Then rub the chicken breast with avocado oil mixture and wrap in the foil.
3. Bake the chicken at 360F for 45 minutes.

Nutritional info per serve: Calories 140, Fat 3.7, Fiber 0.4, Carbs 0.8, Protein 24.2

Cheese Chicken Casserole

Prep time: 15 minutes
Cook time: 50 minutes
Servings: 6
Ingredients:
- 1-pound chicken breast, skinless, boneless, chopped
- 1 cup Cheddar cheese, shredded
- 1 tablespoon butter, softened
- ½ teaspoon chili flakes
- ½ cup of water
- 1 cup bell pepper, chopped

Method:
1. Grease the casserole mold with butter.
2. Then mix chicken breast with chili flakes and put in the casserole mold in one layer.
3. Top it with bell pepper and water.
4. Then add Cheddar cheese and flatten it well.
5. Bake the casserole at 360F for 50 minutes.

Nutritional info per serve: Calories 185, Fat 10.1, Fiber 0.3, Carbs 1.8, Protein 20.9

Lemon Chicken

Prep time: 10 minutes
Cook time: 40 minutes
Servings: 6
Ingredients:
- 6 chicken drumsticks
- ½ lemon, sliced
- 1 teaspoon salt
- 1 tablespoon butter

Method:
1. Grease the baking tray with butter.
2. Sprinkle the chicken drumsticks with salt and put it in the baking tray.
3. Top the chicken with sliced lemon and bake it for 40 minutes at 355F.

Nutritional info per serve: Calories 96, Fat 4.6, Fiber 0.1, Carbs 0.5, Protein 12.7

Italian Style Chicken

Prep time: 10 minutes
Cook time: 35 minutes
Servings: 4
Ingredients:
- 4 chicken drumsticks
- 1 teaspoon dried oregano
- ½ teaspoon dried thyme
- 2 tablespoons avocado oil

Method:
1. Rub the chicken drumsticks with thyme and oregano.
2. Then sprinkle the chicken with avocado oil and put in the baking tray in one layer.
3. Bake the chicken at 360F for 35 minutes.

Nutritional info per serve: Calories 89, Fat 3.6, Fiber 0.5, Carbs 0.7, Protein 12.8

Paprika Chicken Fillet

Prep time: 10 minutes
Cook time: 10 minutes
Servings: 5
Ingredients:
- 1 tablespoon butter
- 1 teaspoon ground paprika
- ½ teaspoon ground turmeric
- 1-pound chicken fillet
- ½ teaspoon keto tomato paste

Method:
1. Melt the butter in the skillet.
2. Meanwhile, slice the chicken fillet and mix it with ground paprika, ground turmeric, and keto tomato paste.
3. Put the chicken in the melted butter and roast it for 5 minutes per side.

Nutritional info per serve: Calories 195, Fat 9.1, Fiber 0.2, Carbs 0.5, Protein 26.4

Coconut Chicken Fillets

Prep time: 10 minutes
Cook time: 20 minutes
Servings: 2
Ingredients:
- 12 oz chicken fillets
- ½ cup coconut cream
- 1 teaspoon ground black pepper
- 1 tablespoon coconut flour
- 1 oz Parmesan, grated
- 1 teaspoon avocado oil

Method:
1. Mix the chicken fillets with ground black pepper and put it in the hot skillet.
2. Add avocado oil and roast the chicken for 4 minutes. Stir it well.
3. Add coconut flour and coconut cream and carefully mix the mixture.
4. Then top it with grated Parmesan and close the lid.
5. Cook the chicken for 15 minutes on low heat.

Nutritional info per serve: Calories 528, Fat 30.6, Fiber 3.2, Carbs 7.1, Protein 55.8

Chicken with Peppers

Prep time: 10 minutes
Cook time: 25 minutes
Servings: 4
Ingredients:
- 12 oz chicken fillet, chopped
- 1 cup bell pepper, roughly chopped
- 1 teaspoon keto tomato paste
- 1 tablespoon coconut oil
- ¼ cup of water
- 1 teaspoon ground black pepper

Method:
1. Mix the chicken fillet with keto tomato paste, ground black pepper, and water and put it in the saucepan.
2. Add coconut oil and bell peppers.
3. Cook the meal on medium heat for 25 minutes. Stir it from time to time.

Nutritional info per serve: Calories 203, Fat 9.8, Fiber 0.8, Carbs 2.8, Protein 25

Chicken Pie

Prep time: 15 minutes
Cook time: 45 minutes
Servings: 6
Ingredients:
- 1 cup coconut flour
- 2 tablespoons butter, softened
- ½ teaspoon ground black pepper
- 1 egg, beaten
- 1 cup ground chicken
- 1 teaspoon dried dill
- 1 oz Parmesan, grated

Method:
1. In the mixing bowl, mix coconut flour with butte. Knead the sough.
2. Then put the dough in the baking pan and flatten it in the shape of the pie crust.
3. After this, mix ground black pepper with ground chicken, dill, and Parmesan.
4. Put the ground chicken over the pie crust, flatten it well.
5. Then pour the beaten egg over the ground chicken.
6. Bake the pie at 355F for 45 minutes.

Nutritional info per serve: Calories 185, Fat 10, Fiber 6.7, Carbs 11.1, Protein 12

Tarragon Chicken

Prep time: 10 minutes
Cook time: 30 minutes
Servings: 4
Ingredients:
- 1-pound chicken breast, skinless, boneless, chopped
- 1 tablespoon dried tarragon
- 1 tablespoon avocado oil

Method:
1. Sprinkle the chicken with dried tarragon and avocado oil.
2. Then put the chicken in the oven and cook it for 30 minutes at 355F.

Nutritional info per serve: Calories 135, Fat 3.3, Fiber 0.2, Carbs 0.4, Protein 24.2

Masala Chicken Thighs

Prep time: 15 minutes
Cook time: 30 minutes
Servings: 3
Ingredients:
- 3 chicken thighs, boneless, skinless
- ¼ cup coconut cream
- 1 teaspoon garam masala
- ½ teaspoon dried thyme
- 1 tablespoon avocado oil

Method:
1. In the mixing bowl, mix garam masala, coconut cream, and dried thyme.
2. Then preheat the avocado oil in the saucepan and add chicken thighs.
3. Roast them for 3 minutes per side.
4. Add coconut cream mixture and close the lid.
5. Simmer the chicken thighs for 30 minutes on low heat.

Nutritional info per serve: Calories 330, Fat 16.2, Fiber 0.7, Carbs 1.5, Protein 42.8

Chicken with Olives

Prep time: 10 minutes
Cook time: 40 minutes
Servings: 2
Ingredients:
- 2 kalamata olives, pitted, sliced
- 2 chicken thighs, skinless, boneless
- 1 teaspoon chili powder
- 1 tablespoon lemon juice
- 1 tablespoon avocado oil

Method:
1. Brush the baking pan with avocado oil.
2. Then mix the chicken thighs with chili powder and lemon juice.
3. Put the chicken inside the baking pan.
4. Top the chicken with Kalamata olives and cover with foil.
5. Bake the meal at 360F for 40 minutes.

Nutritional info per serve: Calories 298, Fat 12.5, Fiber 0.9, Carbs 1.5, Protein 42.6

Cheddar Chicken Thighs

Prep time: 10 minutes
Cook time: 40 minutes
Servings: 4
Ingredients:
- 4 chicken thighs, boneless, skinless
- 5 oz Cheddar cheese, shredded
- 1 tablespoon butter
- 1 teaspoon dried cilantro
- ½ teaspoon cayenne pepper

Method:
1. Mix chicken thighs with dried cilantro and cayenne pepper.
2. Put it in the baking pan.
3. Add butter and shredded cheese.
4. Bake the chicken thighs for 40 minutes at 360F.

Nutritional info per serve: Calories 446, Fat 25.5, Fiber 0.1, Carbs 0.6, Protein 51.1

Lemon Duck Breast

Prep time: 10 minutes
Cook time: 40 minutes
Servings: 4
Ingredients:
- 1-pound duck breast, skinless, boneless, chopped
- 1 lemon, sliced
- 1 tablespoon olive oil

Method:
1. Sprinkle the duck fillet with olive oil and put it in the baking pan.
2. Top it with sliced lemon and cover with foil.
3. Bake the duck breast for 40 minutes at 360F.

Nutritional info per serve: Calories 181, Fat 8.1, Fiber 0.4, Carbs 1.4, Protein 25.1

Parsley Chicken

Prep time: 10 minutes
Cook time: 12 minutes
Servings: 4
Ingredients:
- 1 tablespoon dried parsley
- 1 teaspoon salt
- 1-pound chicken breast, skinless, boneless, chopped
- 1 tablespoon avocado oil

Method:
1. Mix the chicken with dried parsley, salt, and avocado oil.
2. Then put it in the preheated skillet and roast for 6 minutes per side.

Nutritional info per serve: Calories 134, Fat 3.3, Fiber 0.2, Carbs 0.3, Protein 24.1

Duck with Zucchinis

Prep time: 10 minutes
Cook time: 55 minutes
Servings: 2
Ingredients:
- 10 oz duck breast, skinless, boneless
- 1 zucchini, sliced

- 1 teaspoon ground black pepper
- 1 tablespoon avocado oil
- 1 teaspoon keto tomato paste
- 1 teaspoon cayenne pepper
- ¼ cup of water

Method:
1. Mix keto tomato paste with avocado oil, cayenne pepper, and ground black pepper. Add water and whisk well.
2. Then mix duck breast with tomato mixture and transfer in the baking pan.
3. Add zucchini and cover the baking pan with foil.
4. Bake the meal at 360F for 55 minutes.

Nutritional info per serve: Calories 216, Fat 6.9, Fiber 2, Carbs 5.4, Protein 32.8

Oregano Meatballs

Prep time: 10 minutes
Cook time: 10 minutes
Servings: 6
Ingredients:
- 2 cups ground chicken
- 1 tablespoon dried oregano
- 1 teaspoon ground paprika
- 1 teaspoon garlic powder
- 1 tablespoon avocado oil

Method:
1. In the mixing bowl mix ground chicken with dried oregano, ground paprika, and garlic powder.
2. Then make the medium-size meatballs.
3. Preheat the avocado oil well.
4. Put the meatballs in the hot oil and roast for 3 minutes per side.

Nutritional info per serve: Calories 97, Fat 3.9, Fiber 0.1, Carbs 1.2, Protein 13.7

Duck Salad

Prep time: 10 minutes
Cook time: 16 minutes
Servings: 4
Ingredients:
- 8 oz duck fillet
- 1 teaspoon mustard
- 1 teaspoon avocado oil
- 1 teaspoon chili powder
- 2 cups lettuce, chopped
- 2 oz Feta, crumbled
- 1 tablespoon olive oil

Method:
1. Mix the duck fillet with avocado oil and mustard and roast in the skillet for 8 minutes per side.
2. Then slice the duck fillet and put it in the salad bowl.
3. Add chili powder, lettuce, and olive oil.
4. Shake the salad well and top with crumbled feta.

Nutritional info per serve: Calories 149, Fat 7.4, Fiber 0.6, Carbs 2.1, Protein 19.2

Clove Chicken

Prep time: 10 minutes
Cook time: 20 minutes
Servings: 4
Ingredients:
- 4 chicken thighs, skinless, boneless
- 1 teaspoon ground clove
- 1 tablespoon avocado oil
- ½ teaspoon ground black pepper
- 1 teaspoon cayenne pepper

Method:
1. In the shallow bowl, mix cayenne pepper, ground black pepper, and ground clove.
2. Rub the chicken thighs with the spice mixture and sprinkle with avocado oil.
3. Roast it in the preheated skillet for 10 minutes per side.

Nutritional info per serve: Calories 286, Fat 11.5, Fiber 0.5, Carbs 0.9, Protein 42.4

Turkey Bake

Prep time: 10 minutes
Cook time: 45 minutes
Servings: 6
Ingredients:
- 1-pound turkey breast, skinless, boneless, chopped
- ½ cup Cheddar cheese, shredded
- 2 zucchinis, chopped
- 1 teaspoon chili powder
- 1 teaspoon white pepper
- ½ teaspoon dried sage
- 1 tablespoon coconut oil
- 1 teaspoon avocado oil
- ½ cup coconut cream

Method:
1. Mix the turkey breast with chili powder, white pepper, dried sage, and avocado oil.
2. Then put in the baking pan and flatten well.
3. Top the turkey breast with zucchinis, avocado oil, coconut cream, and shredded cheese.
4. Bake the meal at 360F for 45 minutes.

Nutritional info per serve: Calories 196, Fat 11.7, Fiber 1.8, Carbs 7.2, Protein 16.6

Garlic and Curry Chicken

Prep time: 10 minutes
Cook time: 30 minutes
Servings: 4
Ingredients:
- 1-pound chicken breast, skinless, boneless, chopped
- 1 teaspoon curry powder
- 1 cup coconut cream
- 1 teaspoon minced garlic
- 1 tablespoon coconut oil

Method:
1. Mix curry powder with coconut cream, and minced garlic.
2. Pour the liquid in the saucepan.
3. Add chicken breast and coconut oil.
4. Close the lid and cook the chicken on medium-low heat for 30 minutes.

Nutritional info per serve: Calories 299, Fat 20.6, Fiber 1.5, Carbs 3.8, Protein 25.5

Turkey Soup

Prep time: 10 minutes
Cook time: 20 minutes
Servings: 4
Ingredients:
- 1 cup ground turkey
- ½ cup celery stalk, chopped
- 4 cups chicken broth
- 1 teaspoon ground turmeric
- 1 teaspoon dried dill
- ½ teaspoon salt

Method:
1. Bring the chicken broth to boil.
2. Add ground turkey, dill, and ground turmeric.
3. Add salt and boil the soup for 5 minutes.
4. After this, add celery stalk and bring the soup to boil. Switch off the heat.

Nutritional info per serve: Calories 110, Fat 4, Fiber 0.4, Carbs 1.8, Protein 15.2

Cheese Pizza

Prep time: 10 minutes
Cook time: 25 minutes
Servings: 4
Ingredients:
- 1 cup ground chicken
- 1 cup Cheddar cheese, shredded
- ½ teaspoon dried dill
- 1 teaspoon dried basil
- 1 teaspoon butter
- 2 tablespoons almond flour

Method:
1. In the mixing bowl, mix ground chicken with dried dill, basil, and almond flour.
2. Then grease the baking pan with butter and put the ground chicken inside. Flatten it in the shape of the pizza and bake at 360F for 10 minutes
3. Then top the chicken pizza crust with shredded cheese and bake at 360F for 15 minutes.

Nutritional info per serve: Calories 269, Fat 19.9, Fiber 1.5, Carbs 3.4, Protein 20.2

Creamy Turkey

Prep time: 10 minutes
Cook time: 25 minutes
Servings: 8
Ingredients:
- 1 egg, beaten
- 2-pound ground turkey
- 1 tablespoon butter
- 1 teaspoon ground black pepper
- ½ cup coconut cream
- 1 oz Mozzarella, shredded

Method:
1. Mix the ground turkey with ground black pepper and egg.
2. Then melt the butter in the saucepan. Add ground turkey mixture and cook it for 10 minutes on the medium heat. Stir it from time to time.
3. After this, add all remaining ingredients and carefully mix.
4. Close the lid and cook the turkey on medium-low heat for 10 minutes.

Nutritional info per serve: Calories 287, Fat 18.7, Fiber 0.4, Carbs 1.2, Protein 33.1

Cordon Bleu Chicken

Prep time: 15 minutes
Cook time: 30 minutes
Servings: 3
Ingredients:
- 10 oz chicken fillets
- 3 ham slices
- 3 Cheddar cheese slices
- 2 eggs, beaten
- ½ cup almond flour
- 1 tablespoon olive oil

Method:
1. Cut the chicken fillet into 3 servings. Beat the chicken fillet gently.
2. Then top the chicken fillets with ham slices and cheese slices and roll into the rolls. Secure the chicken rolls if needed.
3. After this, dip the chicken rolls in the eggs and coat in the almond flour.
4. Repeat the same steps.
5. Then sprinkle the chicken rolls with olive oil and bake at 360F for 30 minutes.

Nutritional info per serve: Calories 447, Fat 28.6, Fiber 0.9, Carbs 2.7, Protein 43.7

Cumin Stew

Prep time: 10 minutes
Cook time: 35 minutes
Servings: 8
Ingredients:
- 1 cup bell pepper, chopped
- 4 oz leek, chopped
- ½ cup turnip, chopped
- 1 teaspoon cumin seeds
- 1 tablespoon coconut oil
- 1-pound chicken breast, skinless, boneless, chopped
- 3 cups of water

Method:
1. Melt the coconut oil in the saucepan.
2. Add chicken and cumin seeds.
3. Roast the mixture for 10 minutes.
4. Add turnip, leek, bell pepper, and water.
5. Carefully mix the stew and simmer it for 25 minutes on medium heat.

Nutritional info per serve: Calories 96, Fat 3.3, Fiber 0.6, Carbs 3.8, Protein 12.5

Turkey Burgers

Prep time: 10 minutes
Cook time: 20 minutes
Servings: 4
Ingredients:
- 1 cup ground turkey
- 1 ½ tablespoon dried dill
- ½ teaspoon salt

- 1 tablespoon coconut flour
- 1 tablespoon avocado oil
- ½ teaspoon chili powder

Method:
1. In the mixing bowl, mix ground turkey, dried dill, salt, coconut flour, and chili powder.
2. Make 4 burgers.
3. Then brush the baking tray with avocado oil.
4. Put the burgers in the tray and bake at 360F for 10 minutes per side.

Nutritional info per serve: Calories 185, Fat 10.1, Fiber 1.7, Carbs 3, Protein 23.4

Chicken Curry

Prep time: 10 minutes
Cook time: 25 minutes
Servings: 4
Ingredients:
- 1-pound chicken breast, skinless, boneless, chopped
- 1 tablespoon curry paste
- 1 cup of coconut milk
- 1 tablespoon avocado oil
- ½ teaspoon saffron

Method:
1. Roast the chicken in the saucepan with avocado oil for 4 minutes per side.
2. Then add curry paste, coconut milk, and saffron.
3. Close the lid and simmer the meal for 10-15 minutes on medium heat.

Nutritional info per serve: Calories 297, Fat 19.8, Fiber 1.5, Carbs 4.6, Protein 25.7

Chili Chicken

Prep time: 10 minutes
Cook time: 20 minutes
Servings: 3
Ingredients:
- 1-pound chicken breast, skinless, boneless
- 1 tablespoon chili powder
- 1 tablespoon ground paprika
- 1 tablespoon coconut oil
- ¼ cup of water

Method:
1. Mix the chicken breast with chili powder and ground paprika.
2. Then melt the coconut oil in the saucepan. Add chicken breast and roast it for 4 minutes per side.
3. Add water and close the lid.
4. Cook the chicken on medium heat for 10 minutes.

Nutritional info per serve: Calories 226, Fat 9, Fiber 1.7, Carbs 2.7, Protein 32.7

Turkey Salad

Prep time: 10 minutes
Cook time: 10 minutes
Servings: 4
Ingredients:
- 4 cups romaine lettuce leaves, torn
- 12 oz chicken breast, skinless, boneless, chopped
- 1 tablespoon avocado oil
- 1 teaspoon coconut oil
- 1 tablespoon apple cider vinegar
- 1 teaspoon ground black pepper
- 3 oz Feta, crumbled

Method:
1. Put the chicken in the skillet. Add coconut oil and ground black pepper.
2. Roast it for 10 minutes on the medium heat. Stir it from time to time.
3. Then mix lettuce with feta in the salad bowl.
4. Add apple cider vinegar and avocado oil. Shake the mixture and add cooked chicken.

Nutritional info per serve: Calories 177, Fat 8.3, Fiber 0.6, Carbs 3.1, Protein 21.4

Rosemary Chicken

Prep time: 10 minutes
Cook time: 65 minutes
Servings: 7
Ingredients:
- 3-pound whole chicken
- 1 tablespoon dried rosemary
- 1 teaspoon salt
- 3 tablespoons avocado oil

Method:
1. Mix avocado oil with salt and dried rosemary.
2. Then rub the chicken with rosemary mixture and wrap in the foil.
3. Bake the chicken at 365F for 65 minutes.

Nutritional info per serve: Calories 379, Fat 15.2, Fiber 0.5, Carbs 0.6, Protein 56.3

Stuffed Chicken

Prep time: 10 minutes
Cook time: 55 minutes
Servings: 3
Ingredients:
- 12 oz chicken breast, skinless, boneless
- 1 cup spinach, chopped
- 1 tablespoon cream cheese
- 1 oz Parmesan, grated
- 1 tablespoon keto tomato paste
- 1 tablespoon avocado oil
- ½ teaspoon cayenne pepper

Method:
1. Make the lengthwise cut in the chicken breast to get the pocket.
2. Then mix spinach with cream cheese, Parmesan, and cayenne pepper.
3. Fill the chicken breast pocket with spinach mixture. Secure the cut well.
4. Then brush the chicken with avocado oil and keto tomato paste.
5. Wrap it in the foil and bake at 360F for 55 minutes.

Nutritional info per serve: Calories 185, Fat 6.7, Fiber 0.7, Carbs 2.2, Protein 28

Chicken Tortillas

Prep time: 15 minutes
Cook time: 0 minutes
Servings: 4
Ingredients:
- 4 keto tortillas
- 10 oz chicken fillet, boiled, shredded
- 1 tablespoon cream cheese
- ½ teaspoon minced garlic
- 1 teaspoon dried dill
- 1 teaspoon lemon juice

Method:
1. Mix the chicken with cream cheese, minced garlic, dried dill, and lemon juice.
2. Then put the chicken mixture over the keto tortillas and fold them.

Nutritional info per serve: Calories 295, Fat 14.2, Fiber 4.1, Carbs 8.4, Protein 32.8

Dijon Chicken

Prep time: 10 minutes
Cook time: 16 minutes
Servings: 3
Ingredients:
- 1-pound chicken fillet
- 2 tablespoons Dijon mustard
- 1 tablespoon avocado oil
- 1 tablespoon lemon juice
- 1 teaspoon lemon zest, grated

Method:
1. In the mixing bowl, mix Dijon mustard with avocado oil, lemon juice, and lemon zest.
2. Then rub the chicken fillets with mustard mixture.
3. Preheat the skillet well.
4. Put the chicken fillet inside and roast it on medium heat for 8 minutes per side.

Nutritional info per serve: Calories 302, Fat 12.3, Fiber 0.6, Carbs 1.1, Protein 44.3

Chicken and Cream

Prep time: 10 minutes
Cook time: 30 minutes
Servings: 2
Ingredients:
- 8 oz chicken fillet
- 1 teaspoon butter
- 1 tablespoon cream cheese
- ¼ cup heavy cream
- 1 teaspoon ground black pepper
- 1 teaspoon salt

Method:
1. Chop the chicken fillet roughly and put it in the saucepan.
2. Add all remaining ingredients and carefully mix the mixture.
3. Close the lid and cook the meal on medium-low heat for 30 minutes.

Nutritional info per serve: Calories 294, Fat 16, Fiber 0.3, Carbs 1.5, Protein 34.3

Arugula Chicken

Prep time: 10 minutes
Cook time: 16 minutes
Servings: 6
Ingredients:
- 10 oz chicken fillet
- 1 teaspoon coconut oil
- 1 teaspoon lemon juice
- ½ teaspoon lime zest, grated
- 1 teaspoon chili powder
- 3 cups arugula, chopped
- 1 oz Parmesan, shaved
- 1 tablespoon avocado oil

Method:
1. Mix the chicken fillet with chili powder and put it in the skillet.
2. Add avocado oil and roast it for 8 minutes per side.
3. Then slice the chicken and put it in the big bowl.
4. Add all remaining ingredients and carefully mix the mixture.

Nutritional info per serve: Calories 119, Fat 5.7, Fiber 0.4, Carbs 1, Protein 15.5

Cheese Wrapped Chicken Wings

Prep time: 10 minutes
Cook time: 20 minutes
Servings: 5
Ingredients:
- 5 chicken wings, skinless
- 5 Cheddar cheese slices
- 1 teaspoon ground black pepper
- ½ teaspoon salt
- 2 tablespoons coconut oil

Method:
1. Mix the chicken wings with ground black pepper and salt.
2. Then melt the coconut oil in the skillet. Add chicken wings and roast them for 5 minutes per side.
3. After this, cool the chicken wings till room temperature and wrap in the cheese.
4. Bake the chicken at 360F for 10 minutes more.

Nutritional info per serve: Calories 320, Fat 25.4, Fiber 0.3, Carbs 6, Protein 16.8

Grilled Chicken Sausages

Prep time: 10 minutes
Cook time: 10 minutes
Servings: 6
Ingredients:
- 2-pounds chicken sausages
- 1 tablespoon olive oil
- 1 teaspoon dried thyme

Method:
1. Preheat the grill to 400F.
2. Then sprinkle the chicken sausages with dried thyme and olive oil.
3. Grill the meal for 5 minutes per side.

Nutritional info per serve: Calories 347, Fat 24, Fiber 0.1, Carbs 12.4, Protein 20.6

Mushroom Chicken

Prep time: 15 minutes
Cook time: 25 minutes

Servings: 4
Ingredients:
- 1-pound chicken fillet
- ½ cup mushrooms, chopped
- 1 tablespoon coconut oil
- ½ cup heavy cream
- 1 teaspoon salt
- 1 teaspoon ground black pepper

Method:
1. Melt the coconut oil in the saucepan.
2. Slice the chicken fillet and put it in the coconut oil.
3. Add salt and ground black pepper.
4. Then add mushrooms and carefully mix the chicken mixture.
5. Roast it for 10 minutes on medium heat.
6. Then add all remaining ingredients and close the lid. Cook the meal on low for 15 minutes.

Nutritional info per serve: Calories 300, Fat 17.4, Fiber 0.2, Carbs 1.1, Protein 33.5

Mozzarella Chicken

Prep time: 10 minutes
Cook time: 25 minutes
Servings: 8
Ingredients:
- 2-pound chicken breast, skinless, boneless, chopped
- 1 cup mozzarella, shredded
- 1 teaspoon keto tomato paste
- 1 teaspoon lemon juice
- 1 teaspoon avocado oil
- 1 teaspoon butter, softened
- ¼ cup of water

Method:
1. In the shallow bowl, mix keto tomato paste, lemon juice, avocado oil, and butter.
2. Then mix the chopped chicken breast with tomato mixture.
3. Put it in the hot skillet and roast for 10 minutes. Stir the chicken from time to time.
4. Then add water and carefully mix.
5. Top the chicken with mozzarella and close the lid.
6. Cook the meal on medium heat for 10 minutes.

Nutritional info per serve: Calories 145, Fat 4, Fiber 0.1, Carbs 0.3, Protein 25.1

Vinegar Chicken

Prep time: 15 minutes
Cook time: 25 minutes
Servings: 4
Ingredients:
- 1-pound chicken breast, skinless, boneless
- ¼ cup apple cider vinegar
- 1 teaspoon chili flakes
- 2 tablespoons olive oil

Method:
1. Mix the chicken breast with apple cider vinegar and chili flakes.
2. Leave it for 10 minutes to marinate.
3. Then preheat the olive oil in the saucepan.
4. Add chicken breast and roast it on medium-low heat for 12 minutes per side.

Nutritional info per serve: Calories 193, Fat 9.8, Fiber 0, Carbs 0.2, Protein 24.1

Fajita Chicken

Prep time: 10 minutes
Cook time: 20 minutes
Servings: 3
Ingredients:
- 3 chicken thighs, skinless, boneless
- 1 tablespoon fajita seasonings
- 2 tablespoons avocado oil

Method:
1. Preheat the avocado oil well.
2. Then rub the chicken thighs with fajita seasonings and put in the hot avocado oil.
3. Roast the chicken for 10 minutes per side.

Nutritional info per serve: Calories 257, Fat 13.1, Fiber 0, Carbs 0.2, Protein 32.1

Cajun Chicken

Prep time: 10 minutes
Cook time: 20 minutes
Servings: 2
Ingredients:
- 8 oz chicken breast, skinless, boneless
- 1 tablespoon avocado oil
- 1 teaspoon Cajun seasonings

Method:
1. Mix the chicken breast with cajun seasonings and put it in the hot skillet.
2. Add avocado oil and roast the chicken on medium-low heat for 10 minutes per side.

Nutritional info per serve: Calories 139, Fat 3.7, Fiber 0.3, Carbs 0.4, Protein 24.2

Chicken with Sauce

Prep time: 10 minutes
Cook time: 30 minutes
Servings: 4
Ingredients:
- 1-pound chicken fillet, chopped
- ½ cup heavy cream
- ¼ cup of water
- 1 tablespoon keto tomato paste
- 1 teaspoon taco seasonings
- 1 jalapeno pepper, chopped

Method:
1. Mix the chicken fillet with taco seasonings and put it in the hot saucepan.
2. Add water and heavy cream.
3. Then add keto tomato paste and jalapeno pepper. Carefully mix the mixture and simmer it on medium-low heat for 30 minutes.

Nutritional info per serve: Calories 277, Fat 14, Fiber 0.3, Carbs 2.4, Protein 33.3

Lemon Chicken Breast

Prep time: 15 minutes
Cook time: 55 minutes
Servings: 3
Ingredients:

- 1 lemon, sliced
- 1 teaspoon dried cilantro
- 1 teaspoon garlic powder
- 2 tablespoons coconut oil
- 12 oz chicken breast, skinless, boneless

Method:
1. In the shallow bowl, mix coconut oil with garlic powder and dried cilantro.
2. Rub the chicken breast with coconut oil mixture well.
3. Then put the chicken breast in the foil and top with lemon. Wrap the chicken.
4. Bake the chicken breast at 365F for 55 minutes.

Nutritional info per serve: Calories 216, Fat 12, Fiber 0.6, Carbs 2.5, Protein 24.4

Chicken and Broccoli Casserole

Prep time: 10 minutes
Cook time: 60 minutes
Servings: 4
Ingredients:
- 1 cup cheddar cheese, shredded
- 1 cup broccoli, chopped
- 1-pound chicken breast, skinless, boneless, chopped
- 1 teaspoon ground paprika
- 1 teaspoon chili powder
- 1 cup of water
- 1 teaspoon avocado oil

Method:
1. Brush the casserole mold with avocado oil.
2. Then mix chicken breast with ground paprika and chili powder.
3. Put it in the casserole mold and top with broccoli.
4. Then add shredded cheese and water.
5. Cover the casserole with foil and bake it at 365F for 60 minutes.

Nutritional info per serve: Calories 298, Fat 13.2, Fiber 1.1, Carbs 2.6, Protein 40.7

Coconut Chicken

Prep time: 15 minutes
Cook time: 21 minutes
Servings: 6
Ingredients:
- 6 chicken drumsticks
- ½ cup coconut flour
- ½ cup of coconut milk
- 1 teaspoon salt
- 1 teaspoon ground paprika
- ½ teaspoon ground turmeric
- 1 teaspoon onion powder
- 1 teaspoon butter

Method:
1. Mix the chicken drumsticks with salt, ground paprika, ground turmeric, and onion powder.
2. Then coat the chicken in the coconut flour and put it in the hot skillet.
3. Add butter and roast the chicken drumsticks on medium-high heat for 3 minutes per side.
4. After this, add coconut milk and close the lid. Simmer the chicken on medium heat for 15 minutes.

Nutritional info per serve: Calories 172, Fat 9.4, Fiber 4, Carbs 7.1, Protein 14.6

Dill Chicken Soup

Prep time: 10 minutes
Cook time: 35 minutes
Servings: 4
Ingredients:
- 1 tablespoon fresh dill, chopped
- 1-pound chicken breast, skinless, boneless, chopped
- 5 cups of water
- 1 teaspoon peppercorns
- 1 teaspoon salt

Method:
1. Pour water in the pan and bring ti to boil.
2. Add chicken breast and boil it for 15 minutes.
3. Then add all remaining ingredients and close the lid.
4. Cook the chicken soup on medium heat for 20 minutes.

Nutritional info per serve: Calories 133, Fat 2.9, Fiber 0.3, Carbs 0.8, Protein 24.3

Chicken Meatballs with Turmeric

Prep time: 10 minutes
Cook time: 25 minutes
Servings: 2
Ingredients:
- 7 oz ground chicken
- 1 teaspoon ground turmeric
- 1 teaspoon onion powder
- 1 teaspoon dried parsley
- ¼ teaspoon salt
- 1 tablespoon almond flour

Method:
1. Put all ingredients in the mixing bowl and carefully mix.
2. Then make the chicken meatballs.
3. Line the baking tray with baking paper. Put the chicken meatballs inside.
4. Bake the meal at 360F for 25 minutes or until the chicken meatballs are light brown.

Nutritional info per serve: Calories 217, Fat 9.2, Fiber 0.7, Carbs 2.5, Protein 29.7

Chicken Pancakes

Prep time: 10 minutes
Cook time: 25 minutes
Servings: 8
Ingredients:
- 4 eggs, beaten
- ½ cup coconut flour
- 2 cups ground chicken
- 1 teaspoon ground black pepper
- ½ teaspoon dried parsley
- 1 tablespoon coconut oil

Method:
1. Melt the coconut oil in the skillet.

2. Meanwhile, mix all ingredients in the mixing bowl and stir until homogenous.
3. Then pour the small amount of chicken batter in the hot skillet and flatten in the shape of a pancake.
4. Roast the pancake for 3 minutes per side or until it is light brown. Repeat the same steps with the remaining batter.
Nutritional info per serve: Calories 143, Fat 7.5, Fiber 2.6, Carbs 4.4, Protein 13.9

Butter Chicken

Prep time: 10 minutes
Cook time: 25 minutes
Servings: 4
Ingredients:
- ½ teaspoon cayenne pepper
- ½ teaspoon salt
- 1 teaspoon ground paprika
- 1-pound chicken breast, skinless, boneless, chopped
- ½ cup butter

Method:
1. Melt the butter in the saucepan.
2. Add ground paprika, salt, cayenne pepper, and chicken breast.
3. Stir the mixture well and cook it with the closed lid for 25 minutes.
Nutritional info per serve: Calories 335, Fat 26, Fiber 0.3, Carbs 0.5, Protein 24.4

Monterey Jack Cheese Chicken

Prep time: 10 minutes
Cook time: 30 minutes
Servings: 4
Ingredients:
- 4 chicken thighs, skinless, boneless
- ½ cup Cheddar cheese, shredded
- 1 teaspoon butter
- ½ teaspoon taco seasonings
- 1/3 cup heavy cream

Method:
1. Mix chicken thighs with taco seasonings and put in the hot saucepan.
2. Add butter and roast the chicken on medium heat for 4 minutes per side.
3. Then add heavy cream and simmer the chicken for 20 minutes.
4. Add cheddar cheese and carefully mix the mixture.
5. Cook it for 2-3 minutes more or until the chicken is soft.
Nutritional info per serve: Calories 380, Fat 20.2, Fiber 0, Carbs 1, Protein 46

Jalapeno Chicken Chowder

Prep time: 10 minutes
Cook time: 15 minutes
Servings: 4
Ingredients:
- 1 oz bacon, chopped, cooked
- 4 chicken wings, skinless, boneless
- 4 cups of water
- 1 jalapeno, chopped
- ½ cup cauliflower, chopped
- ½ cup heavy cream
- 1 teaspoon salt

Method:
1. Put all ingredients in the saucepan and bring to boil.
2. Simmet the chowder for 10 minutes on medium heat.
Nutritional info per serve: Calories 204, Fat 11.4, Fiber 0.3, Carbs 1.2, Protein 23

Bacon-Wrapped Chicken

Prep time: 15 minutes
Cook time: 45 minutes
Servings: 4
Ingredients:
- 4 bacon slices
- 4 chicken drumsticks
- 1 teaspoon white pepper
- 1 teaspoon apple cider vinegar
- 1 teaspoon olive oil

Method:
1. Mix the chicken drumsticks with white pepper and apple cider vinegar.
2. Then wrap them in the bacon slices and brush in the olive oil.
3. Put the wrapped chicken drumsticks in the baking tray and roast them for 45 minutes at 365F.
Nutritional info per serve: Calories 192, Fat 11.8, Fiber 0.1, Carbs 0.6, Protein 19.8

Tender Chicken Fillets

Prep time: 10 minutes
Cook time: 10 minutes
Servings: 2
Ingredients:
- 6 oz chicken fillet
- ½ cup apple cider vinegar
- 2 tablespoons coconut oil
- 1 teaspoon ground black pepper

Method:
1. Slice the chicken fillets and mix them with ground black pepper and apple cider vinegar.
2. Then melt the coconut oil in the skillet and preheat it well.
3. Add the sliced chicken fillets and roast them for 5 minutes per side on medium-low heat.
Nutritional info per serve: Calories 294, Fat 19.9, Fiber 0.3, Carbs 1.2, Protein 24.7

Basil Chicken

Prep time: 10 minutes
Cook time: 25 minutes
Servings: 4
Ingredients:
- 1-pound chicken breast, skinless, boneless
- 1 tablespoon dried basil
- 2 tablespoon butter
- 1 teaspoon salt

Method:
1. Melt the butter in the saucepan.

2. Add chicken breast and sprinkle it with salt and dried basil.
3. Then carefully mix the chicken and roast it for 10 minutes per side on medium heat.
Nutritional info per serve: Calories 180, Fat 8.6, Fiber 0, Carbs 0, Protein 24.1

Chicken Meatloaf
Prep time: 15 minutes
Cook time: 45 minutes
Servings: 6
Ingredients:
- 2 cups ground chicken
- 1 egg, beaten
- 1 teaspoon onion powder
- 1 teaspoon dried parsley
- 1 teaspoon chili flakes
- 1 teaspoon olive oil
- ¼ cup coconut flour

Method:
1. Brush the loaf pan with olive oil from inside.
2. Then mix all remaining ingredients in the mixing bowl. Transfer the mixture in the loaf mold and flatten well.
3. Bake it at 365F for 45 minutes.
Nutritional info per serve: Calories 127, Fat 5.6, Fiber 1.7, Carbs 3.1, Protein 15.1

Orange Chicken
Prep time: 10 minutes
Cook time: 40 minutes
Servings: 4
Ingredients:
- 4 chicken thighs, skinless, boneless
- 1 orange, sliced
- 4 teaspoons butter
- 1 teaspoon onion powder
- ½ teaspoon chili powder

Method:
1. Rub the chicken thighs with onion powder and chili powder and put in the baking pan.
2. Top the chicken thighs with butter and sliced orange and bake them at 365F for 40 minutes.
Nutritional info per serve: Calories 336, Fat 14.8, Fiber 1.2, Carbs 6.1, Protein 42.8

Sage Chicken
Prep time: 15 minutes
Cook time: 35 minutes
Servings: 4
Ingredients:
- 1-pound chicken breast, skinless, boneless
- 1 teaspoon dried sage
- 1 tablespoon avocado oil
- 1 teaspoon apple cider vinegar

Method:
1. Mix apple cider vinegar with avocado oil and dried sage.
2. Then mix chicken breast with the sage mixture and leave for 10-15 minutes to marinate.
3. Bake the marinated chicken for 35 minutes.

Nutritional info per serve: Calories 135, Fat 3.3, Fiber 0.2, Carbs 0.3, Protein 24.1

Crustless Chicken Pie
Prep time: 10 minutes
Cook time: 40 minutes
Servings: 4
Ingredients:
- 1 cup ground chicken
- 1 cup Mozzarella, shredded
- 1 jalapeno, chopped
- ¼ cup coconut flour
- 1 teaspoon chili flakes
- 1 teaspoon dried cilantro
- 1 teaspoon avocado oil

Method:
1. Brush the baking pan with avocado oil.
2. Then mix ground chicken with chopped jalapeno, coconut flour, chili flakes, and dried cilantro.
3. Put the mixture in the baking pan and flatten well in the shape of the pie crust.
4. Then top it with Mozzarella and cover with foil.
5. Bake the chicken pie for 40 minutes at 360F.
Nutritional info per serve: Calories 119, Fat 5, Fiber 2.7, Carbs 4.6, Protein 13.2

Coriander Chicken
Prep time: 10 minutes
Cook time: 45 minutes
Servings: 2
Ingredients:
- 2 chicken thighs, skinless, boneless
- 1 teaspoon ground coriander
- 2 teaspoons avocado oil

Method:
1. Rub the chicken thighs with coriander and sprinkle with avocado oil.
2. Put the chicken thighs in the tray and bake at 360F for 45 minutes.
Nutritional info per serve: Calories 284, Fat 11.4, Fiber 0.2, Carbs 0.3, Protein 42.3

Scallions Chicken
Prep time: 10 minutes
Cook time: 20 minutes
Servings: 4
Ingredients:
- 1-pound chicken breast, skinless, boneless, chopped
- 2 oz scallions, chopped
- 1 tablespoon coconut oil
- 1 teaspoon ground ginger

Method:
1. Mix the chicken breast with ground ginger and put it in the skillet.
2. Add coconut oil and roast the chicken for 20 minutes on medium heat. Stir ti from time to time.
3. Then sprinkle the chicken with chopped scallions and carefully mix.
Nutritional info per serve: Calories 165, Fat 6.3, Fiber 0.4, Carbs 1.4, Protein 24.3

Seasoned Chicken

Prep time: 15 minutes
Cook time: 25 minutes
Servings: 4
Ingredients:
- 1 tablespoon ghee
- 1 teaspoon taco seasoning
- 8 chicken wings, skinless, boneless

Method:
1. Melt the gree in the skillet.
2. Then mix chicken wings with taco seasonings and put in the melted ghee.
3. Roast the chicken for 10 minutes per side on the medium-low heat.

Nutritional info per serve: Calories 252, Fat 8.9, Fiber 0, Carbs 0.5, Protein 39.6

Sweet Chicken Wings

Prep time: 10 minutes
Cook time: 16 minutes
Servings: 4
Ingredients:
- 3 pounds chicken wings, skinless, boneless
- 1 tablespoon Erythritol
- 1 teaspoon white pepper
- 1 teaspoon chili pepper
- 1 tablespoon butter
- 1 teaspoon avocado oil

Method:
1. In the shallow bowl, mix Erythritol, white pepper, and chili pepper.
2. Rub the chicken wings with the sweet spice mixture and put in the skillet.
3. Add avocado oil and butter and roast the chicken wings for 8 minutes per side on the medium heat.

Nutritional info per serve: Calories 67,5 Fat 28.3, Fiber 0.2, Carbs 0.5, Protein 98.5

Sour Duck Breast

Prep time: 20 minutes
Cook time: 55 minutes
Servings: 6
Ingredients:
- 16 oz duck breast, skinless, boneless
- ½ cup Greek yogurt
- 1 teaspoon dried thyme
- 1 teaspoon ground cumin
- 1 teaspoon salt
- 1 tablespoon avocado oil
- 3 tablespoons lemon juice

Method:
1. In the mixing bowl, mix Greek yogurt, dried thyme, ground cumin, and salt.
2. Then mix greek yogurt mixture with duck breast and leave it for 10 minutes to marinate.
3. After this, transfer the chicken in the tray.
4. Add lemon juice and avocado oil and bake it at 365F for 55 minutes.

Nutritional info per serve: Calories 117, Fat 3.8, Fiber 0.2, Carbs 1.2, Protein 18.5

Cardamom Chicken

Prep time: 10 minutes
Cook time: 20 minutes
Servings: 4
Ingredients:
- 4 chicken thighs, skinless, boneless
- 1 teaspoon ground cardamom
- 1 teaspoon dried cilantro
- 1 teaspoon dried thyme
- 3 tablespoons butter

Method:
1. Rub the chicken thighs with ground cardamom. Dried cilantro, and dried thyme.
2. Then melt the butter in the skillet.
3. Add chicken thighs and roast them for 10 minutes per side on the medium-low heat.

Nutritional info per serve: Calories 356, Fat 19.5, Fiber 0.2, Carbs 0.5, Protein 42.4

Garlic Duck Bites

Prep time: 10 minutes
Cook time: 35 minutes
Servings: 2
Ingredients:
- 1 teaspoon minced garlic
- 1 teaspoon olive oil
- 1 teaspoon chili flakes
- 8 oz duck fillet, roughly chopped

Method:
1. Mix the olive oil with minced garlic and chili flakes.
2. Then mix duck fillet with garlic mixture and leave it for 10-51 minutes to marinate.
3. Put the duck in the baking tray and bake it at 360F for 35 minutes.

Nutritional info per serve: Calories 163, Fat 3, Fiber 0, Carbs 0.5, Protein 33.6

Chicken in Parmesan Sauce

Prep time: 10 minutes
Cook time: 25 minutes
Servings: 4
Ingredients:
- ½ cup heavy cream
- 2 oz Parmesan
- 1 teaspoon cayenne pepper
- 4 chicken thighs
- 1 tablespoon butter

Method:
1. Melt the butter in the skillet.
2. Add chicken thighs and roast them for 3 minutes per side on high heat.
3. After this, sprinkle the chicken thighs with cayenne pepper and add heavy cream.
4. Simmer the meal for 10 minutes and top with Parmesan.
5. Close the lid and cook the meal on medium heat for 4 minutes.

Nutritional info per serve: Calories 402, Fat 22.4, Fiber 0.1, Carbs 1.2, Protein 47.2

Saffron Duck

Prep time: 10 minutes
Cook time: 30 minutes

Servings: 4
Ingredients:
- 1-pound duck breast, skinless, boneless, chopped
- 1 teaspoon saffron
- 1 cup of coconut milk
- 2 spring onions, diced
- 1 teaspoon ground turmeric
- 1 tablespoon coconut oil
- 1 teaspoon salt

Method:
1. Melt the coconut oil in the saucepan.
2. Add spring onion, ground turmeric, salt, and saffron.
3. Roast the onion for 2-3 minutes and add duck breast. Stir the mixture well.
4. Then add coconut milk and carefully mix the meal.
5. Close the lid and cook it on medium heat for 20 minutes.

Nutritional info per serve: Calories 310, Fat 20.6, Fiber 2, Carbs 6.4, Protein 25.8

Chicken under Onion Blanket

Prep time: 10 minutes
Cook time: 45 minutes
Servings: 4
Ingredients:
- 4 chicken thighs, skinless, boneless
- 1 spring onion, sliced
- 1 tablespoon butter
- 1 teaspoon ground black pepper
- ¼ cup of water

Method:
1. Mix butter, onion, and ground black pepper.
2. Pour water and add chicken thighs in the baking pan. Top the chicken with spring onion mixture.
3. Bake the chicken at 360F for 45 minutes.

Nutritional info per serve: Calories 315, Fat 13.8, Fiber 0.7, Carbs 2.9, Protein 42.6

Oregano Duck

Prep time: 3 hours
Cook time: 35 minutes
Servings: 6
Ingredients:
- 2-pounds duck breast, skinless, boneless
- 1 tablespoon dried oregano
- 1 teaspoon peppercorns
- 3 cups of water
- 1 teaspoon salt

Method:
1. Pour water in the saucepan and bring it to boil.
2. Add duck breast, dried oregano, peppercorns, and salt. Boil the duck for 30 minutes.
3. Then cover the saucepan with duck with a towel and leave for 3 hours.
4. Remove the duck breast from the saucepan and slice into servings.

Nutritional info per serve: Calories 210, Fat 9.2, Fiber 0.5, Carbs 1.9, Protein 28.4

Marjoram Chicken Breast

Prep time: 15 minutes
Cook time: 60 minutes
Servings: 4
Ingredients:
- 1-pound chicken breast, skinless, boneless
- 2 tablespoons butter, softened
- 1 tablespoon dried marjoram
- ½ teaspoon salt

Method:
1. Rub the chicken breast with salt and marjoram.
2. Then grease it with butter and wrap in the foil.
3. Bake the chicken breast at 360F for 60 minutes.

Nutritional info per serve: Calories 181, Fat 8.6, Fiber 0.2, Carbs 0.3, Protein 24.2

Turmeric Chicken Skin

Prep time: 10 minutes
Cook time: 10 minutes
Servings: 4
Ingredients:
- 9 oz chicken skin
- 1 teaspoon ground turmeric
- ½ teaspoon salt
- 1 tablespoon avocado oil

Method:
1. Preheat the skillet well.
2. Meanwhile, mix ground turmeric with salt and chicken skin.
3. Put the chicken skin mixture in the hot skillet and roast it for 5 minutes per side or until the chicken skin is lightly crunchy.

Nutritional info per serve: Calories 296, Fat 26.4, Fiber 0.3, Carbs 0.6, Protein 13.1

Thyme Sausages

Prep time: 10 minutes
Cook time: 20 minutes
Servings: 5
Ingredients:
- 16 oz chicken sausages
- 1 tablespoon dried thyme
- 2 tablespoons olive oil
- 1 teaspoon lemon juice
- 1 teaspoon keto tomato paste

Method:
1. In the mixing bowl, mix keto tomato paste with lemon juice, thyme, and olive oil.
2. Mix the chicken sausages with keto tomato paste mixture and transfer in the hot skillet.
3. Roast the sausages for 10 minutes per side on the medium heat.

Nutritional info per serve: Calories 222, Fat 15.6, Fiber 0.8, Carbs 6.7, Protein 11.9

Strawberries Chicken

Prep time: 10 minutes
Cook time: 35 minutes
Servings: 4

Ingredients:
- 1-pound chicken breast, skinless, boneless, chopped
- 1 oz strawberries, chopped
- 1 tablespoon butter, softened
- 1 teaspoon chili powder

Method:
1. Mix the chicken breast with chili powder, strawberries, and butter.
2. Put the mixture in the baking tray and bake at 365F for 35 minutes.

Nutritional info per serve: Calories 159, Fat 5.9, Fiber 0.4, Carbs 0.9, Protein 24.2

Parmesan Chicken Thighs

Prep time: 10 minutes
Cook time: 25 minutes
Servings: 4
Ingredients:
- 4 chicken thighs, skinless, boneless
- 2 oz Parmesan, grated
- 1 tablespoon butter
- 1 teaspoon dried rosemary
- ¼ cup of water

Method:
1. Rub the chicken thighs with rosemary and put in the saucepan.
2. Add butter and roast the chicken thighs on high heat for 5 minutes per side.
3. Then add water and close the lid.
4. Simmer the chicken for 10 minutes.
5. Add Parmesan and cook the chicken or 5 minutes more.

Nutritional info per serve: Calories 349, Fat 16.8, Fiber 0.1, Carbs 0.7, Protein 46.8

Chicken Spread

Prep time: 15 minutes
Cook time: 30 minutes
Servings: 6
Ingredients:
- 4 tablespoons butter, softened
- 1-pound chicken liver
- 1 teaspoon salt
- 1 teaspoon peppercorns
- 1 bay leaf
- 2 cups of water

Method:
1. Bring the water to boil.
2. Add bay leaf and peppercorns.
3. Then add the chicken liver and simmer it for 15 minutes.
4. After this, drain the water and transfer the liver in the food processor. Add butter and blend the mixture until smooth.
5. Transfer the cooked spread in the bowl and store it in the fridge for up to 5 days.

Nutritional info per serve: Calories 233, Fat 11.2, Fiber 0.1, Carbs 0.5, Protein 31.2

Macadamia Chicken

Prep time: 10 minutes
Cook time: 35 minutes
Servings: 4
Ingredients:
- 1 teaspoon ground black pepper
- 1 teaspoon cayenne pepper
- 3 tablespoons butter
- 1 oz macadamia nuts, chopped
- 4 chicken thighs, skinless, boneless

Method:
1. Mix the ground black pepper with cayenne pepper and macadamia nuts.
2. Then coat the chicken thighs in the spices.
3. Preheat the skillet well.
4. Add butter and coated chicken thighs. Roast them for 2 minutes per side on high heat.
5. Then transfer the chicken thighs in the preheated to 360F oven and cook for 30 minutes.

Nutritional info per serve: Calories 349, Fat 16.8, Fiber 0.1, Carbs 0.7, Protein 46.8

Duck Spread

Prep time: 15 minutes
Cook time: 0 minutes
Servings: 6
Ingredients:
- 1/3 cup heavy cream
- 1 teaspoon dried thyme
- ½ teaspoon salt
- 1-pound duck liver, boiled
- ¼ teaspoon chili powder

Method:
1. Put all ingredients in the food processor and blend until smooth.
2. Transfer the mixture in the bowl and flatten the surface of the duck spread well.

Nutritional info per serve: Calories 127, Fat 6, Fiber 0.1, Carbs 3, Protein 14.3

Tomato Chicken

Prep time: 10 minutes
Cook time: 40 minutes
Servings: 6
Ingredients:
- 6 chicken thighs, skinless, boneless
- 1 tablespoon keto tomato paste
- 1 tablespoon avocado oil
- 1 teaspoon onion powder
- ½ teaspoon ground black pepper
- 1 tablespoon lemon juice

Method:
1. Mix the chicken thighs with keto tomato paste, avocado oil, onion powder, ground black pepper, and lemon juice.
2. Then transfer the chicken thighs in the baking tray and bake at 365F for 40 minutes.

Nutritional info per serve: Calories 285, Fat 11.2, Fiber 0.3, Carbs 1.1, Protein 42.5

Cinnamon Chicken Drumsticks

Prep time: 10 minutes
Cook time: 60 minutes
Servings: 2
Ingredients:
- 1 teaspoon ground cinnamon

- 1 tablespoon butter, softened
- 4 chicken drumsticks
- ½ teaspoon salt

Method:
1. In the mixing bowl, mix softened butter with salt and ground cinnamon.
2. Then rub the chicken drumsticks with butter mixture and put in the baking tray.
3. Bake the chicken drumsticks for 60 minutes at 355F.

Nutritional info per serve: Calories 209, Fat 11, Fiber 0.6, Carbs 0.9, Protein 25.4

Coated Chicken

Prep time: 10 minutes
Cook time: 40 minutes
Servings: 4
Ingredients:
- 4 chicken thighs, skinless, boneless
- 2 oz pork rinds
- 2 eggs, beaten
- ½ teaspoon ground black pepper
- ½ teaspoon cayenne pepper
- ½ teaspoon salt
- 1 tablespoon avocado oil

Method:
1. In the shallow bowl, mix ground black pepper, cayenne pepper, and salt.
2. Then rub the chicken thighs with the spices and dip in the beaten eggs.
3. After this, coat the chicken thighs in the pork rinds.
4. Preheat the avocado oil in the skillet and put the chicken thighs in hot oil.
5. Roast the chicken thighs on high heat for 3 minutes per side. Then bake the chicken in the oven at 360F for 30 minutes.

Nutritional info per serve: Calories 396, Fat 18.6, Fiber 0.3, Carbs 0.7, Protein 54.2

Jalapeno Chicken

Prep time: 10 minutes
Cook time: 45 minutes
Servings: 4
Ingredients:
- 2 jalapeno peppers, minced
- 4 chicken thighs, skinless, boneless
- 3 tablespoons apple cider vinegar
- 1 teaspoon ground paprika
- 1 teaspoon ground turmeric
- 1 tablespoon olive oil

Method:
1. Brush the baking pan with olive oil.
2. Then rub the chicken thighs with minced jalapeno peppers. Apple cider vinegar, ground paprika, and ground turmeric.
3. Put the chicken thighs in the prepared baking pan and cook them in the preheated to 365F oven for 45 minutes.

Nutritional info per serve: Calories 316, Fat 14.5, Fiber 0.6, Carbs 1.3, Protein 42.5

Chicken Calzone

Prep time: 30 minutes
Cook time: 20 minutes
Servings: 4
Ingredients:
- 1 egg, beaten
- 1 cup almond flour
- 2 tablespoons coconut oil
- 10 oz chicken fillet, cooked, shredded
- 1 oz bacon, chopped, cooked
- 1 oz scallions, chopped
- 1 teaspoon avocado oil

Method:
1. In the mixing bowl mix almond flour with coconut oil, and egg. Knead the dough.
2. Then cut it into 4 pieces and roll up into 4 rounds.
3. Mix scallions with chopped bacon, and shredded chicken.
4. Put the mixture on the ½ part of every dough round and fold the dough. Secure the edges of the calzones and brush them with avocado oil.
5. Bake the calzones for 20 minutes at 350F or until they are light brown.

Nutritional info per serve: Calories 291, Fat 19.8, Fiber 1, Carbs 2.3, Protein 26.2

Shredded Chicken Pancakes

Prep time: 10 minutes
Cook time: 30 minutes
Servings: 4
Ingredients:
- 7 oz chicken fillet, boiled, shredded
- 1 teaspoon cayenne pepper
- 3 eggs, beaten
- 1 tablespoon coconut flour
- 1 tablespoon coconut oil
- 1 oz Parmesan, grated

Method:
1. Melt the coconut oil in the skillet.
2. Meanwhile, mix all remaining ingredients in the mixing bowl and carefully stir until you get a homogenous batter.
3. After this, pour the small amount of batter in the hot skillet with help of the ladle and flatten it in the shape of a pancake.
4. Roast the pancakes for 3 minutes per side on low heat.

Nutritional info per serve: Calories 291, Fat 19.8, Fiber 1, Carbs 2.3, Protein 26.2

Chicken Cream Soup

Prep time: 10 minutes
Cook time: 40 minutes
Servings: 6
Ingredients:
- 1-pound chicken breast, skinless, boneless
- 7 cups of water
- 1 cup heavy cream
- 1 cup turnip, chopped
- 1 teaspoon ground black pepper
- 1 teaspoon salt
- 1 cup Cheddar cheese, shredded

Method:

1. Put all ingredients except Cheddar cheese in the saucepan and boil for 20 minutes.
2. Then remove the chicken breast from the liquid.
3. Add cheddar cheese in the hot soup liquid and simmer it until cheese is melted.
4. After this, blend the soup with the help of the immersion blender.
5. Shred the chicken and add it in the soup.
Nutritional info per serve: Calories 238, Fat 15.6, Fiber 0.5, Carbs 2.4, Protein 21.4

Crunchy Chicken Wings

Prep time: 15 minutes
Cook time: 45 minutes
Servings: 6
Ingredients:
- 6 chicken wings
- ½ cup coconut shred
- 3 eggs, beaten
- 1 teaspoon ground paprika
- 1 teaspoon salt

Method:
1. Mix the chicken wings with ground paprika and salt and then dip in the eggs.
2. After this, coat every chicken wing in coconut shred and transfer in the baking tray in one layer.
3. Bake the chicken wings at 365F for 45 minutes or until they are golden brown.
Nutritional info per serve: Calories 258, Fat 19.6, Fiber 1.6, Carbs 8.4, Protein 12.6

Sriracha Chicken

Prep time: 10 minutes
Cook time: 40 minutes
Servings: 2
Ingredients:
- 2 tablespoon sriracha
- 2 chicken thighs, skinless, boneless
- 1 tablespoon avocado oil
- ½ teaspoon lemon juice

Method:
1. Mix avocado oil with lemon juice and sriracha.
2. Then brush chicken thighs with sriracha mixture well.
3. Lune the baking tray with baking paper and put the prepared chicken thighs inside.
4. Bake the meal at 360F for 40 minutes.
Nutritional info per serve: Calories 302, Fat 11.7, Fiber 0.3, Carbs 3.4, Protein 42.3

Indian Style Chicken

Prep time: 10 minutes
Cook time: 30 minutes
Servings: 4
Ingredients:
- ½ cup of coconut milk
- 1 teaspoon garam masala
- 1 teaspoon dried oregano
- 1 tablespoon coconut oil
- 4 chicken thighs, skinless, boneless

Method:
1. Rub the chicken thighs with garam masala, dried oregano, and put in the hot saucepan.
2. Roast the chicken for 1 minute per side.
3. Add coconut oil and coconut milk.
4. Close the lid and cook the chicken thighs for 30 minutes on medium-low heat.
Nutritional info per serve: Calories 377, Fat 21.4, Fiber 0.8, Carbs 1.9, Protein 43

Greens and Chicken Bowl

Prep time: 10 minutes
Cook time: 15 minutes
Servings: 4
Ingredients:
- 1 cup arugula, chopped
- 1-pound chicken fillet, chopped
- 1 teaspoon ground paprika
- 1 tablespoon avocado oil
- 1 teaspoon chili flakes
- 2 tablespoons lemon juice
- 1 cup lettuce, chopped
- 1 teaspoon olive oil

Method:
1. Mix chicken with chili flakes, avocado oil, and ground paprika.
2. Roast the chicken in the skillet for 15 minutes. Stir ti from time to time.
3. Meanwhile, mix all remaining ingredients in the bowl and carefully mix.
4. When the chicken is cooked, put it over the arugula mixture.
Nutritional info per serve: Calories 237, Fat 10.2, Fiber 0.6, Carbs 1.3, Protein 33.2

Chicken Roast

Prep time: 15 minutes
Cook time: 30 minutes
Servings: 4
Ingredients:
- 1-pound chicken breast, roughly chopped
- 1 tablespoon olive oil
- 1 teaspoon chili powder
- 1 teaspoon salt

Method:
1. Mix chicken breast with olive oil, chili powder, and salt.
2. Put it in the baking tray and cook at 365F in the oven for 30 minutes. Stir it from time to time to avoid burning.
Nutritional info per serve: Calories 161, Fat 6.5, Fiber 0.2, Carbs 0.4, Protein 24.1

Cream Cheese Chicken

Prep time: 10 minutes
Cook time: 30 minutes
Servings: 4
Ingredients:
- 2 tablespoons cream cheese
- 1 teaspoon minced garlic
- 1 tablespoon coconut milk
- ½ teaspoon dried dill
- 4 chicken thighs, skinless, boneless

- 1 tablespoon avocado oil

Method:
1. In the mixing bowl, mix minced garlic with coconut milk, dried dill, and cream cheese.
2. Put the chicken inside the coconut mixture and leave for 10-15 minutes to marinate.
3. After this, preheat the saucepan well, add avocado oil and chicken thighs.
4. Roast them on high heat for 5 minutes per side.
5. Then add remaining coconut milk mixture and simmer the meal on medium heat for 20 minutes.

Nutritional info per serve: Calories 310, Fat 13.9, Fiber 0.3, Carbs 0.8, Protein 42.8

Chili Chicken Ground

Prep time: 10 minutes
Cook time: 15 minutes
Servings: 4
Ingredients:
- 1 teaspoon chili flakes
- 1 chili pepper, chopped
- 1 tablespoon coconut oil
- 2 cups ground chicken
- 1 teaspoon keto tomato paste
- ½ teaspoon salt

Method:
1. Melt the coconut oil in the saucepan.
2. Add all remaining ingredients and carefully mix the mixture.
3. Cook it on medium heat for 15 minutes, stir it from time to time.

Nutritional info per serve: Calories 164, Fat 8.6, Fiber 0.1, Carbs 0.4, Protein 20.3

Yogurt Chicken

Prep time: 15 minutes
Cook time: 35 minutes
Servings: 4
Ingredients:
- 1-pound chicken breast, skinless, boneless, chopped
- 1 cup plain yogurt
- 1 teaspoon lemon zest, grated
- 1 tablespoon apple cider vinegar
- ½ teaspoon ground paprika
- 1 teaspoon butter, melted

Method:
1. Mix all ingredients in the big bowl and leave for 10 minutes to marinate.
2. Then transfer the mixture in the saucepan and close the lid.
3. Simmer the chicken on medium-low heat for 35 minutes or until the chicken is soft.

Nutritional info per serve: Calories 183, Fat 4.6, Fiber 0.1, Carbs 4.6, Protein 27.6

Leek Chicken

Prep time: 10 minutes
Cook time: 25 minutes
Servings: 2
Ingredients:
- 2 chicken thighs, skinless, boneless
- ½ cup leek, chopped
- 1 tablespoon butter
- ½ teaspoon ground black pepper
- ½ cup chicken broth

Method:
1. Mix the chicken thighs with ground black pepper and put it in the saucepan.
2. Roast the chicken thighs for 1 minute per side.
3. Add leek and chicken broth. Cook the chicken on medium heat for 20 minutes.

Nutritional info per serve: Calories 353, Fat 17, Fiber 0.5, Carbs 3.7, Protein 43.9

Stuffed Chicken with Olives

Prep time: 10 minutes
Cook time: 40 minutes
Servings: 4
Ingredients:
- 1-pound chicken fillet
- 2 kalamata olives, pitted, sliced
- ½ cup plain yogurt
- 1 teaspoon chili powder
- 1 teaspoon salt

Method:
1. Make the lengthwise cut in the chicken fillet.
2. Then mix olives with chili powder and salt.
3. Fill the chicken fillet with olive mixture and secure the cut with toothpicks.
4. After this, brush the chicken in the plain yogurt and wrap in the foil.
5. Bake the chicken in the oven at 360F for 40 minutes.

Nutritional info per serve: Calories 242, Fat 9.1, Fiber 0.3, Carbs 2.7, Protein 34.7

Dill Chicken Muffins

Prep time: 10 minutes
Cook time: 25 minutes
Servings: 4
Ingredients:
- 1 cup ground chicken
- 3 tablespoons coconut shred
- 1 teaspoon dried dill
- 1 egg, beaten
- ½ teaspoon chili flakes
- 4 teaspoons butter, softened

Method:
1. In the mixing bowl, mix all ingredients.
2. Then put the mixture in the muffin molds.
3. Bake the muffins at 360F for 25 minutes.

Nutritional info per serve: Calories 154, Fat 11.3, Fiber 0.8, Carbs 1.7, Protein 11.6

Chicken with Crumbled Cheese

Prep time: 10 minutes
Cook time: 25 minutes
Servings: 6
Ingredients:
- 2-pounds chicken fillet
- 6 oz Blue cheese, crumbled
- ½ cup heavy cream
- 1 teaspoon ground black pepper

- ½ teaspoon ground coriander
- 1 teaspoon avocado oil

Method:
1. Rub the chicken fillet with ground coriander and ground black pepper.
2. Then put in the hot skillet and roast for 2 minutes per side.
3. Then add avocado oil and heavy cream. Cook the chicken for 10 minutes.
4. Add crumbled cheese and carefully mix the mixture.
5. Cook the meal on medium heat for 10 minutes.

Nutritional info per serve: Calories 424, Fat 23.2, Fiber 0.1, Carbs 1.2, Protein 50.1

Chicken Lettuce Wraps

Prep time: 10 minutes
Cook time: 0 minutes
Servings: 4
Ingredients:
- 1-pound chicken fillet, boiled, shredded
- 2 tablespoons plain yogurt
- 1 teaspoon chives, chopped
- 1 cup lettuce leaves

Method:
1. In the mixing bowl, mix shredded chicken with yogurt and chives.
2. Then fill the lettuce leaves with chicken mixture.

Nutritional info per serve: Calories 223, Fat 8.5, Fiber 0.1, Carbs 1, Protein 33.3

Chicken in Avocado

Prep time: 10 minutes
Cook time: 0 minutes
Servings: 2
Ingredients:
- 1 avocado, pitted, halved
- 8 oz chicken fillet, boiled, shredded
- 1 tablespoon cream cheese
- 1 teaspoon cayenne pepper
- ½ teaspoon lemon juice

Method:
1. In the mixing bowl, mix cream cheese with cayenne pepper, lemon juice, and shredded chicken.
2. Then remove ½ part of all avocado meat.
3. Fill the avocado with a chicken mixture.

Nutritional info per serve: Calories 446, Fat 17.1, Fiber 0.2, Carbs 1.9, Protein 66.6

Duck Casserole

Prep time: 10 minutes
Cook time: 45 minutes
Servings: 5
Ingredients:
- 1-pound ground duck
- 1 cup Monterey Jack cheese, shredded
- 1 cup bell pepper, chopped
- ½ cup of water
- 1 teaspoon Italian seasonings
- 1 teaspoon salt

Method:
1. Mix ground duck with Italian seasonings and salt.
2. Then put it in the casserole mold and flatten well.
3. Top the duck with bell pepper, water, and Monterey Jack cheese.
4. Cover the casserole with foil and bake at 360F for 45 minutes.

Nutritional info per serve: Calories 224, Fat 14.5, Fiber 0.3, Carbs 2.1, Protein 21.6

Mozzarella Chicken

Prep time: 10 minutes
Cook time: 40 minutes
Servings: 4
Ingredients:
- 4 oz Mozzarella, sliced
- 1 tomato, sliced
- 16 oz chicken fillet, sliced
- 1 tablespoon coconut oil
- ¼ cup of water

Method:
1. Melt the coconut oil and pour it in the baking pan.
2. Add water and chicken fillets.
3. Then top the chicken with sliced tomato and sliced mozzarella.
4. Bake the chicken for 40 minutes at 350F.

Nutritional info per serve: Calories 328, Fat 16.8, Fiber 0.2, Carbs 1.6, Protein 41

Aromatic Cumin Chicken

Prep time: 10 minutes
Cook time: 20 minutes
Servings: 4
Ingredients:
- 1 teaspoon cumin seeds
- 1 tablespoon avocado oil
- 1-pound chicken fillet, chopped
- ½ teaspoon dried parsley

Method:
1. Pour avocado oil in the skillet and add cumin seeds. Roast them for 1 minute.
2. Add chicken fillet and dried parsley.
3. Roast the chicken for 15 minutes on medium heat. Stir it from time to time.

Nutritional info per serve: Calories 222, Fat 9, Fiber 0.2, Carbs 0.4, Protein 32.9

Cilantro Chicken

Prep time: 10 minutes
Cook time: 30 minutes
Servings: 4
Ingredients:
- ¼ cup fresh cilantro, chopped
- 1-pound chicken breast, skinless, boneless, chopped
- 1 tablespoon keto tomato paste
- ¼ cup of coconut milk
- 1 teaspoon cayenne pepper

Method:

1. Mix cayenne pepper with keto tomato paste and coconut milk. Add cilantro and transfer the liquid in the saucepan.
2. Add chicken breast and simmer the chicken for 30 minutes on low heat.
Nutritional info per serve: Calories 255, Fat 12.1, Fiber 0.6, Carbs 1.9, Protein 33.4

Bacon Chicken

Prep time: 10 minutes
Cook time: 30 minutes
Servings: 3
Ingredients:
- 3 oz bacon, chopped
- 6 chicken drumsticks
- 1 tablespoon coconut oil
- 1 teaspoon dried rosemary

Method:
1. Rub the chicken drumsticks with the dried rosemary and coconut oil.
2. Then wrap them in the bacon and bake in the preheated to 365F oven for 30 minutes.
Nutritional info per serve: Calories 262, Fat 16.3, Fiber 0.1, Carbs 0.5, Protein 26.9

Herbed Ginger Chicken

Prep time: 10 minutes
Cook time: 30 minutes
Servings: 5
Ingredients:
- 1-pound chicken breast, skinless, boneless, chopped
- 1 teaspoon minced garlic
- 1 teaspoon Italian seasonings
- ½ cup plain yogurt
- ¼ cup of water

Method:
1. Mix plain yogurt with Italian seasonings and minced garlic.
2. Then pour water in the saucepan and bring it to boil.
3. Add chicken breast and yogurt mixture and close the lid.
4. Cook the chicken on medium heat for 30 minutes, stir it from time to time.
Nutritional info per serve: Calories 125, Fat 2.9, Fiber 0, Carbs 2, Protein 20.7

Jalapeno Chicken with Cream Cheese

Prep time: 10 minutes
Cook time: 30 minutes
Servings: 4
Ingredients:
- 2 jalapenos, sliced
- 2 tablespoons cream cheese
- ½ teaspoon garlic powder
- 4 chicken thighs, skinless, boneless
- ¼ cup of water

Method:
1. Mix cream cheese with garlic powder.
2. Rub the chicken thighs with cream cheese mixture and put in the casserole mold.
3. Add water and sliced bacon. Cover the casserole mold with foil and bake at 365F for 30 minutes.
Nutritional info per serve: Calories 298, Fat 12.6, Fiber 0.2, Carbs 0.8, Protein 42.8

Chicken and Leek Stew

Prep time: 10 minutes
Cook time: 30 minutes
Servings: 4
Ingredients:
- 7 oz leek, chopped
- 2 tablespoons butter
- 1 cup of water
- 1-pound chicken breast, skinless, boneless, chopped
- 1 teaspoon keto tomato paste
- 1 tablespoon plain yogurt

Method:
1. Put all ingredients in the saucepan and carefully mix.
2. Then close the lid and cook the stew on medium-low heat for 30 minutes.
Nutritional info per serve: Calories 214, Fat 8.8, Fiber 0.9, Carbs 7.5, Protein 25.1

Fennel Chicken

Prep time: 10 minutes
Cook time: 15 minutes
Servings: 1
Ingredients:
- 4 oz chicken fillet
- 1 teaspoon fennel seeds
- 1 tablespoon coconut oil
- ½ teaspoon salt

Method:
1. Melt the coconut oil in the saucepan.
2. Add fennel seeds and roast them for 2-3 minutes.
3. After this, add chicken fillet and salt.
4. Roast the chicken for 6 minutes per side.
Nutritional info per serve: Calories 340, Fat 22.3, Fiber 0.8, Carbs 1.1, Protein 33.1

Chicken with Asparagus Blanket

Prep time: 10 minutes
Cook time: 30 minutes
Servings: 6
Ingredients:
- 6 chicken thighs, skinless, boneless
- 7 oz asparagus, chopped
- 1 cup Cheddar cheese, shredded
- ½ cup coconut cream
- 1 teaspoon ground black pepper
- 1 teaspoon chili flakes
- 1 teaspoon coconut oil

Method:
1. Grease the baking pan with coconut oil.
2. Then mix chicken thighs with ground black pepper and chili flakes.
3. Put the chicken thighs in the prepared baking pan.

4.   Top it with asparagus, coconut cream, and cheddar cheese.
5.   Bake the chicken at 365F in the oven for 30 minutes.
Nutritional info per serve: Calories 413, Fat 22.6, Fiber 1.2, Carbs 2.9 Protein 48.2

BBQ Shredded Chicken
Prep time: 10 minutes
Cook time: 10 minutes
Servings: 3
Ingredients:
- 10 oz chicken breast, skinless, boneless, boiled, shredded
- ½ cup Keto Keto BBQ sauce
- ¼ cup chicken broth

Method:
1.   Bring the chicken broth to boil and add Keto BBQ sauce. Carefully mix the liquid.
2.   Add shredded chicken, stir it well, and simmer for 2 minutes.
Nutritional info per serve: Calories 173, Fat 2.6, Fiber 0.3, Carbs 15.2, Protein 20.4

KETOGENIC MEAT RECIPES

Lemon Pork Belly

Prep time: 10 minutes
Cook time: 30 minutes
Servings: 6
Ingredients:
- 1-pound pork belly
- 2 cups of water
- 1 teaspoon dried thyme
- 1 teaspoon salt
- 1 teaspoon peppercorn
- 2 tablespoons lemon juice

Method:
1. Bring the water to boil and add peppercorn, salt, and dried thyme.
2. Then add the pork belly and boil it for 30 minutes.
3. After this, remove the cooked pork belly from the water and slice.
4. Sprinkle the pork belly with lemon juice.

Nutritional info per serve: Calories 352, Fat 20.4, Fiber 0.2, Carbs 0.5, Protein 35

Ground Pork Pie

Prep time: 15 minutes
Cook time: 25 minutes
Servings: 6
Ingredients:
- 1 cup coconut flour
- 3 tablespoons Psyllium husk
- 2 tablespoons butter, softened
- 1 cup ground pork
- 2 oz scallions, chopped
- 1 tablespoon almond flour
- 1 teaspoon chili powder
- 1 teaspoon avocado oil

Method:
1. In the mixing bowl, mix coconut flour, psyllium husk, butter, and almond flour. Knead the dough.
2. After this, put the dough in the baking pan and flatten in the shape of the pie crust with the help of the finger palms.
3. After this, in the mixing bowl, mix ground pork with scallions, chili powder, and avocado oil.
4. Put the mixture over the pie crust and flatten well.
5. Bake the ground pork pie for 25 minutes at 355F.

Nutritional info per serve: Calories 341, Fat 18.8, Fiber 22.8, Carbs 31.1, Protein 18

Lemon Stuffed Pork

Prep time: 10 minutes
Cook time: 30 minutes
Servings: 4
Ingredients:
- 1-pound pork loin
- ½ lemon, sliced
- 1 teaspoon dried rosemary
- ½ teaspoon ground paprika
- 2 tablespoons avocado oil

Method:
1. Slice the pork loin into 4 fillets. Beat the pork fillets with the help of the kitchen hammer.
2. After this, rub the meat with dried rosemary and ground pork.
3. Put the lemon slices on the pork fillets and fold them. Secure the meat with toothpicks and brush with avocado oil.
4. Bake the meat at 360F for 30 minutes. Flip the meat on another side during cooking to avoid burning.

Nutritional info per serve: Calories 288, Fat 16.8, Fiber 0.7, Carbs 1.4, Protein 31.2

Beef and Vegetables Stew

Prep time: 10 minutes
Cook time: 55 minutes
Servings: 4
Ingredients:
- 1-pound beef sirloin, chopped
- 1 cup bell pepper, chopped
- 4 cups of water
- 1 tablespoon keto tomato paste
- 1 teaspoon ground coriander
- ½ teaspoon salt
- 1 teaspoon dried sage

Method:
1. Put all ingredients in the saucepan and carefully stir.
2. Bring the mixture to boil, close the lid, and simmer it for 45 minutes on the low heat.

Nutritional info per serve: Calories 224, Fat 7.2, Fiber 0.6, Carbs 3.1, Protein 34.9

Marinated Pork

Prep time: 25 minutes
Cook time: 20 minutes
Servings: 3
Ingredients:
- 16 oz pork loin, chopped
- ½ cup apple cider vinegar
- 1 tablespoon avocado oil
- 1 teaspoon ground coriander

Method:
1. Mix apple cider vinegar with ground coriander.
2. Put the pork loin in the apple cider vinegar liquid and marinate it for 20 minutes.
3. After this, preheat the skillet well.
4. Add avocado oil and marinated meat.
5. Roast the meat for 20 minutes on the medium heat; stir it from time to time.

Nutritional info per serve: Calories 381, Fat 21.6, Fiber 0.2, Carbs 0.6, Protein 41.4

Cheese and Pork Casserole

Prep time: 10 minutes
Cook time: 40 minutes
Servings: 5
Ingredients:
- 2 cups ground pork

- 1 cup Cheddar cheese, shredded
- ½ cup coconut cream
- 1 teaspoon dried cilantro
- ½ teaspoon chili powder
- 1 tablespoon butter, softened

Method:
1. Grease the casserole mold with butter.
2. After this, mix ground pork with dried cilantro, coconut cream, and chili powder.
3. Put the mixture in the casserole mold, flatten it in one layer, and top with Cheddar cheese.
4. Bake the casserole in the oven at 360F for 40 minutes.

Nutritional info per serve: Calories 539, Fat 41.6, Fiber 0.6, Carbs 1.8, Protein 38.4

Pork and Cream Cheese Rolls

Prep time: 10 minutes
Cook time: 30 minutes
Servings: 6
Ingredients:
- 3 tablespoons cream cheese
- 2 oz bacon, chopped, cooked
- 1-pound pork sirloin
- 1 teaspoon apple cider vinegar
- 1 teaspoon white pepper
- 1 tablespoon avocado oil

Method:
1. In the mixing bowl, mix cream cheese with chopped bacon and white pepper.
2. Then slice the pork sirloin into 6 servings.
3. Spread every meat serving with cream cheese mixture and roll.
4. Secure the rolls with the help of the toothpicks if needed.
5. Brush the baking pan with avocado oil and put the meat rolls inside.
6. Bake the meat rolls at 360F for 30 minutes.

Nutritional info per serve: Calories 200, Fat 12.7, Fiber 0.2, Carbs 0.6, Protein 19.3

Leek Stuffed Beef

Prep time: 15 minutes
Cook time: 20 minutes
Servings: 2
Ingredients:
- 8 oz beef tenderloin
- 4 oz leek, chopped
- 1 teaspoon coconut oil
- ½ teaspoon salt
- 1 tablespoon dried parsley
- 1 oz bacon, chopped
- 1 teaspoon avocado oil

Method:
1. Cut the beef tenderloin into 2 servings.
2. Then mix leek with salt, dried parsley, and chopped bacon.
3. Spread the mixture over the beef tenderloins. Fold the meat and secure with the help of the toothpicks.
4. Then melt the coconut oil in the skillet. Add avocado oil.
5. After this, add beef rolls in the hot oil and roast them for 10 minutes per side on the low heat.

Nutritional info per serve: Calories 368, Fat 19, Fiber 1.2, Carbs 8.5, Protein 39

Garlic Pork Loin

Prep time: 10 minutes
Cook time: 50 minutes
Servings: 4
Ingredients:
- 1 teaspoon garlic powder
- 1 garlic clove, diced
- 1-pound pork loin
- 2 tablespoons avocado oil
- ½ teaspoon salt

Method:
1. Rub the pork loin with salt, diced garlic, and garlic powder.
2. Then sprinkle the meat with avocado oil and wrap in the foil.
3. Bake the pork loin in the preheated to 360F oven for 50 minutes.

Nutritional info per serve: Calories 340, Fat 22.8, Fiber 0.1, Carbs 0.8, Protein 31.2

Butter Pork

Prep time: 10 minutes
Cook time: 45 minutes
Servings: 4
Ingredients:
- 1-pound pork tenderloin
- ¼ cup butter
- 1 teaspoon dried rosemary

Method:
1. Rub the pork tenderloin with rosemary and put in the baking tray.
2. Add butter and bake the meat in the oven at 360F for 45 minutes.

Nutritional info per serve: Calories 265, Fat 15.5, Fiber 0.1, Carbs 0.2, Protein 29.8

Almond Pork

Prep time: 10 minutes
Cook time: 20 minutes
Servings: 4
Ingredients:
- ½ cup organic almond milk
- 1-pound pork loin, sliced
- 1 teaspoon ground paprika
- 1 teaspoon ground nutmeg
- 1 tablespoon coconut oil

Method:
1. In the shallow bowl, mix ground paprika and ground nutmeg.
2. Then sprinkle the pork loin with spices and transfer in the skillet.
3. Add coconut oil and roast the pork for 5 minutes per side.
4. After this, add almond milk and carefully mix the meat.
5. Close the lid and cook the pork on medium-low heat for 10 minutes.

Cumin Meatballs

Prep time: 15 minutes
Cook time: 10 minutes
Servings: 2
Ingredients:
- 1 cup ground beef
- 1 teaspoon ground cumin
- ½ teaspoon chili powder
- 1 teaspoon dried cilantro
- 1 teaspoon minced garlic
- 1 tablespoon olive oil

Method:
1. In the mixing bowl, mix ground beef with ground cumin, chili powder, dried cilantro, and minced garlic.
2. Then make the medium-size meatballs.
3. Preheat the olive oil in the skillet well.
4. Put the meatballs in the hot oil and roast them for 5 minutes per side on the medium heat.

Nutritional info per serve: Calories 198, Fat 15.5, Fiber 0.4, Carbs 1.3, Protein 13.4

Sweet Pork

Prep time: 10 minutes
Cook time: 20 minutes
Servings: 4
Ingredients:
- 1-pound pork loin, chopped
- 1 tablespoon Erythritol
- 1 tablespoon butter
- 1 teaspoon onion powder
- ½ teaspoon lemon juice

Method:
1. Mix the pork loin with Erythritol, onion powder, and lemon juice.
2. Then melt the butter in the saucepan and add pork.
3. Carefully mix the mixture and roast it for 20 minutes on the medium-high heat. Stir the meat from time to time.

Nutritional info per serve: Calories 306, Fat 18.7, Fiber 0, Carbs 2.8, Protein 31.1

Curry Meatballs

Prep time: 15 minutes
Cook time: 10 minutes
Servings: 6
Ingredients:
- 2 cups ground pork
- 1 teaspoon curry powder
- 1 teaspoon dried thyme
- 1 tablespoon coconut oil

Method:
1. Mix ground pork with curry powder and dried thyme.
2. Make the meatballs.
3. Then toss the coconut oil in the skillet and preheat it well.
4. Add the meatballs in the hot coconut oil and roast them for 4 minutes per side pr until the meatballs are tender and cooked.

Nutritional info per serve: Calories 176, Fat 13.2, Fiber 0.2, Carbs 0.3, Protein 13.5

Thyme Pork Chops

Prep time: 10 minutes
Cook time: 10 minutes
Servings: 4
Ingredients:
- 4 pork chops
- 1 tablespoon dried thyme
- 2 tablespoons olive oil
- 1 teaspoon salt

Method:
1. Rub the pork chops with dried thyme and salt.
2. Then preheat the skillet well, add olive oil and pork chops.
3. Roast the pork chops on medium-high heat for 5 minutes per side.

Nutritional info per serve: Calories 318, Fat 26.9, Fiber 0.3, Carbs 0.4, Protein 18

Fajita Pork

Prep time: 10 minutes
Cook time: 20 minutes
Servings: 6
Ingredients:
- 2 cups ground pork
- 1 teaspoon Fajita seasonings
- 2 spring onions, chopped
- 1 tablespoon coconut oil
- ¼ cup of water

Method:
1. Mix the ground pork with Fajita seasonings and chopped onion.
2. Then melt the coconut oil in the saucepan.
3. Add ground pork mixture and roast it for 10 minutes. Stir it from time to time.
4. After this, add water and carefully mix the mixture.
5. Cook the meal on medium heat for 10 minutes more.

Nutritional info per serve: Calories 339, Fat 24, Fiber 0.4, Carbs 2.1, Protein 27

Oregano Pork Chops

Prep time: 10 minutes
Cook time: 30 minutes
Servings: 4
Ingredients:
- 2 tablespoons butter
- 1 tablespoon dried oregano
- 1 tablespoon lemon juice
- 1 tablespoon sesame oil
- 4 pork chops

Method:
1. Brush the baking tray with sesame oil.
2. Then rub the pork chops with dried oregano and sprinkle with lemon juice.

3. Put the pork chops in the prepared baking tray and top them with butter.
4. Bake the pork chops in the oven at 360F for 30 minutes. Flip the pork chops on another side during cooking if needed.
Nutritional info per serve: Calories 341, Fat 29.2, Fiber 0.5, Carbs 0.8, Protein 18.2

Chili Pork Skewers

Prep time: 10 minutes
Cook time: 10 minutes
Servings: 4
Ingredients:
- 1-pound pork loin, cubed
- 1 teaspoon chili powder
- 1 tablespoon sesame oil
- ½ teaspoon ground paprika

Method:
1. Mix the pork cubes with chili powder, ground paprika, and sesame oil.
2. Then string the meat into skewers and grill it at 400F for 5 minutes per side.
Nutritional info per serve: Calories 307, Fat 19.3, Fiber 0.3, Carbs 0.5, Protein 31.1

Rosemary Pork Tenderloin

Prep time: 10 minutes
Cook time: 50 minutes
Servings: 4
Ingredients:
- 1-pound pork tenderloin
- 1 teaspoon dried rosemary
- 3 tablespoons butter

Method:
1. Chop the pork tenderloin roughly and put it in the pot.
2. Add dried rosemary and butter.
3. Bake the meat in the preheated to 360F oven for 50 minutes.
Nutritional info per serve: Calories 240, Fat 12.7, Fiber 0.1, Carbs 0.2, Protein 29.8

Paprika Pork Strips

Prep time: 10 minutes
Cook time: 20 minutes
Servings: 2
Ingredients:
- 10 oz pork loin, cut into strips
- 1 teaspoon ground paprika
- ½ teaspoon onion powder
- 1 tablespoon sesame oil
- ¼ teaspoon dried oregano

Method:
1. Preheat the sesame oil in the skillet.
2. Add pork loin strips and sprinkle them with ground paprika, onion powder, and dried oregano.
3. Roast the pork strips on medium heat for 15-18 minutes, stir them occasionally.
Nutritional info per serve: Calories 409, Fat 26.7, Fiber 0.5, Carbs 1.2, Protein 39

Jalapeno Pork Chops

Prep time: 10 minutes
Cook time: 35 minutes
Servings: 4
Ingredients:
- 4 pork chops
- 2 jalapenos, sliced
- ½ teaspoon salt
- 2 tablespoons coconut oil
- ½ teaspoon ground black pepper

Method:
1. In the mixing bowl, mix ground black pepper with coconut oil, salt, and sliced jalapeno.
2. Then line the baking tray with baking paper. Put the pork chops inside the tray.
3. After this, top every pork chop with coconut oil mixture.
4. Bake the pork chops in the preheated to 360F oven for 35 minutes.
Nutritional info per serve: Calories 317, Fat 26.7, Fiber 0.3, Carbs 0.6, Protein 18.1

Beef Lasagna

Prep time: 15 minutes
Cook time: 55 minutes
Servings: 6
Ingredients:
- 2 zucchinis, sliced
- 1 cup Cheddar cheese, shredded
- 1 tablespoon keto tomato paste
- 1 cup of water
- 1 teaspoon butter, softened
- 1 teaspoon dried basil
- 2 cups ground beef
- 1 teaspoon chili powder

Method:
1. Grease the casserole mold with butter.
2. Then make the layer from zucchini.
3. Mix ground beef with chili powder and keto tomato paste and put the mixture over the zucchinis.
4. After this, top the ground beef mixture with the layer of zucchinis and sprinkle with cheese and dried basil.
5. Add water and cover the casserole mold with foil.
6. Bake the lasagna at 360F for 55 minutes.
Nutritional info per serve: Calories 182, Fat 12.5, Fiber 1, Carbs 3.2, Protein 14.4

Nutmeg Pork Chops

Prep time: 10 minutes
Cook time: 25 minutes
Servings: 4
Ingredients:
- 4 pork chops
- 1 teaspoon ground nutmeg
- 2 scallions, sliced
- 1 tablespoon coconut oil

Method:
1. Melt the coconut oil in the skillet.
2. Sprinkle the pork chops with ground nutmeg and put in the hot coconut oil.
3. Roast the pork chops for 3 minutes per side.

4. Then add sliced scallions and close the lid.
5. Cook the pork chops for 15 minutes on the medium-low heat.
Nutritional info per serve: Calories 299, Fat 23.5, Fiber 0.7, Carbs 2.8, Protein 18.3

Chili Ground Pork

Prep time: 10 minutes
Cook time: 25 minutes
Servings: 2
Ingredients:
- 1 cup ground pork
- 1 chili pepper, chopped
- 1 tablespoon sesame oil
- ½ teaspoon keto tomato paste
- ¼ cup of water

Method:
1. Pour the sesame oil in the saucepan and preheat it well.
2. Add ground pork and chili pepper. Roast the meat for 5 minutes on the medium heat.
3. Then add keto tomato paste and water. Carefully mix the mixture and close the lid.
4. Simmer the meal on medium heat for 15 minutes.
Nutritional info per serve: Calories 527, Fat 39.3, Fiber 0.1, Carbs 0.4, Protein 40.3

Thai Style Pork

Prep time: 10 minutes
Cook time: 25 minutes
Servings: 6
Ingredients:
- 1-pound pork loin, sliced
- 1 teaspoon curry powder
- 1 teaspoon cayenne pepper
- 1 teaspoon chili flakes
- 2 tablespoons butter
- ¼ cup of water

Method:
1. Melt the butter in the saucepan.
2. Add sliced pork loin. Sprinkle the meat with curry powder, cayenne pepper, and chili flakes. Carefully mix the meat and cook it for 10 minutes.
3. Then add water and carefully mix the mixture.
4. Close the lid and cook the pork on medium heat for 10 minutes.
Nutritional info per serve: Calories 219, Fat 14.5, Fiber 0.2, Carbs 0.4, Protein 20.8

2-Meat Stew

Prep time: 10 minutes
Cook time: 50 minutes
Servings: 3
Ingredients:
- 7 oz beef sirloin, chopped
- 4 oz pork tenderloin, chopped
- 4 cups of water
- 2 oz leek, chopped
- ½ cup celery stalk, chopped
- 1 teaspoon keto tomato paste
- 1 teaspoon dried thyme

Method:
1. Put all ingredients in the saucepan and carefully mix.
2. Close the lid and cook the stew on medium-low heat for 50 minutes.
Nutritional info per serve: Calories 194, Fat 5.6, Fiber 0.8, Carbs 3.7, Protein 30.5

Pork and Vegetable Meatballs

Prep time: 10 minutes
Cook time: 25 minutes
Servings: 6
Ingredients:
- ½ cup cauliflower, shredded
- 2 cups ground pork
- 1 tablespoon almond flour
- 1 egg, beaten
- 1 teaspoon dried basil
- 1 teaspoon onion powder

Method:
1. In the mixing bowl, mix shredded cauliflower with ground pork, and almond flour.
2. Then add egg, dried basil, and onion powder.
3. Make the small meatballs from the meat mixture.
4. Line the baking tray with baking paper.
5. Put the meatballs in the tray and bake them at 360F for 25 minutes or until the meatballs are light brown.
Nutritional info per serve: Calories 351, Fat 24.7, Fiber 0.7, Carbs 1.8, Protein 28.9

Spring Onion Cubes

Prep time: 10 minutes
Cook time: 25 minutes
Servings: 4
Ingredients:
- 1-pound pork loin, cubed
- 3 spring onions, diced
- 1 tablespoon coconut oil
- 1 teaspoon cayenne pepper
- 1 teaspoon salt

Method:
1. Mix the pork loin cubes with cayenne pepper and salt.
2. Then melt the coconut oil in the saucepan.
3. Add pork loin cubes and roast them for 5 minutes per side.
4. Add diced spring onion and carefully mix the meat mixture.
5. Cook the meal on medium-low heat for 10 minutes more.
Nutritional info per serve: Calories 316, Fat 19.3, Fiber 0.7, Carbs 2.8, Protein 31.3

Pork and Mushrooms Roast

Prep time: 10 minutes
Cook time: 30 minutes
Servings: 6
Ingredients:
- 3½ pounds beef roast, chopped
- 1 cup mushrooms, chopped

- 1 teaspoon ground coriander
- 1 teaspoon ground nutmeg
- ½ teaspoon salt
- 2 tablespoons coconut oil

Method:
1. Grease the baking tray with coconut oil.
2. Then mix beef roast with ground coriander, ground nutmeg, and salt.
3. Put the meat in the baking tray and add mushrooms.
4. Bake the mixture in the preheated to 360F oven for 30 minutes. Stir the mixture from time to time to avoid burning.

Nutritional info per serve: Calories 535, Fat 21.2, Fiber 0.2, Carbs 0.6, Protein 80.7

Turmeric Beef Tenders

Prep time: 10 minutes
Cook time: 25 minutes
Servings: 4
Ingredients:
- 1-pound beef tenderloin, cut into tenders
- 1 teaspoon ground turmeric
- 1 tablespoon apple cider vinegar
- 1 teaspoon keto tomato paste
- 2 tablespoons coconut oil

Method:
1. Melt the coconut oil in the skillet.
2. Then put the meat in the hot oil and sprinkle it with ground turmeric, apple cider vinegar, and keto tomato paste.
3. Carefully mix the mixture and roast it on medium-low heat for 20 minutes.

Nutritional info per serve: Calories 296, Fat 17.2, Fiber 0.2, Carbs 0.6, Protein 32.9

Beef and Zucchini Muffins

Prep time: 10 minutes
Cook time: 25 minutes
Servings: 4
Ingredients:
- ½ cup zucchini, grated
- 1 cup ground beef
- 1 teaspoon ground black pepper
- 1 teaspoon garlic powder
- 1 tablespoon coconut flour
- 1 teaspoon salt
- 1 egg, beaten

Method:
1. In the mixing bowl, mix grated zucchini with ground beef, ground black pepper, garlic powder, salt, coconut flour, and egg.
2. After this, transfer the mixture in the muffin molds.
3. Bake the muffins for 25 minutes at 355F.

Nutritional info per serve: Calories 87, Fat 5.3, Fiber 0.4, Carbs 1.5, Protein 8.3

Tomato Pork Ribs

Prep time: 20 minutes
Cook time: 35 minutes
Servings: 6
Ingredients:
- 2-pound pork ribs, roughly chopped
- 1 tablespoon keto tomato paste
- 1 teaspoon cayenne pepper
- 3 tablespoons lemon juice
- 1 tablespoon avocado oil

Method:
1. In the mixing bowl, mix avocado oil with lemon juice, cayenne pepper, and keto tomato paste.
2. Then coat the pork ribs in the tomato mixture and leave for 10-15 minutes to marinate.
3. Roast the pork ribs in the preheated to 365F oven for 35 minutes. Flip the ribs on another side in halfway of cooking.

Nutritional info per serve: Calories 421, Fat 27.2, Fiber 0.3, Carbs 1, Protein 40.3

Pork Balls Bake

Prep time: 10 minutes
Cook time: 40 minutes
Servings: 8
Ingredients:
- 2 cups ground pork
- 1 teaspoon dried basil
- 1 teaspoon ground black pepper
- 1 teaspoon chili powder
- 1 cup Mozzarella, shredded
- ½ cup of coconut milk
- 1 teaspoon sesame oil

Method:
1. In the mixing bowl, mix ground pork, dried basil, ground black pepper, and chili powder.
2. Make the small meatballs from the mixture.
3. Brush the casserole mold with sesame oil and put the meatballs inside.
4. Add coconut milk and Mozzarella.
5. Bake the meal for 40 minutes at 355F.

Nutritional info per serve: Calories 284, Fat 21.1, Fiber 0.5, Carbs 1.3, Protein 21.5

Sage Pork Chops

Prep time: 10 minutes
Cook time: 15 minutes
Servings: 7
Ingredients:
- 7 pork chops
- 1 tablespoon dried sage
- ½ teaspoon salt
- 2 tablespoons coconut oil, melted

Method:
1. Rub the pork chops with dried sage and salt.
2. Then melt the coconut oil in the skillet.
3. Put the pork chops inside and cook them for 6 minutes per side.

Nutritional info per serve: Calories 290, Fat 23.8, Fiber 0.1, Carbs 0.2, Protein 18

Beef Stuffed Avocado

Prep time: 15 minutes
Cook time: 0 minutes
Servings: 2
Ingredients:
- 7 oz beef loin, boiled, shredded

- 1 teaspoon plain yogurt
- 1 garlic clove, diced
- 1 avocado, halved, pitted
- 1 pecan, chopped

Method:
1. Scoop ½ part of all avocado flesh and mash it.
2. Then mix mashed avocado flesh with pecan, garlic, and plain yogurt. Add shredded beef loin.
3. Fill the avocado halves with beef mixture.

Nutritional info per serve: Calories 438, Fat 32.9, Fiber 7.5, Carbs 10.3, Protein 29.5

Tomato Pulled Pork

Prep time: 15 minutes
Cook time: 50 minutes
Servings: 4
Ingredients:
- 1-pound pork shoulder
- 4 cups of water
- 1 teaspoon peppercorn
- 1 teaspoon cayenne pepper
- 1 tablespoon keto tomato paste

Method:
1. Mix water with pork shoulder and bring the mixture to boil. Add peppercorn, and cayenne pepper. Simmer it for 45 minutes.
2. After this, remove the pork shoulder from the liquid and shred it.
3. Mix the shredded pork with ½ part of the remaining liquid and keto tomato paste. Bring the mixture to boil and carefully mix.

Nutritional info per serve: Calories 337, Fat 24.4, Fiber 0.4, Carbs 1.4, Protein 26.7

Beef with Pickled Chilies

Prep time: 10 minutes
Cook time: 20 minutes
Servings: 4
Ingredients:
- 2 oz chilies, chopped, pickled
- 1 jalapeno, chopped
- 1-pound beef loin, sliced
- 1 tablespoon coconut oil
- 1 teaspoon ground paprika

Method:
1. Toss the coconut oil in the skillet.
2. Add sliced beef loin and roast it for 2 minutes per side.
3. Then sprinkle the meat with ground paprika, jalapeno, and chilies.
4. Carefully mix the meal and cook it for 15 minutes on medium heat. Stir it from time to time.

Nutritional info per serve: Calories 284, Fat 13.8, Fiber 4.4, Carbs 10.4, Protein 32

Almond Meatballs

Prep time: 15 minutes
Cook time: 15 minutes
Servings: 4
Ingredients:
- 1 cup ground beef
- 1 tablespoon almond flour
- 1 oz almonds, grinded
- 1 oz Parmesan, grated
- 1 tablespoon coconut oil

Method:
1. Mix ground beef with almond flour, almonds, and grated cheese.
2. Make the meatballs from the meat mixture.
3. Preheat the coconut oil well.
4. Put the meatballs in the hot oil and roast them for 4 minutes per side on medium heat.

Nutritional info per serve: Calories 182, Fat 15, Fiber 1.6, Carbs 3.3, Protein 10.5

Scallions Beef Meatloaf

Prep time: 10 minutes
Cook time: 50 minutes
Servings: 6
Ingredients:
- 2 oz scallions, diced
- 1 egg, beaten
- 1 teaspoon salt
- 1 teaspoon dried basil
- 2 cups ground beef
- 1 teaspoon butter, softened

Method:
1. Grease the loaf mold with butter from inside.
2. Then mix all remaining ingredients in the mixing bowl.
3. Transfer the mixture in the loaf mold and flatten well.
4. Bake the meatloaf for 50 minutes at 360F.

Nutritional info per serve: Calories 89, Fat 5.4, Fiber 0.4, Carbs 1.8, Protein 8.1

Bacon Beef

Prep time: 15 minutes
Cook time: 55 minutes
Servings: 4
Ingredients:
- 1-pound beef brisket
- 2 oz bacon, sliced
- 1 teaspoon ground cardamom
- 1 tablespoon olive oil
- 1 teaspoon salt

Method:
1. Rub the beef brisket with ground cardamom and salt.
2. Then wrap the beef in the bacon and brush with olive oil.
3. Wrap the meat in the foil and bake at 360F for 55 minutes.

Nutritional info per serve: Calories 134, Fat 8.1, Fiber 0.6, Carbs 2.7, Protein 12.2

Beef Sauce with Broccoli

Prep time: 10 minutes
Cook time: 35 minutes
Servings: 6
Ingredients:
- 1 cup broccoli, shredded
- 1-pound beef loin, diced
- 2 spring onions, diced

- 1 tablespoon keto tomato paste
- 2 cups of water
- 1 tablespoon coconut flour
- 1 teaspoon salt
- ½ teaspoon cayenne pepper

Method:
1. Mix water with beef loin in the saucepan and bring it to boil.
2. Add all remaining ingredients and carefully mix until homogenous.
3. Simmer the meal on medium heat for 25 minutes.

Nutritional info per serve: Calories 163, Fat 6.8, Fiber 1.8, Carbs 4.6, Protein 21.3

Parsley Taco Beef

Prep time: 10 minutes
Cook time: 15 minutes
Servings: 4
Ingredients:
- 1 teaspoon taco seasonings
- 1 teaspoon dried parsley
- 1-pound beef loin
- 1 tablespoon coconut oil

Method:
1. Chop the beef loin and mix it with parsley and taco seasonings.
2. Then put the meat in the hot skillet.
3. Add coconut oil and roast it for 15 minutes on medium heat. Stir the meat every 3 minutes during cooking.

Nutritional info per serve: Calories 238, Fat 12.9, Fiber 0, Carbs 0.5, Protein 30.3

Meatballs in Coconut Sauce

Prep time: 10 minutes
Cook time: 15 minutes
Servings: 6
Ingredients:
- 2 cups ground beef
- 1 teaspoon dried cilantro
- 1 teaspoon chili powder
- 1 teaspoon minced garlic
- 1 cup coconut cream
- 1 teaspoon ground turmeric
- 1 teaspoon ground coriander
- 1 tablespoon butter

Method:
1. Mix ground beef with all ingredients except butter and coconut cream.
2. Make the meatballs.
3. Melt the butter in the saucepan.
4. Add meatballs and roast them for 3 minutes per side on medium heat.
5. Then add coconut cream and close the lid.
6. Simmer the meatballs on medium heat for 10 minutes.

Nutritional info per serve: Calories 178, Fat 15.6, Fiber 1.1, Carbs 2.9, Protein 8.1

Pork Rolls

Prep time: 10 minutes
Cook time: 30 minutes
Servings: 4
Ingredients:
- 4 white cabbage leaves
- 1 cup ground pork
- 1 garlic clove, diced
- 1 teaspoon cayenne pepper
- 1 cup chicken broth
- 1 teaspoon dried dill

Method:
1. In the mixing bowl, mix ground pork with diced garlic, cayenne pepper, and dried dill.
2. Then fill the cabbage leaves with ground pork mixture and roll them.
3. Put the rolls in the casserole mold, add chicken broth, and bake at 360F for 30 minutes.

Nutritional info per serve: Calories 74, Fat 4.5, Fiber 0.6, Carbs 1.7, Protein 6.6

White Beef Soup

Prep time: 10 minutes
Cook time: 30 minutes
Servings: 8
Ingredients:
- 1 cup of coconut milk
- ½ cup fresh parsley, chopped
- 1-pound beef loin, chopped
- ½ cup celery stalk, chopped
- 1 teaspoon salt
- 1 teaspoon white pepper

Method:
1. Put all ingredients in the saucepan and stir well.
2. Simmer the soup on medium-high heat for 30 minutes.

Nutritional info per serve: Calories 156, Fat 11.3, Fiber 1, Carbs 2.9, Protein 11.3

Cardamom Sausages

Prep time: 10 minutes
Cook time: 15 minutes
Servings: 4
Ingredients:
- 1-pound pork sausages
- 1 teaspoon ground cardamom
- 1 teaspoon sesame oil
- 1 tablespoon plain yogurt

Method:
1. Mix pork sausages with plain yogurt and ground cardamom.
2. Then preheat the skillet well. Add sesame oil.
3. Add the pork sausages and roast them for 6 minutes per side.

Nutritional info per serve: Calories 399, Fat 33.4, Fiber 0.1, Carbs 0.6, Protein 22.3

Spicy Ground Beef Casserole

Prep time: 10 minutes
Cook time: 40 minutes
Servings: 6
Ingredients:
- 1 cup Mozzarella, shredded
- 1 cup ground beef

- 1 teaspoon Cajun seasonings
- 1 teaspoon sesame oil
- 1 cup asparagus, chopped
- ½ cup chicken broth

Method:
1. Brush the casserole mold with sesame oil.
2. Then mix ground beef with Cajun seasonings. Put the meat mixture in the casserole mold and flatten it gently.
3. Then top the meat with asparagus and shredded Mozzarella.
4. Add chicken broth.
5. Cook the casserole in the preheated to 360F oven for 40 minutes.

Nutritional info per serve: Calories 61, Fat 3.7, Fiber 0.5, Carbs 1.1, Protein 5.7

Marjoram Pork Tenderloin

Prep time: 10 minutes
Cook time: 40 minutes
Servings: 4
Ingredients:
- 1-pound pork tenderloin
- 1 teaspoon dried marjoram
- 1 teaspoon ground coriander
- 1 tablespoon coconut oil
- 2 tablespoons apple cider vinegar

Method:
1. Mix ground coriander with dried marjoram.
2. Then rub the pork tenderloin with the spice mixture and sprinkle with apple cider vinegar.
3. Grease the baking pan with coconut oil and put the pork tenderloin inside.
4. Cook the meat at 360F for 40 minutes in the oven.

Nutritional info per serve: Calories 193, Fat 7.4, Fiber 0.1, Carbs 0.2, Protein 29.7

Beef with Noodles

Prep time: 10 minutes
Cook time: 20 minutes
Servings: 5
Ingredients:
- 9 oz ground beef
- 1 teaspoon keto tomato paste
- 1 teaspoon ground turmeric
- 1 teaspoon ground paprika
- 1 tablespoon butter
- ½ cup of coconut milk
- 2 zucchinis, spiralized

Method:
1. Toss butter in the saucepan and melt it.
2. Add ground beef, turmeric, and paprika. Stir the mixture and cook it for 10 minutes.
3. Then mix it carefully and add keto tomato paste and coconut milk. Simmer the mixture for 5 minutes.
4. Add spiralized zucchinis and cook the meal for 3 minutes on medium heat.

Nutritional info per serve: Calories 187, Fat 11.4, Fiber 1.7, Carbs 4.7, Protein 17.1

Smoked Paprika Pork

Prep time: 10 minutes
Cook time: 45 minutes
Servings: 6
Ingredients:
- 2-pound pork butt shoulder
- 1 tablespoon smoked paprika
- 1 tablespoon sesame oil

Method:
1. Rub the pork with smoked paprika and brush it with sesame oil.
2. Wrap the meat in the foil and bake in the oven at 360F for 45 minutes.

Nutritional info per serve: Calories 419, Fat 27.6, Fiber 0.4, Carbs 0.6, Protein 39.8

Sweet Pork Belly

Prep time: 10 minutes
Cook time: 50 minutes
Servings: 4
Ingredients:
- 10 oz pork belly
- 1 tablespoon Erythritol
- 1 tablespoon butter
- 1 teaspoon chili powder

Method:
1. Melt the butter in the skillet.
2. Add pork belly and cook it for 4 minutes per side on high heat.
3. Then sprinkle the pork belly with Erythritol and chili powder and bake it in the oven at 360F for 40 minutes.

Nutritional info per serve: Calories 355, Fat 22.1, Fiber 0.2, Carbs 0.4, Protein 32.8

Dill Beef Patties

Prep time: 10 minutes
Cook time: 10 minutes
Servings: 6
Ingredients:
- 1 teaspoon ground coriander
- 1 teaspoon dried dill
- 1 teaspoon onion powder
- 2 cups ground beef
- 3 eggs, beaten
- 1 tablespoon coconut oil

Method:
1. Melt the coconut oil in the skillet.
2. Meanwhile, mix all remaining ingredients in the mixing bowl.
3. Make the patties with the help of the fingertips and put them in the hot coconut oil.
4. Roast the patties for 4 minutes per side on the medium heat.

Nutritional info per serve: Calories 152, Fat 8.4, Fiber 0, Carbs 0.6, Protein 17.8

Beef Saute

Prep time: 15 minutes
Cook time: 60 minutes
Servings: 4
Ingredients:
- 1 cup white cabbage, shredded
- 2 cups of water

- 1 teaspoon keto tomato paste
- 1 teaspoon cayenne pepper
- 1 teaspoon ground nutmeg
- 1-pound beef tenderloin, chopped
- 1 tablespoon coconut oil

Method:
1. Melt the coconut oil in the saucepan.
2. Add chopped beef and roast it for 5 minutes. Stir it well.
3. Then add all remaining ingredients and carefully mix.
4. Close the lid and cook the saute on medium-low heat for 55 minutes.

Nutritional info per serve: Calories 273, Fat 14.1, Fiber 0.7, Carbs 1.8, Protein 33.2

Beef and Broccoli Stew

Prep time: 10 minutes
Cook time: 55 minutes
Servings: 5
Ingredients:
- 2 cups broccoli, chopped
- 1-pound beef tenderloin, chopped
- 2 cups chicken broth
- 2 garlic cloves, peeled
- 1 teaspoon ground cinnamon
- 1 tablespoon sesame oil

Method:
1. Roast the beef tenderloin in the saucepan with sesame oil for 2 minutes per side.
2. Then add all remaining ingredients and carefully mix.
3. Close the lid and simmer the stew on medium-low heat for 50 minutes.

Nutritional info per serve: Calories 242, Fat 11.7, Fiber 1.3, Carbs 3.6, Protein 29.3

Cinnamon Beef Stew

Prep time: 10 minutes
Cook time: 50 minutes
Servings: 3
Ingredients:
- 8 oz beef fillet, chopped
- 1 teaspoon ground cinnamon
- 1 teaspoon chili powder
- ½ cup of coconut milk
- 1 teaspoon ground paprika
- 1 cup radish, chopped
- 1 cup of water

Method:
1. Put all ingredients in the saucepan and carefully mix.
2. Close the lid and cook the stew on medium heat for 50 minutes.

Nutritional info per serve: Calories 189, Fat 13.2, Fiber 2.5, Carbs 6.4, Protein 13.6

Beef and Eggplant Stew

Prep time: 15 minutes
Cook time: 45 minutes
Servings: 4
Ingredients:
- 1 eggplant, chopped
- 3 spring onions, chopped
- 1-pound beef loin, chopped
- 1 teaspoon keto tomato paste
- 1 teaspoon chili flakes
- 2 cups of water
- 1 teaspoon sesame oil

Method:
1. Preheat the sesame oil in the saucepan and add eggplant.
2. Roast it for 2 minutes per side and add spring onion and beef loin.
3. Stir the mixture and cook it for 6 minutes.
4. Add chili flakes, keto tomato paste, and water. Carefully mix the stew and close the lid.
5. Cook the stew on medium heat for 35 minutes.

Nutritional info per serve: Calories 220, Fat 9.5, Fiber 4.7, Carbs 10.9, Protein 22.4

Beef Rolls

Prep time: 15 minutes
Cook time: 50 minutes
Servings: 6
Ingredients:
- 1-pound beef loin
- 2 oz bacon, sliced
- 1 teaspoon cream cheese
- 1 teaspoon dried parsley
- 2 oz mozzarella, sliced
- ½ cup of water

Method:
1. Beat the beef loin with the help of the kitchen hammer to get the flat fillet.
2. Then rub the meat with dried parsley.
3. Mix cream cheese with mozzarella and put this mixture over the meat.
4. Roll the meat into a roll and wrap in the bacon.
5. Secure the meat roll with the toothpicks if needed and put in the baking pan.
6. Add water and cook the meal in the oven at 360F for 50 minutes.

Nutritional info per serve: Calories 217, Fat 12.1, Fiber 0, Carbs 0.5, Protein 26.4

Mint Lamb Chops

Prep time: 10 minutes
Cook time: 10 minutes
Servings: 4
Ingredients:
- 1 teaspoon dried mint
- 4 lamb chops
- ½ teaspoon salt
- 1 tablespoon avocado oil

Method:
1. Preheat the avocado oil well.
2. Rub the lamb chops with dried mint and salt.
3. Then put the meat in the hot oil and roast them for 5 minutes per side on the medium heat.

Nutritional info per serve: Calories 163, Fat 6.7, Fiber 0.2, Carbs 0.2, Protein 23.9

Chipotle Lamb Ribs

Prep time: 15 minutes
Cook time: 20 minutes
Servings: 6
Ingredients:
- 2-pound lamb ribs
- 1 tablespoon chipotle pepper, minced
- 2 tablespoons sesame oil
- 1 teaspoon apple cider vinegar

Method:
1. Mix lamb ribs with all ingredients and leave to marinate for 10 minutes.
2. Then transfer the lamb ribs and all marinade in the baking tray and cook the meat in the oven at 360F for 40 minutes. Flip the ribs on another side after 20 minutes of cooking.

Nutritional info per serve: Calories 392, Fat 24.7, Fiber 0, Carbs 0.2, Protein 39.6

Lamb and Pecan Salad

Prep time: 10 minutes
Cook time: 10 minutes
Servings: 4
Ingredients:
- 2 lamb chops
- 1 tablespoon sesame oil
- 2 pecans, chopped
- 2 cups lettuce, chopped
- 1 teaspoon cayenne pepper
- 1 tablespoon avocado oil

Method:
1. Sprinkle the lamb chops with cayenne pepper and put in the hot skillet.
2. Add sesame oil and roast the meat for 4 minutes per side.
3. Then chops the lamb chops and put them in the salad bowl.
4. Add all remaining ingredients and carefully mix the salad.

Nutritional info per serve: Calories 168, Fat 12.1, Fiber 1., Carbs 2.3, Protein 12.9

Lime Ribs

Prep time: 10 minutes
Cook time: 10 minutes
Servings: 6
Ingredients:
- 3-pounds pork ribs, chopped
- 2 tablespoons lime juice
- 1 teaspoon lime zest, grated
- 2 tablespoons sesame seeds
- ½ teaspoon salt
- ½ teaspoon ground black pepper

Method:
1. In the shallow bowl, mix lime juice, lime zest, sesame seeds, salt, and ground black pepper.
2. Mix the pork ribs with lime juice mixture and grill in the preheated to 390F grill for 5 minutes per side.

Nutritional info per serve: Calories 638, Fat 41.7, Fiber 0.5, Carbs 1.2, Protein 60.6

Hot Sauce Lamb

Prep time: 10 minutes
Cook time: 35 minutes
Servings: 4
Ingredients:
- 2 teaspoons paprika
- 1-pound lamb fillet, chopped
- 1 tablespoon coconut oil
- 4 tablespoons keto hot sauce
- ½ cup of water

Method:
1. Pour water in the saucepan and bring it to boil.
2. Add lamb and boil it for 20 minutes.
3. After this, preheat the skillet well.
4. Add boiled lamb fillet, coconut oil, and paprika.
5. Roast the ingredients for 6 minutes per side or until the meat is light brown.
6. Then add hot sauce and carefully mix the meal.

Nutritional info per serve: Calories 245, Fat 11.9, Fiber 0.4, Carbs 0.8, Protein 32.1

Paprika Beef Steaks

Prep time: 15 minutes
Cook time: 15 minutes
Servings: 2
Ingredients:
- 2 beef steaks (7 oz each)
- 1 teaspoon smoked paprika
- 1 tablespoon olive oil
- 1 teaspoon dried basil

Method:
1. Rub the beef steaks with smoked paprika, dried basil, and olive oil.
2. Then preheat the skillet well.
3. Roast the beef steaks for 6 minutes per side.

Nutritional info per serve: Calories 432, Fat 19.5, Fiber 0.4, Carbs 0.6, Protein 60.4

Mustard Lamb Chops

Prep time: 10 minutes
Cook time: 40 minutes
Servings: 4
Ingredients:
- 1 cup spinach
- 3 tablespoons mustard
- 2 tablespoons sesame oil
- ½ teaspoon ground turmeric
- 4 lamb chops

Method:
1. Blend the spinach and mix it with mustard, sesame oil, and ground turmeric.
2. Then rub the lamb chops with the mustard mixture and put in the baking pan.
3. Bake the meat at 355F for 40 minutes. Flip the meat after 20 minutes of cooking.

Nutritional info per serve: Calories 102, Fat 9.3, Fiber 1.5, Carbs 3.4, Protein 2.3

Masala Ground Pork

Prep time: 10 minutes
Cook time: 15 minutes

Servings: 4
Ingredients:
- 2 cups ground pork
- 1 teaspoon garam masala
- 1 tablespoon avocado oil
- ½ cup plain yogurt

Method:
1. Mix garam masala with plain yogurt.
2. Preheat the avocado oil in the saucepan well.
3. Add ground pork and cook it for 5 minutes.
4. Then add yogurt mixture, carefully mix it, and simmer for 10 minutes on medium heat.

Nutrition value/serving Calories 141, Fat 8.8, Fiber 0.2, Carbs 2.4, Protein 11.8

Ginger Lamb Chops

Prep time: 15 minutes
Cook time: 30 minutes
Servings: 6
Ingredients:
- 6 lamb chops
- 1 tablespoon keto tomato paste
- 1 teaspoon minced ginger
- 2 tablespoons avocado oil
- 1 teaspoon plain yogurt

Method:
1. Mix plain yogurt with keto tomato paste and minced ginger.
2. Then put the lamb chops in the yogurt mixture and marinate for 10-15 minutes.
3. After this, transfer the mixture in the tray, add avocado oil, and cook the meat at 360F in the oven for 30 minutes.

Nutritional info per serve: Calories 330, Fat 26.6, Fiber 0.4, Carbs 1, Protein 19.3

Parmesan Lamb

Prep time: 10 minutes
Cook time: 20 minutes
Servings: 4
Ingredients:
- 4 lamb chops
- 2 oz Parmesan, grated
- ½ cup plain yogurt
- 3 scallions, sliced
- 1 tablespoon butter, softened

Method:
1. Melt the butter in the saucepan. Add scallions and roast it for 3-4 minutes.
2. Then stir the scallions and add lamb chops.
3. Roast them for 2 minutes per side.
4. Add yogurt and close the lid. Cook the meat for 10 minutes.
5. After this, top the meat with Parmesan and cook it for 2 minutes more.

Nutritional info per serve: Calories 262, Fat 12.6, Fiber 0.6, Carbs 5.2, Protein 30.5

Clove Lamb

Prep time: 10 minutes
Cook time: 25 minutes
Servings: 4
Ingredients:
- 1 teaspoon ground clove
- 2 tablespoons butter
- 1 teaspoon ground paprika
- 1 teaspoon dried rosemary
- ¼ cup of water
- 12 oz lamb fillet

Method:
1. In the shallow bowl, mix ground clove with ground paprika, and dried rosemary.
2. Rub the lamb fillet with spices and grease with butter.
3. Then put the meat in the hot skillet and roast it for 5 minutes per side on the low heat.
4. Add water. Close the lid and cook the lamb on medium heat for 15 minutes.

Nutritional info per serve: Calories 55, Fat 6, Fiber 0.5, Carbs 0.8, Protein 0.2

Carrot Lamb Roast

Prep time: 10 minutes
Cook time: 40 minutes
Servings: 4
Ingredients:
- 1-pound lamb loin
- 1 carrot, chopped
- 1 teaspoon dried thyme
- 2 tablespoons coconut oil
- 1 teaspoon salt

Method:
1. Put all ingredients in the baking tray, mix well.
2. Bake the mixture in the preheated to 360F oven for 40 minutes.

Nutritional info per serve: Calories 295, Fat 17.9, Fiber 0.5, Carbs 1.7, Protein 30.3

Lamb and Celery Casserole

Prep time: 10 minutes
Cook time: 45 minutes
Servings: 2
Ingredients:
- ¼ cup celery stalk, chopped
- 2 lamb chops, chopped
- ½ cup Mozzarella, shredded
- 1 teaspoon butter
- ¼ cup coconut cream
- 1 teaspoon taco seasonings

Method:
1. Mix lamb chops with taco seasonings and put in the casserole mold.
2. Add celery stalk, coconut cream, and shredded mozzarella.
3. Then add butter and cook the casserole in the preheated to 360F oven for 45 minutes.

Nutritional info per serve: Calories 283, Fat 19.3, Fiber 0.9, Carbs 3.3, Protein 24.8

Lamb in Almond Sauce

Prep time: 10 minutes
Cook time: 30 minutes
Servings: 6
Ingredients:

- 14 oz lamb fillet, cubed
- 1 cup organic almond milk
- 1 teaspoon almond flour
- 1 teaspoon ground nutmeg
- ½ teaspoon ground cardamom
- 1 tablespoon olive oil
- 1 tablespoon lemon juice
- 1 tablespoon butter
- ½ teaspoon minced garlic

Method:
1. Preheat the olive oil in the saucepan.
2. Meanwhile, mix lamb, ground nutmeg, ground cardamom, and minced garlic.
3. Put the lamb in the hot olive oil. Roast the meat for 2 minutes per side.
4. Then add butter, lemon juice, and almond milk. Carefully mix the mixture.
5. Cook the meal for 15 minutes on medium heat.
6. Then add almond flour, stir well and simmer the meal for 10 minutes more.

Nutritional info per serve: Calories 258, Fat 19, Fiber 1.1, Carbs 2.7, Protein 19.7

Sweet Leg of Lamb

Prep time: 10 minutes
Cook time: 45 minutes
Servings: 6
Ingredients:
- 2 pounds lamb leg
- 1 tablespoon Erythritol
- 3 tablespoons coconut milk
- 1 teaspoon chili flakes
- 1 teaspoon ground turmeric
- 1 teaspoon cayenne pepper
- 3 tablespoons coconut oil

Method:
1. In the shallow bowl, mix cayenne pepper, ground turmeric, chili flakes, and Erythritol.
2. Rub the lamb leg with spices.
3. Melt the coconut oil in the saucepan.
4. Add lamb leg and roast it for 10 minutes per side on low heat.
5. After this, add coconut milk and cook the meal for 30 minutes on low heat. Flip the meat on another side from time to time.

Nutritional info per serve: Calories 350, Fat 18.8, Fiber 0.3, Carbs 0.8, Protein 42.8

Coconut Lamb Shoulder

Prep time: 10 minutes
Cook time: 75 minutes
Servings: 5
Ingredients:
- 2-pound lamb shoulder
- 1 teaspoon ground cumin
- 2 tablespoons butter
- ¼ cup of coconut milk
- 1 teaspoon coconut shred
- ½ cup kale, chopped

Method:
1. Put all ingredients in the saucepan and mix well.
2. Close the lid and cook the meal on low heat for 75 minutes.

Nutritional info per serve: Calories 414, Fat 21.2, Fiber 0.5, Carbs 1.7, Protein 51.5

Lavender Lamb

Prep time: 10 minutes
Cook time: 35 minutes
Servings: 4
Ingredients:
- 4 lamb chops
- 1 teaspoon dried lavender
- 2 tablespoons butter
- 1 teaspoon cumin seeds
- 1 cup of water

Method:
1. Toss the butter in the saucepan and melt it.
2. Add lamb chops and roast them for 3 minutes.
3. Then add dried lavender, cumin seeds, and water.
4. Close the lid and cook the meat for 30 minutes on medium-low heat.

Nutritional info per serve: Calories 211, Fat 12.1, Fiber 0.1, Carbs 0.2, Protein 24

Dill Lamb Shank

Prep time: 10 minutes
Cook time: 40 minutes
Servings: 3
Ingredients:
- 3 lamb shanks (4 oz each)
- 1 tablespoon dried dill
- 1 teaspoon peppercorns
- 3 cups of water
- 1 carrot, chopped
- 1 teaspoon salt

Method:
1. Bring the water to boil.
2. Add lamb shank, dried dill, peppercorns, carrot, and salt.
3. Close the lid and cook the meat in medium heat for 40 minutes.

Nutritional info per serve: Calories 224, Fat 84, Fiber 0.8, Carbs 3, Protein 32.3

Mexican Lamb Chops

Prep time: 10 minutes
Cook time: 15 minutes
Servings: 4
Ingredients:
- 4 lamb chops
- 1 tablespoon Mexican seasonings
- 2 tablespoons sesame oil
- 1 teaspoon butter

Method:
1. Rub the lamb chops with Mexican seasonings.
2. Then melt the butter in the skillet. Add sesame oil.
3. Then add lamb chops and roast them for 7 minutes per side on medium heat.

Nutritional info per serve: Calories 323, Fat 14, Fiber 0, Carbs 1.1, Protein 24.1

Tender Lamb Stew

Prep time: 10 minutes
Cook time: 60 minutes
Servings: 4
Ingredients:
- 1-pound lamb fillet, chopped
- 3 cups of water
- 1 zucchini, chopped
- ½ cup leek, chopped
- 1 teaspoon ground paprika
- 1 teaspoon cayenne pepper
- 1 teaspoon salt
- 1 teaspoon butter

Method:
1. Put all ingredients in the saucepan. Mix the mixture and close the lid.
2. Cook the stew on medium-low heat for 60 minutes.

Nutritional info per serve: Calories 237, Fat 9.5, Fiber 1.1, Carbs 3.8, Protein 32.7

Lime Lamb

Prep time: 10 minutes
Cook time: 40 minutes
Servings: 4
Ingredients:
- 2 lamb shanks
- ½ lime
- 1 teaspoon salt
- 1 teaspoon Erythritol
- 3 tablespoons butter

Method:
1. Melt the butter in the saucepan.
2. Add lamb shanks in the hot butter and roast them for 5 minutes per side on the medium heat.
3. Then sprinkle the meat with salt and Erythritol.
4. Close the lid and simmer the meat on low heat for 30 minutes.

Nutritional info per serve: Calories 158, Fat 11.8, Fiber 0.2, Carbs 2.1, Protein 12.1

Basil Meatloaf

Prep time: 10 minutes
Cook time: 40 minutes
Servings: 8
Ingredients:
- 2-pounds ground beef
- 2 eggs, beaten
- 1 teaspoon dried basil
- ½ teaspoon salt
- 3 tablespoons almond flour
- 1 teaspoon butter, softened

Method:
1. Grease the loaf mold with butter.
2. Then mix all remaining ingredients in the mixing bowl.
3. Transfer the meat mixture into the mold and flatten the surface of it.
4. Bake the meatloaf for 40 minutes at 360F.

Nutritional info per serve: Calories 246, Fat 10, Fiber 0.3, Carbs 0.6, Protein 36.4

Lamb Saute with Mint and Lemon

Prep time: 10 minutes
Cook time: 45 minutes
Servings: 4
Ingredients:
- 1-pound lamb fillet
- 1 teaspoon dried mint
- 1 teaspoon lemon zest, grated
- 2 cups of water
- 1 carrot, chopped
- 1 teaspoon keto tomato paste
- 1 teaspoon cayenne pepper

Method:
1. Chop the lamb fillet roughly and put it in the saucepan.
2. Roast the meat for 2 minutes per side.
3. Add dried mint, lemon zest, carrot, keto tomato paste, and cayenne pepper.
4. Then add water and carefully stir the ingredients.
5. Close the lid and cook the saute on medium heat for 40 minutes.

Nutritional info per serve: Calories 220, Fat 8.4, Fiber 0.6, Carbs 2.1, Protein 32.1

Pancetta Lamb

Prep time: 10 minutes
Cook time: 35 minutes
Servings: 5
Ingredients:
- 1-pound lamb fillet
- 2 oz pancetta, sliced
- 1 teaspoon chili powder
- 1 teaspoon ground turmeric
- 1 tablespoon coconut oil

Method:
1. Cut the lamb fillet into 5 servings.
2. Then mix meat with chili powder and ground turmeric.
3. After this, wrap every lamb fillet with pancetta.
4. Preheat the coconut oil in the skillet.
5. Add meat and roast it for 3 minutes.
6. After this, transfer the meat in the preheated to 360F oven and cook for 30 minutes.

Nutritional info per serve: Calories 257, Fat 14.2, Fiber 0.3, Carbs 0.7, Protein 29.8

Sweet Lamb with Oregano

Prep time: 10 minutes
Cook time: 25 minutes
Servings: 4
Ingredients:
- 1-pound lamb fillet, sliced
- 1 teaspoon dried oregano
- 1 teaspoon Erythritol
- 3 tablespoons butter
- 1 tablespoon apple cider vinegar

Method:
1. Melt butter in the saucepan.

2. Add dried oregano, Erythritol, and apple cider vinegar. Bring the liquid to boil.
3. Add sliced lamb fillet and roast it for 20 minutes. Stir the meat from time to time.
Nutritional info per serve: Calories 289, Fat 17, Fiber 0.2, Carbs 1.5, Protein 32

Keto Pie

Prep time: 10 minutes
Cook time: 40 minutes
Servings: 8
Ingredients:
- 15 oz pork steak, cubed
- 2 spring onions, diced
- 1 tablespoon coconut oil
- 1 teaspoon salt
- 1 teaspoon chili flakes
- ½ teaspoon smoked paprika
- ¾ cup coconut cream
- 1 cup coconut flour
- 1 egg, beaten
- 4 tablespoons organic almond milk
- 1 teaspoon sesame oil
- 1 teaspoon ground coriander

Method:
1. Melt the coconut oil in the skillet.
2. Then mix pork with diced spring onion, salt, chili flakes, and smoked paprika. Put the meat in the hot coconut oil and roast for 10 minutes on the medium heat.
3. Meanwhile, make the dough: mix coconut flour with coconut cream, egg, and ground coriander. Knead the dough.
4. After this, transfer the dough in the non-stick baking pan and flatten in the shape of the pie crust.
5. Then sprinkle the pie crust with sesame oil and put the meat mixture inside. Add organic almond milk.
6. Bake the pie at 355F for 40 minutes.
Nutritional info per serve: Calories 173, Fat 12.3, Fiber 1.5, Carbs 3.7, Protein 12

Veal and Cabbage Salad

Prep time: 10 minutes
Cook time: 0 minutes
Servings: 4
Ingredients:
- 1-pound veal, boiled, chopped
- 1 cup white cabbage, shredded
- 1 tablespoon olive oil
- 1 teaspoon apple cider vinegar
- 1 teaspoon dried dill
- 1 teaspoon salt

Method:
1. Put all ingredients in the salad bowl.
2. Carefully mix the salad.
Nutritional info per serve: Calories 230, Fat 12.1, Fiber 0.5, Carbs 1.2, Protein 27.9

Nutmeg Lamb

Prep time: 15 minutes
Cook time: 25 minutes
Servings: 4
Ingredients:
- 13 oz rack of lamb
- 1 teaspoon ground nutmeg
- 1 tablespoon coconut oil
- ½ teaspoon ground black pepper

Method:
1. Rub the lamb with ground nutmeg and ground black pepper.
2. Then melt the coconut oil in the skillet.
3. Add rack of lamb and roast it on medium heat for 10 minutes per side.
Nutritional info per serve: Calories 188, Fat 11.8, Fiber 0.2, Carbs 0.4, Protein 18.8

Thyme Beef

Prep time: 10 minutes
Cook time: 40 minutes
Servings: 8
Ingredients:
- 3-pounds beef brisket, chopped
- 1 tablespoon dried thyme
- 3 tablespoons avocado oil
- 1 tablespoon apple cider vinegar

Method:
1. Mix the beef brisket with dried thyme, avocado oil, and apple cider vinegar. Wrap the meat in the foil.
2. Bake the meal at 360F for 40 minutes.
3. Then slice the cooked beef.
Nutritional info per serve: Calories 324, Fat 11.3, Fiber 0.4, Carbs 0.5, Protein 51.7

Sausage Casserole

Prep time: 10 minutes
Cook time: 40 minutes
Servings: 6
Ingredients:
- 1-pound beef sausages, chopped
- 2 scallions, sliced
- 1 chili pepper, chopped
- 1 tablespoon butter, softened
- 1 teaspoon chili powder
- 2 oz Parmesan, grated
- ½ cup chicken broth

Method:
1. Grease the casserole mold with butter and put the sausages inside.
2. Then top the sausages with scallions, chili pepper, and chicken broth.
3. Add Parmesan and bake the casserole in the preheated to 365F oven for 40 minutes.
Nutritional info per serve: Calories 432, Fat 15.1, Fiber 0.5, Carbs 0.7, Protein 68.9

Onion Beef Roast

Prep time: 10 minutes
Cook time: 55 minutes
Servings: 8
Ingredients:
- 5-pound beef loin, chopped
- 2 spring onions, sliced
- 2 tablespoons coconut oil

- 1 teaspoon ginger powder
- 1 teaspoon dried oregano

Method:
1. Grease the baking tray with coconut oil and put the chopped beef inside.
2. Then sprinkle the beef with sliced spring onion, ginger powder, and dried oregano.
3. Cover the ingredients with foil and bake in the oven at 360F for 55 minutes.

Nutritional info per serve: Calories 458, Fat 23.7, Fiber 0.4, Carbs 4.9, Protein 52.5

Cajun Pork

Prep time: 10 minutes
Cook time: 20 minutes
Servings: 4
Ingredients:
- 1-pound pork tenderloin, sliced
- 1 teaspoon Cajun seasonings
- 1 teaspoon keto tomato paste
- 2 tablespoons coconut oil, melted

Method:
1. Mix the pork tenderloin with Cajun seasonings and put in the preheated skillet.
2. Add coconut oil and roast the meat for 10 minutes. Stir it from time to time.
3. Then add keto tomato paste and carefully mix the meat.
4. Roast the Cajun pork for 10 minutes more over the medium-high heat.

Nutritional info per serve: Calories 222, Fat 10.8, Fiber 0.1, Carbs 0.3, Protein 29.8

Beef and Chili

Prep time: 10 minutes
Cook time: 25 minutes
Servings: 4
Ingredients:
- 2 chili peppers, chopped
- 1-pound beef tenderloin, chopped
- 1 teaspoon garlic powder
- 1 tablespoon butter
- ½ teaspoon chili powder

Method:
1. Melt butter in the saucepan and add chopped beef.
2. Then sprinkle the meat with chili powder and garlic powder; roast the meat for 10 minutes on the medium heat. Stir it from time to time.
3. Then add chili peppers and carefully mix the meal. Close the lid.
4. Cook the meal on medium heat for 10 minutes.

Nutritional info per serve: Calories 263, Fat 13.3, Fiber 0.3, Carbs 0.9, Protein 33.1

Beef Loin in Parmesan Sauce

Prep time: 10 minutes
Cook time: 25 minutes
Servings: 4
Ingredients:
- 1 oz Parmesan, grated
- ½ cup coconut cream
- ½ teaspoon ground black pepper
- ½ teaspoon onion powder
- 1 tablespoon avocado oil
- 1-pound beef loin, cubed
- ½ teaspoon dried rosemary

Method:
1. Mix beef loin with dried rosemary and avocado oil.
2. Roast the meat for 10 minutes on medium heat.
3. Add coconut cream, ground black pepper, and onion powder. Stir the meal and close the lid.
4. Simmer the meat on medium heat for 15 minutes, stir it from time to time.

Nutritional info per serve: Calories 305, Fat 18.6, Fiber 1, Carbs 2.6, Protein 33.4

Coconut Pork Bowl

Prep time: 10 minutes
Cook time: 25 minutes
Servings: 4
Ingredients:
- 1-pound pork loin, sliced
- 1 tablespoon coconut shred
- 1 teaspoon onion powder
- 1 tablespoon coconut oil
- ¼ cup of coconut milk
- 1 teaspoon ground cumin

Method:
1. Put all ingredients in the saucepan and carefully mix.
2. Close the lid and cook the meal on medium-high heat for 25 minutes.

Nutritional info per serve: Calories 305, Fat 18.6, Fiber 1, Carbs 2.6, Protein 33.4

BBQ Pork Ribs

Prep time: 15 minutes
Cook time: 25 minutes
Servings: 4
Ingredients:
- 3 oz Keto BBQ sauce
- 1-pound pork ribs, chopped
- 1 tablespoon olive oil

Method:
1. Roast the pork ribs in the olive oil for 5 minutes per side.
2. Then add Keto BBQ sauce and carefully mix the pork ribs.
3. Bake them in the oven at 360F for 15 minutes.

Nutritional info per serve: Calories 371, Fat 23.6, Fiber 0.1, Carbs 7.7, Protein 30

Sausage Stew with Turnip

Prep time: 10 minutes
Cook time: 35 minutes
Servings: 4
Ingredients:
- 1-pound pork sausages, chopped
- ½ cup chicken broth
- ½ cup turnip, chopped
- 1 tablespoon sesame oil

- 1 teaspoon ground paprika
- 1 teaspoon dried basil

Method:
1. Roast the pork sausages in the sesame oil for 5 minutes per side.
2. Then add all remaining ingredients and close the lid.
3. Cook the stew on medium heat for 30 minutes.

Nutritional info per serve: Calories 425, Fat 35.8, Fiber 0.5, Carbs 1.5, Protein 22.9

Butter Beef

Prep time: 10 minutes
Cook time: 30 minutes
Servings: 2
Ingredients:
- 8 oz beef loin, sliced
- 4 tablespoons butter
- 1 teaspoon ground black pepper
- 1 teaspoon salt

Method:
1. Melt the butter in the saucepan.
2. Add beef loin, ground black pepper, and salt.
3. Simmer the beef for 30 minutes on medium heat. Stir it from time to time during cooking.

Nutritional info per serve: Calories 413, Fat 32.5, Fiber 0.3, Carbs 0.7, Protein 30.7

Spicy Beef

Prep time: 10 minutes
Cook time: 50 minutes
Servings: 7
Ingredients:
- 2-pound beef chuck roast, cubed
- 1 teaspoon dried sage
- 1 teaspoon dried rosemary
- ½ teaspoon ground cardamom
- 3 tablespoons butter

Method:
1. Rub the beef chuck roast with dried sage, dried rosemary, and ground cardamom.
2. Then put the meat in the roast pan. Add butter.
3. Bake the meat at 360F for 50 minutes.

Nutritional info per serve: Calories 515, Fat 41, Fiber 0.2, Carbs 0.3, Protein 34

Tender Indian Pork

Prep time: 10 minutes
Cook time: 35 minutes
Servings: 2
Ingredients:
- 1 teaspoon curry paste
- 8 oz pork loin, chopped
- 2 tablespoons coconut cream
- ¼ teaspoon minced garlic
- 1 teaspoon avocado oil

Method:
1. Roast the pork loin in avocado oil for 2 minutes per side.
2. Then sprinkle it with coconut cream, minced garlic, and curry paste. Carefully mix the meat mixture.
3. Close the lid and cook the pork on medium-high heat for 30 minutes.

Nutritional info per serve: Calories 329, Fat 21.1, Fiber 0.4, Carbs 1.8, Protein 31.5

Keto Beef

Prep time: 10 minutes
Cook time: 14 minutes
Servings: 8
Ingredients:
- 2-pounds beef loin, chopped
- 1 tablespoon keto seasonings
- 2 tablespoons avocado oil

Method:
1. Mix the beef loin with keto seasonings and sprinkle with avocado oil.
2. Grilled the chopped meat in the preheated to 400F grill for 7 minutes per side.

Nutritional info per serve: Calories 173, Fat 8.5, Fiber 0.2, Carbs 1.6, Protein 21

Bergamot Pork

Prep time: 10 minutes
Cook time: 25 minutes
Servings: 4
Ingredients:
- 1 teaspoon ground bergamot
- 2 tablespoons butter
- ½ teaspoon salt
- ½ teaspoon chili flakes
- 1-pound pork tenderloin, sliced

Method:
1. Melt the butter. Add bergamot and bring the butter to boil.
2. Add salt, chili flakes, and sliced pork tenderloin.
3. Roast the meat for 5 minutes per side.
4. Then close the lid and cook it for 10 minutes on low heat.

Nutritional info per serve: Calories 213, Fat 9.7, Fiber 0, Carbs 0, Protein 29.7

Wrapped Ham Bites

Prep time: 10 minutes
Cook time: 0 minutes
Servings: 6
Ingredients:
- 6 ham slices, cooked
- 6 Cheddar cheese slices
- 1 teaspoon lemon juice

Method:
1. Wrap the ham slices in the cheese slices and secure with toothpicks.
2. Sprinkle the ham bites with lemon juice before serving.

Nutritional info per serve: Calories 159, Fat 11.7, Fiber 0.4, Carbs 1.5, Protein 11.6

Avocado and Meat Salad

Prep time: 10 minutes

Cook time: 0 minutes
Servings: 4
Ingredients:
- 1 avocado, sliced
- 10 oz pork loin, boiled, chopped
- 1 cup baby spinach, chopped
- 1 teaspoon mustard
- 2 tablespoons coconut cream
- ¼ teaspoon minced garlic

Method:
1. Put all ingredients in the salad bowl.
2. Shake the salad until homogenous.

Nutritional info per serve: Calories 297, Fat 21.7, Fiber 3.8, Carbs 5.4, Protein 20.9

Tender Veal

Prep time: 8 hours
Cook time: 40 minutes
Servings: 5
Ingredients:
- 1-pound veal
- 2 cups of water
- 1 teaspoon garam masala
- ½ teaspoon salt

Method:
1. Pour water in the saucepan.
2. Add salt, garam masala, and veal.
3. Close the lid and cook the veal for 30 minutes.
4. Then cover the saucepan with a towel and leave for 8 hours.

Nutritional info per serve: Calories 156, Fat 6.8, Fiber 0, Carbs 0, Protein 22.1

Oil and Herbs Lamb

Prep time: 10 minutes
Cook time: 65 minutes
Servings: 4
Ingredients:
- 11 oz rack of lamb, trimmed
- 3 tablespoons olive oil
- 1 tablespoon Italian seasonings

Method:
1. Mix the Italian seasonings with olive oil.
2. Then sprinkle the rack of lamb with oily mixture and bake in the oven at 360F for 65 minutes.
3. Slice the cooked lamb.

Nutritional info per serve: Calories 232, Fat 18.4, Fiber 0, Carbs 0.4, Protein 15.9

Sage Beef

Prep time: 10 minutes
Cook time: 35 minutes
Servings: 4
Ingredients:
- 1-pound beef brisket, chopped
- 1 tablespoon dried sage
- ¼ cup of water
- 1 tablespoon avocado oil

Method:
1. Roast the beef brisket in avocado oil for 5 minutes per side.
2. Then add dried sage and water.
3. Close the lid and simmer the meat for 25 minutes on medium heat.

Nutritional info per serve: Calories 217, Fat 17.6, Fiber 0.4, Carbs 0.5, Protein 34.5

Anise Beef

Prep time: 10 minutes
Cook time: 15 minutes
Servings: 4
Ingredients:
- 1-pound beef brisket, sliced
- 1 tablespoon ground anise
- 3 tablespoons butter
- ½ teaspoon salt

Method:
1. Melt the butter in the saucepan.
2. Add ground anise and salt.
3. Then add beef brisket and carefully mix.
4. Roast the beef for 7 minutes per side on medium heat.

Nutritional info per serve: Calories 287, Fat 15.7, Fiber 0, Carbs 0, Protein 34.5

Spearmint Veal

Prep time: 10 minutes
Cook time: 45 minutes
Servings: 6
Ingredients:
- 1 tablespoon dried spearmint
- 1 teaspoon ground turmeric
- ½ teaspoon onion powder
- 1-pound veal, sliced
- 3 cups of water
- 1 tablespoon sesame oil

Method:
1. Roast the veal in sesame oil for 2 minutes per side.
2. Add all remaining ingredients and close the lid.
3. Cook the veal on medium heat for 40 minutes.

Nutritional info per serve: Calories 152, Fat 8, Fiber 0.2, Carbs 0.5, Protein 18.5

Garlic Pork Ribs

Prep time: 10 minutes
Cook time: 15 minutes
Servings: 4
Ingredients:
- 1-pound pork baby back ribs
- 1 tablespoon minced garlic
- 4 tablespoons butter
- 1 tablespoon dried dill

Method:
1. Rub the pork ribs with minced garlic and dried dill and put in a hot skillet.
2. Roast the pork ribs for 2 minutes per side.
3. Then add butter and cook the pork ribs for 5 minutes per side.

Nutritional info per serve: Calories 521, Fat 45.3, Fiber 0.2, Carbs 1.1, Protein 26.1

Veal and Sorrel Saute

Prep time: 10 minutes
Cook time: 65 minutes
Servings: 2
Ingredients:
- 8 oz veal, chopped
- 1 cup sorrel, chopped
- 1 cup of water
- 1 teaspoon keto tomato paste
- 1 teaspoon cayenne pepper
- 1 teaspoon salt
- 1 spring onion, sliced

Method:
1. Put all ingredients in the pot and gently mix.
2. Close the lid and bake the saute in the preheated to 360F oven for 65 minutes.

Nutritional info per serve: Calories 225, Fat 9.2, Fiber 2.9, Carbs 5.7, Protein 29.5

Creamy Pork Skewers

Prep time: 15 minutes
Cook time: 10 minutes
Servings: 4
Ingredients:
- 1 teaspoon chili powder
- ¼ cup coconut cream
- 1 teaspoon mustard
- 12 oz pork tenderloin, roughly cubed
- 1 teaspoon avocado

Method:
1. Mix pork tenderloin with avocado oil, mustard, coconut cream, and chili powder.
2. Then string the pork into the skewers and grill in the preheated to 360F grill for 5 minutes per side.

Nutritional info per serve: Calories 164, Fat 7.1, Fiber 0.7, Carbs 1.6, Protein 22.9

Grilled Pork Sausage

Prep time: 10 minutes
Cook time: 10 minutes
Servings: 6
Ingredients:
- 2-pounds pork sausages
- ½ teaspoon ground coriander
- 1 tablespoon avocado oil

Method:
1. Sprinkle the pork sausages with ground coriander and avocado oil.
2. Grill the sausages for 5 minutes per side at 400F.

Nutritional info per serve: Calories 516, Fat 43.2, Fiber 0.1, Carbs 0.1, Protein 29.4

Allspice Pork

Prep time: 10 minutes
Cook time: 20 minutes
Servings: 1
Ingredients:
- 5 oz pork tenderloin, chopped
- 1 teaspoon allspices
- 1 tablespoon coconut oil

Method:
1. Melt the coconut oil in the skillet. Add pork tenderloin and allspices and roast the meat for 20 minutes on the medium heat. Stir the meat from time to time to avoid burning.

Nutritional info per serve: Calories 325, Fat 18.8, Fiber 0.4, Carbs 1.4, Protein 37.2

Hot Sauce Sausage

Prep time: 10 minutes
Cook time: 25 minutes
Servings: 4
Ingredients:
- 1-pound pork sausages
- 1 teaspoon chili powder
- 1 teaspoon keto tomato paste
- 1 tablespoon avocado oil
- ½ teaspoon minced garlic
- ¼ cup of water

Method:
1. Mix avocado oil with minced garlic, water, keto tomato paste, and chili powder.
2. Then pour the liquid in the saucepan and bring to boil.
3. Add pork sausages and simmer them for 25 minutes on medium heat.

Nutritional info per serve: Calories 393, Fat 32.7, Fiber 0.4, Carbs 0.9, Protein 22.2

Tomato Beef Bake

Prep time: 15 minutes
Cook time: 50 minutes
Servings: 4
Ingredients:
- 1-pound beef tenderloin
- 1 tablespoon coconut oil
- 1 teaspoon ground black pepper
- 1 tomato, sliced
- ½ cup Cheddar cheese, shredded

Method:
1. Grease the ramekins with coconut oil.
2. Then chop the beef tenderloin and mix it with ground black pepper.
3. Put the beef in the ramekins and top with sliced tomato and cheese.
4. Bake the beef in the preheated to 360F oven for 50 minutes.

Nutritional info per serve: Calories 324, Fat 18.5, Fiber 0.3, Carbs 1.1, Protein 36.6

Pork with Gouda Cheese

Prep time: 10 minutes
Cook time: 75 minutes
Servings: 4
Ingredients:
- 1-pound pork loin, cubed
- 2 oz Gouda cheese, shredded
- 1 tablespoon coconut oil
- 1 teaspoon chili flakes
- 1 teaspoon coconut milk

Method:
1. Put all ingredients in the casserole mold and stir until homogenous.

2. Bake the meat in the preheated to 360F for 75 minutes.
Nutritional info per serve: Calories 364, Fat 24.2, Fiber 0, Carbs 0.3, Protein 34.6

Prosciutto Wrap
Prep time: 15 minutes
Cook time: 60 minutes
Servings: 4
Ingredients:
- 10 oz pork loin
- 3 oz prosciutto, sliced
- 1 teaspoon sesame oil
- ½ teaspoon chili flakes

Method:
1. Sprinkle the pork loin with chili flakes and wrap in the prosciutto.
2. Then brush it with sesame oil and roast in the oven at 365F for 60 minutes.
Nutritional info per serve: Calories 212, Fat 12.2, Fiber 0, Carbs 0.3, Protein 23.8

Sausage and Asparagus Bowl
Prep time: 10 minutes
Cook time: 50 minutes
Servings: 4
Ingredients:
- 8 pork sausage links, sliced
- 1 cup asparagus, chopped
- 1 teaspoon sesame oil
- 1 teaspoon sesame seeds
- 2 tablespoons lemon juice

Method:
1. Mix all ingredients in the baking tray and flatten in one layer.
2. Cook the meal in the preheated to 360F oven for 50 minutes. Stir the ingredients from time to time.
Nutritional info per serve: Calories 111, Fat 9, Fiber 0.8, Carbs 1.6, Protein 6

Garlic Pork Ribs
Prep time: 15 minutes
Cook time: 75 minutes
Servings: 4
Ingredients:
- 1-pound pork ribs, chopped
- 1 tablespoon garlic, minced
- 2 teaspoons sesame oil

Method:
1. Mix all ingredients in the mixing bowl.
2. Then transfer them in the roasting pan and cook in the oven at 360F for 75 minutes.
3. Flip the pork ribs on another side after 40 minutes of cooking.
Nutritional info per serve: Calories 333, Fat 22.4, Fiber 0, Carbs 0.7, Protein 30.2

Smoked Paprika Sausage Soup
Prep time: 10 minutes
Cook time: 20 minutes
Servings: 6
Ingredients:
- 1-pound beef sausages, chopped
- 1 tablespoon smoked paprika
- ½ cup asparagus, chopped
- 1 tablespoon avocado oil
- ½ cup plain yogurt
- 6 cups of water

Method:
1. Put all ingredients in the saucepan and bring to boil.
2. Close the lid and simmer the soup for 20 minutes on low heat.
Nutritional info per serve: Calories 323, Fat 28.1, Fiber 0.8, Carbs 4.7, Protein 12

Tomato Lamb Ribs
Prep time: 10 minutes
Cook time: 30 minutes
Servings: 4
Ingredients:
- 11 oz lamb ribs, roughly chopped
- 2 teaspoons keto tomato paste
- 2 tablespoons sesame oil
- 1 teaspoon cayenne pepper
- 1 tablespoon apple cider vinegar

Method:
1. Roast lamb ribs in the sesame oil for 4 minutes per side.
2. Then add keto tomato paste, cayenne pepper, apple cider vinegar, and keto tomato paste.
3. Carefully stir the lamb ribs and close the lid.
4. Cook the lamb ribs on medium heat for 20 minutes.
Nutritional info per serve: Calories 222, Fat 14.5, Fiber 0.2, Carbs 0.8, Protein 20.9

Beef Soup with Spinach
Prep time: 10 minutes
Cook time: 47 minutes
Servings: 6
Ingredients:
- 6 cups of water
- 2 cups spinach, chopped
- 1-pound beef loin, chopped
- 1 teaspoon chili pepper
- 1 spring onion, diced
- 1 tablespoon coconut oil

Method:
1. Melt the coconut oil in the saucepan.
2. Add beef loin and roast it for 3 minutes per side.
3. Then add chili pepper, diced spring onion, and water.
4. Cook the mixture for 30 minutes.
5. Then add spinach and cook the soup for 10 minutes more.
Nutritional info per serve: Calories 142, Fat 7.7, Fiber 0.7, Carbs 3.1, Protein 14.5

KETOGENIC VEGETABLE RECIPES

Bacon Broccoli Mash

Prep time: 10 minutes
Cook time: 0 minutes
Servings: 5
Ingredients:
- 2-pounds broccoli, boiled
- 2 oz bacon, chopped, roasted
- ¼ cup coconut cream
- 1 teaspoon salt

Method:
1. Put the cooked broccoli in the food processor.
2. Add coconut cream and salt. Blend the mixture until smooth.
3. Then add bacon and mix the cooked mash.

Nutritional info per serve: Calories 134, Fat 7.8, Fiber 4.8, Carbs 10.4, Protein 8.1

Parsley Asparagus

Prep time: 10 minutes
Cook time: 20 minutes
Servings: 4
Ingredients:
- 1-pound asparagus
- 1 teaspoon dried parsley
- ½ teaspoon salt
- 1 tablespoon coconut oil

Method:
1. Mix the asparagus with dried parsley and salt.
2. Put the vegetables in the baking tray. Add coconut oil.
3. Cook the asparagus in the oven at 360F for 20 minutes.

Nutritional info per serve: Calories 52, Fat 3.5, Fiber 2.4, Carbs 4.4, Protein 2.5

Marinated Broccoli

Prep time: 10 minutes
Cook time: 20 minutes
Servings: 4
Ingredients:
- 2 cups broccoli, chopped, boiled
- 3 tablespoons apple cider vinegar
- 1 teaspoon chili flakes
- 1 tablespoon olive oil
- ½ teaspoon salt

Method:
1. Mix the broccoli with apple cider vinegar, chili flakes, and olive oil.
2. Add salt and mix the broccoli well. Leave it in the fridge for 20 minutes to marinate.

Nutritional info per serve: Calories 48, Fat 3.7, Fiber 1.2, Carbs 3.1, Protein 1.3

Lemon Bell Peppers

Prep time: 10 minutes
Cook time: 8 minutes
Servings: 2
Ingredients:
- 1 cup bell pepper, trimmed
- 1 teaspoon minced garlic
- 1 tablespoon avocado oil
- 1 tablespoon lemon juice

Method:
3. Pierce the bell peppers with the help of the knife and put in the hot skillet.
4. Roast the bell peppers for 4 minutes per side.
5. After this, peel the peppers and slice them.
6. Add avocado oil, lemon juice, and minced garlic. Mix the bell peppers.

Nutritional info per serve: Calories 32, Fat 1.1, Fiber 1.2, Carbs 5.5, Protein 0.8

Watercress Soup

Prep time: 10 minutes
Cook time: 15 minutes
Servings: 4
Ingredients:
- 2 spring onions, chopped
- 6 oz watercress, chopped
- 4 cups chicken broth
- 1 teaspoon ground black pepper
- 1 teaspoon olive oil

Method:
1. Roast the spring onion with olive oil in the saucepan for 2 minutes per side.
2. Add watercress, chicken broth, ground black pepper, and close the lid.
3. Simmer the soup for 10 minutes on medium heat.

Nutritional info per serve: Calories 69, Fat 2.8, Fiber 1.2, Carbs 4, Protein 6.4

Garlic Cauliflower Fritters

Prep time: 15 minutes
Cook time: 10 minutes
Servings: 5
Ingredients:
- 1 cup cauliflower, shredded
- 1 egg, beaten
- 1 oz Cheddar cheese, shredded
- 1 teaspoon minced garlic
- 2 tablespoons almond flour
- 1 tablespoon coconut oil

Method:
1. Mix shredded cauliflower with egg, cheese, minced garlic, and almond flour.
2. Make the fritters and roast them in the hot coconut oil for 5 minutes per side.

Nutritional info per serve: Calories 129, Fat 11.1, Fiber 1.7, Carbs 3.8, Protein 5.4

Coconut Mushroom Cream Soup

Prep time: 10 minutes
Cook time: 25 minutes
Servings: 4
Ingredients:
- 3 oz Parmesan, grated
- 1 cup of coconut milk

- 3 cups of water
- 2 scalllions, diced
- 1 tablespoon avocado oil
- 2 cups mushrooms, chopped

Method:
1. Pour the avocado oil in the saucepan and preheat.
2. Add mushrooms and scallions. Roast the vegetables for 10 minutes on the medium heat.
3. After this, add water, coconut milk, and Parmesan. Stir the soup and bring to boil.
4. Simmer the soup for 10 minutes. Then blend it until smooth with the help of the immersion blender.

Nutritional info per serve: Calories 161, Fat 13.9, Fiber 2.1, Carbs 4.7, Protein 6.7

Rosemary Grilled Peppers

Prep time: 10 minutes
Cook time: 5 minutes
Servings: 4
Ingredients:
- 1 cup bell peppers, roughly chopped
- 1 teaspoon dried rosemary
- 1 tablespoon avocado oil
- ½ teaspoon salt

Method:
7. Mix the bell peppers with dried rosemary, avocado oil, and salt.
8. Then preheat the grill to 400F.
9. Put the bell peppers in the frill and roast them for 2 minutes per side.

Nutritional info per serve: Calories 15, Fat 0.6, Fiber 0.7, Carbs 2.6, Protein 0.4

Roasted Bok Choy

Prep time: 10 minutes
Cook time: 10 minutes
Servings: 2
Ingredients:
- 10 oz bok choy, roughly sliced
- 2 oz pancetta, chopped
- 1 teaspoon coconut oil
- ½ teaspoon dried thyme

Method:
1. Put the pancetta in the skillet and roast it for 2 minutes per side.
2. Add coconut oil and melt it.
3. Then add bok choy and dried thyme. Roast the vegetables for 1 minute per side.

Nutritional info per serve: Calories 192, Fat 14.4, Fiber 1.5, Carbs 3.7, Protein 12.7

Baked Rutabaga

Prep time: 10 minutes
Cook time: 10 minutes
Servings: 4
Ingredients:
- 2 cups rutabaga, chopped
- 1 tablespoon coconut oil
- 1 teaspoon ground coriander
- ½ teaspoon salt

Method:
1. Mix rutabaga with coconut oil, ground coriander, and salt.
2. Put the vegetables in the baking pan and bake them in the preheated to 360F oven for 10 minutes.

Nutritional info per serve: Calories 55, Fat 3.5, Fiber 1.8, Carbs 5.7, Protein 0.8

Celery Cream Soup

Prep time: 10 minutes
Cook time: 20 minutes
Servings: 4
Ingredients:
- 1 cup celery stalk, chopped
- ½ cup leek, chopped
- 2 tablespoons coconut oil
- ½ teaspoon cayenne pepper
- 4 cups chicken broth
- ¼ cup coconut cream

Method:
1. Melt coconut oil in the saucepan and add leek. Roast the leek for 5 minutes on medium heat.
2. Add all remaining ingredients and close the lid.
3. Simmer the soup for 10 minutes. Then blend the soup until smooth.

Nutritional info per serve: Calories 143, Fat 11.9, Fiber 1, Carbs 4.2, Protein 5.6

Lettuce Sandwich

Prep time: 10 minutes
Cook time: 0 minutes
Servings: 2
Ingredients:
- 4 lettuce leaves
- 2 Cheddar cheese slices
- 2 teaspoons cream cheese
- 1 teaspoon chives, chopped

Method:
1. Mix cream cheese with chives.
2. Put the chives mixture in 2 lettuce leaves.
3. Add Cheddar cheese slices.
4. Cover the cheese with the remaining lettuce.

Nutritional info per serve: Calories 126, Fat 10.5, Fiber 0.1, Carbs 0.8, Protein 7.3

Fenugreek Celery Stalks

Prep time: 10 minutes
Cook time: 5 minutes
Servings: 8
Ingredients:
- 8 celery stalks
- 1 teaspoon fenugreek powder
- 1 tablespoon butter
- ½ teaspoon salt

Method:
1. Melt the butter in the skillet.
2. Add celery stalks and roast them for 1 minute per side.
3. Then sprinkle the celery stalks with salt and fenugreek powder.
4. Roast the vegetables for 2 minutes more.

Nutritional info per serve: Calories 15, Fat 1.5, Fiber 0.3, Carbs 0.5, Protein 0.1

Cauliflower Cream

Prep time: 10 minutes
Cook time: 15 minutes
Servings: 4
Ingredients:
- 1 cup organic almond milk
- 1 teaspoon salt
- ¼ cup provolone cheese, shredded
- ½ teaspoon chili powder
- 1 cup cauliflower, chopped
- 1 spring onion, diced
- 1 teaspoon coconut oil

Method:
1. Mix cauliflower with almond milk and boil the mixture for 10 minutes.
2. Then add salt, provolone cheese, chili powder, spring onion, and coconut oil. Simmer the meal for 5 minutes more.
3. Blend the cooked meal until smooth.

Nutritional info per serve: Calories 61, Fat 4.2, Fiber 1, Carbs 3, Protein 3.1

Celery Cream Soup

Prep time: 10 minutes
Cook time: 25 minutes
Servings: 6
Ingredients:
- 2 cups of coconut milk
- 2 cups celery stalk, chopped
- 1 spring onion, diced
- 1 teaspoon coconut oil
- 2 oz Parmesan, grated
- 1 teaspoon chili powder

Method:
1. Roast the spring onion with coconut oil in the saucepan until tender.
2. Then add celery stalk, coconut milk, and chili powder.
3. Boil the soup for 15 minutes on medium heat.
4. Then blend the mixture until you get the creamy texture. Add Parmesan and stir the soup well.

Nutritional info per serve: Calories 231, Fat 22, Fiber 2.7, Carbs 6.9, Protein 5.3

Broccoli Spread

Prep time: 15 minutes
Cook time: 0 minutes
Servings: 6
Ingredients:
- 2 cups broccoli, boiled
- 1 oz macadamia nuts, grinded
- 2 tablespoons cream cheese
- ½ teaspoon ground paprika
- ½ cup Cheddar cheese, shredded

Method:
1. Mash the broccoli with the help of the potato masher until smooth.
2. Then add macadamia nuts, cream cheese, ground paprika, and Cheddar cheese.
3. Carefully mix the broccoli spread.

Nutritional info per serve: Calories 94, Fat 8, Fiber 1.3, Carbs 3, Protein 3.9

Cheese and Spinach Cream

Prep time: 10 minutes
Cook time: 10 minutes
Servings: 8
Ingredients:
- 3 cups fresh spinach, chopped
- 1 cup Cheddar cheese, shredded
- 2 tablespoons butter
- 1 teaspoon coconut shred
- 1 teaspoon ground paprika
- ½ teaspoon cayenne pepper
- ¼ cup of water

Method:
1. Melt the butter in the saucepan and add spinach. Roast it for 2 minutes.
2. Then stir it and add coconut shred, ground paprika, and cayenne pepper.
3. Add water and simmer the spinach for 5 minutes.
4. Add cheese and carefully mix the cooked meal.

Nutritional info per serve: Calories 88, Fat 7.9, Fiber 0.4, Carbs 0.9, Protein 3.9

Brussel Sprouts Fritters

Prep time: 10 minutes
Cook time: 10 minutes
Servings: 6
Ingredients:
- 1 cup Brussel Sprouts, shredded
- 2 eggs, beaten
- 2 tablespoons coconut flour
- 1 teaspoon ground turmeric
- 1 teaspoon ground black pepper
- 1 oz Parmesan, grated
- 1 tablespoon coconut oil

Method:
1. Mix Brussel sprouts with eggs, coconut flour, ground turmeric, ground black pepper, and Parmesan.
2. Make the fritters from the vegetable mixture.
3. Then melt the coconut oil in the skillet.
4. Add fritters and roast them for 4 minutes per side on the medium heat.

Nutritional info per serve: Calories 74, Fat 5.2, Fiber 1.6, Carbs 3.4, Protein 4.3

Lemon Greens

Prep time: 7 minutes
Cook time: 10 minutes
Servings: 4
Ingredients:
- 1 cup collard greens, chopped
- 1 tablespoon butter
- 1 teaspoon lemon zest, grated
- 1 tablespoon lemon juice
- ½ teaspoon smoked paprika

Method:

1. Melt the butter in the skillet.
2. Add all remaining ingredients and mix.
3. Cook the greens on medium heat for 5 minutes.
Nutritional info per serve: Calories 31, Fat 3, Fiber 0.5, Carbs 0.9, Protein 0.4

Garlic Mash

Prep time: 10 minutes
Cook time: 0 minutes
Servings: 3
Ingredients:
- 1 cup cauliflower, boiled, mashed
- 1 teaspoon minced garlic
- 2 tablespoons butter
- ¼ cup of coconut milk

Method:
1. Put all ingredients in the mixing bowl.
2. Carefully mix the garlic mash.
Nutritional info per serve: Calories 124, Fat 12.5, Fiber 1.3, Carbs 3.2, Protein 1.3

Buttered Onion

Prep time: 5 minutes
Cook time: 10 minutes
Servings: 4
Ingredients:
- 3 spring onions, sliced
- 3 tablespoons butter
- ½ teaspoon Erythritol

Method:
1. Melt the butter in the skillet.
2. Add spring onion and cook it for 4 minutes on medium heat.
3. Then add Erythritol and carefully mix the onion.
4. Cook it on low heat for 5 minutes more.
Nutritional info per serve: Calories 87, Fat 8.7, Fiber 0.6, Carbs 2.6, Protein 0.4

Broccoli Curry

Prep time: 10 minutes
Cook time: 15 minutes
Servings: 4
Ingredients:
- 2 cups broccoli florets
- 1 tablespoon curry powder
- ½ cup of coconut milk
- 1 tablespoon coconut oil

Method:
1. Mix curry powder with coconut milk.
2. Melt the coconut oil in the skillet. Add broccoli florets and roast them for 3 minutes per side.
3. Then add coconut milk liquid and carefully mix the broccoli.
4. Close the lid and simmer the broccoli for 8 minutes on medium heat.
Nutritional info per serve: Calories 119, Fat 10.9, Fiber 2.4, Carbs 5.6, Protein 2.2

Keto Tomatoes

Prep time: 10 minutes
Cook time: 0 minutes
Servings: 2
Ingredients:
- 1 tomato, roughly sliced
- 1 teaspoon sesame oil
- ½ teaspoon sesame seeds
- ¼ teaspoon salt

Method:
1. Put the sliced tomato in the plate in one layer.
2. Then sprinkle it with sesame oil, salt, and sesame seeds.
Nutritional info per serve: Calories 30, Fat 2.7, Fiber 0.5, Carbs 1.4, Protein 0.4

Lime Green Beans

Prep time: 10 minutes
Cook time: 25 minutes
Servings: 4
Ingredients:
- 2 cups green beans
- 1 teaspoon lime zest, grated
- 1 tablespoon lime juice
- 2 tablespoons coconut oil
- ¼ cup of water

Method:
1. Roast the green beans in the coconut oil for 3 minutes per side.
2. Then sprinkle the green beans with line juice and lime zest.
3. Add water and close the lid.
4. Cook the green beans on medium heat for 15 minutes.
Nutritional info per serve: Calories 76, Fat 6.9, Fiber 1.9, Carbs 4, Protein 1

Mustard Asparagus

Prep time: 5 minutes
Cook time: 20 minutes
Servings: 4
Ingredients:
- 1-pound asparagus, roughly chopped
- 1 cup of water
- 1 tablespoon mustard
- 1 teaspoon avocado oil
- ½ teaspoon sesame oil

Method:
1. Roast asparagus in avocado oil for 5 minutes per side on low heat.
2. Then add water and boil the asparagus for 10 minutes.
3. Remove the asparagus from the water and sprinkle with sesame oil and mustard.
4. Shake the vegetables before serving.
Nutritional info per serve: Calories 42, Fat 1.7, Fiber 2.8, Carbs 5.5, Protein 3.2

Baked Kale

Prep time: 10 minutes
Cook time: 15 minutes
Servings: 6
Ingredients:
- 5 cups kale, roughly chopped
- 1 teaspoon olive oil

- 1 teaspoon smoked paprika
- 2 oz Parmesan, grated

Method:
1. Brush the baking pan with olive oil.
2. Then mix kale with smoked paprika and Parmesan.
3. Put the mixture in the baking pan and bake it for 15 minutes at 360F.

Nutritional info per serve: Calories 66, Fat 2.8, Fiber 1, Carbs 6.4, Protein 4.8

Asparagus Soup

Prep time: 10 minutes
Cook time: 20 minutes
Servings: 4
Ingredients:
- 4 cups chicken broth
- ½ cup of coconut milk
- 10 oz asparagus, chopped
- 1 teaspoon butter
- ½ carrot, diced
- 1 teaspoon dried oregano
- 1 teaspoon garlic powder

Method:
1. Put the butter in the saucepan. Melt it.
2. Add asparagus and roast it for 5 minutes.
3. Then add all remaining ingredients.
4. Simmer the soup for 15 minutes on medium heat.

Nutritional info per serve: Calories 137, Fat 9.6, Fiber 2.6, Carbs 6.8, Protein 7.3

Parmesan Artichokes

Prep time: 10 minutes
Cook time: 20 minutes
Servings: 4
Ingredients:
- 2 artichokes, halved
- 1 teaspoon allspices
- 1 oz Parmesan, grated
- 1 teaspoon sesame oil

Method:
1. Rub the artichokes with sesame oil and allspices.
2. Then top them with Parmesan and bake in the oven at 360F for 20 minutes.

Nutritional info per serve: Calories 72, Fat 2.8, Fiber 4.5, Carbs 9.1, Protein 5

Mustard Greens Soup

Prep time: 10 minutes
Cook time: 30 minutes
Servings: 4
Ingredients:
- 2 cups mustard greens, chopped
- 2 cups collard greens, chopped
- 3 quarts vegetable stock
- 1 onion, peeled and chopped
- Salt and ground black pepper, to taste
- 2 tablespoons coconut aminos
- 2 teaspoons fresh ginger, grated

Method:
1. Put the stock into a saucepan and bring to a simmer over medium-high heat.
2. Add mustard, collard greens, onion, salt, pepper, coconut aminos, ginger, stir, cover the pan, and cook for 30 minutes.
3. Blend the soup using an immersion blender, add more salt, and pepper, heat up over medium heat, ladle into soup bowls, and serve.

Nutritional info per serve: Calories 35, Fat 0.4, Fiber 2.8, Carbs 7, Protein 1.9

Rutabaga Cakes

Prep time: 15 minutes
Cook time: 25 minutes
Servings: 4
Ingredients:
- 8 oz rutabaga, diced
- 2 eggs, beaten
- 1 teaspoon ground coriander
- 3 tablespoons almond flour
- 1 teaspoon ground paprika
- 1 tablespoon coconut oil
- ¼ cup coconut cream

Method:
1. Mix rutabaga with eggs, ground coriander, almond flour, ground paprika, and coconut cream.
2. Then grease the baking pan with coconut oil.
3. Make the small cakes from the rutabaga mixture and put them in the prepared baking pan.
4. Bake the rutabaga cakes at 365F for 25 minutes.

Nutritional info per serve: Calories 147, Fat 12, Fiber 2.5, Carbs 7, Protein 5

Greens Soup

Prep time: 5 minutes
Cook time: 20 minutes
Servings: 6
Ingredients:
- 6 cups chicken broth
- 2 cups fresh spinach, chopped
- 1 teaspoon ginger powder
- ½ cup turnip, chopped
- ½ cup coconut cream
- ½ teaspoon dried oregano
- ½ teaspoon salt

Method:
1. Put all ingredients in the saucepan and mix.
2. Close the lid and boil the soup for 20 minutes on medium-low heat.

Nutritional info per serve: Calories 91, Fat 6.2, Fiber 1, Carbs 3.4, Protein 5.7

Cheese Edamame Beans

Prep time: 10 minutes
Cook time: 15 minutes
Servings: 2
Ingredients:
- 1 cup edamame beans, cooked
- ¼ cup Provolone cheese, shredded
- 1 teaspoon coconut oil
- ¼ teaspoon ground black pepper

- ½ teaspoon apple cider vinegar

Method:
1. Roast the edamame beans with coconut oil for 2 minutes.
2. Then add ground black pepper and apple cider vinegar. Mix the vegetables.
3. Add Provolone cheese and close the lid.
4. Cook the meal on medium heat for 10 minutes.

Nutritional info per serve: Calories 137, Fat 7, Fiber 3.8, Carbs 11, Protein 8.2

Cilantro Asparagus

Prep time: 10 minutes
Cook time: 20 minutes
Servings: 3
Ingredients:
- 1 asparagus bunch, trimmed
- 3 teaspoons sesame oil
- 1 teaspoon apple cider vinegar
- 1 tablespoon dried oregano

Method:
1. Roast the asparagus in the sesame oil for 4 minutes per side.
2. Then add dried oregano and apple cider vinegar. Stir the asparagus.
3. Close the lid and cook it for 10 minutes on low heat.

Nutritional info per serve: Calories 54, Fat 4.7, Fiber 1.6, Carbs 2.7, Protein 1.2

Sauteed Collard Greens

Prep time: 10 minutes
Cook time: 10 minutes
Servings: 2
Ingredients:
- 1 cup Collard Greens
- 1 teaspoon apple cider vinegar
- 1 teaspoon ground black pepper
- ½ cup of coconut milk

Method:
1. Pour coconut milk in the saucepan and bring it to boil.
2. Add collard greens and ground black pepper. Boil the greens for 5 minutes.
3. Then add apple cider vinegar and remove the meal from the heat.

Nutritional info per serve: Calories 147, Fat 14.5, Fiber 2.4, Carbs 5.3, Protein 2

Spinach Fritters

Prep time: 10 minutes
Cook time: 10 minutes
Servings: 2
Ingredients:
- 2 cups spinach, chopped
- 2 eggs, beaten
- 2 oz Cheddar cheese, shredded
- 2 tablespoons coconut flour
- ½ teaspoon chili powder
- 1 tablespoon sesame oil

Method:
1. Mix spinach with eggs, Cheddar cheese, coconut flour, and chili powder.
2. Then preheat the sesame oil in the skillet well.
3. Make the fritters from the spinach mixture and put them in the hot oil.
4. Roast the fritters for 5 minutes per side on the medium heat.

Nutritional info per serve: Calories 281, Fat 22.1, Fiber 3.9, Carbs 6.7, Protein 15

Oregano Eggplants

Prep time: 10 minutes
Cook time: 10 minutes
Servings: 3
Ingredients:
- 2 eggplants, sliced
- 1 teaspoon salt
- 1 tablespoon coconut oil
- 1 tablespoon dried oregano

Method:
1. Mix the eggplants with salt and dried oregano.
2. Then melt the coconut oil in the skillet.
3. Add the eggplants. Flatten in one layer and roast them for 2 minutes per side.

Nutritional info per serve: Calories 86, Fat 7.6, Fiber 0.6, Carbs 1.2, Protein 3.9

Yogurt Asparagus

Prep time: 10 minutes
Cook time: 15 minutes
Servings: 4
Ingredients:
- ½ cup Plain yogurt
- 1 teaspoon chili flakes
- 1-pound asparagus, chopped
- ½ cup of water
- ½ teaspoon salt

Method:
1. Mix plain yogurt with chili flakes, water, and salt and pour in the saucepan.
2. Add asparagus and simmer the vegetables for 15 minutes on medium-high heat.

Nutritional info per serve: Calories 45, Fat 0.5, Fiber 2.4, Carbs 6.6, Protein 4.2

Avocado and Walnut Bowl

Prep time: 10 minutes
Cook time: 0 minutes
Servings: 2
Ingredients:
- 1 avocado, pitted, halved, chopped
- 1 oz walnuts, chopped
- 1 oz Parmesan, chopped
- 1 teaspoon olive oil
- 1 teaspoon Italian seasonings

Method:
1. Put the avocado in the bowl.
2. Add walnuts, Parmesan, olive oil, and Italian seasonings.
3. Shake the ingredient well.

Nutritional info per serve: Calories 365, Fat 34, Fiber 7.7, Carbs 10.8, Protein 9.9

Greens Omelette

Prep time: 10 minutes
Cook time: 10 minutes
Servings: 4
Ingredients:
- ½ cup of coconut milk
- 4 eggs, beaten
- 1 cup spinach, chopped
- ¼ cup asparagus, chopped
- 1 tablespoon butter
- ½ teaspoon salt

Method:
1. Mix eggs with coconut milk and salt.
2. Then melt butter in the skillet.
3. Add egg mixture and spinach.
4. Close the lid and cook the omelet for 10 minutes on low heat.

Nutritional info per serve: Calories 161, Fat 14.4, Fiber 1, Carbs 2.6, Protein 6.7

Asparagus Masala

Prep time: 10 minutes
Cook time: 20 minutes
Servings: 4
Ingredients:
- 1-pound asparagus, chopped
- 1 cup coconut cream
- 1 teaspoon butter
- 1 teaspoon garam masala

Method:
1. Melt the butter in the saucepan.
2. Add asparagus and roast it for 3 minutes per side.
3. Add garam masala and coconut cream.
4. Close the lid and cook the vegetables for 10 minutes.

Nutritional info per serve: Calories 169, Fat 15.4, Fiber 3.7, Carbs 7.7, Protein 3.9

Monterey Jack Cheese Asparagus

Prep time: 10 minutes
Cook time: 25 minutes
Servings: 3
Ingredients:
- 10 oz asparagus, chopped
- ½ cup Monterey Jack Cheese, shredded
- 1 tablespoon cream cheese
- 1 teaspoon mustard
- 1 teaspoon butter, softened
- ¼ cup of water

Method:
1. Grease the baking pan with butter and put asparagus inside.
2. Add mustard, cream cheese, and water.
3. Then add Monterey Jack cheese and bake the meal in the oven at 365F for 25 minutes.

Nutritional info per serve: Calories 117, Fat 8.6, Fiber 2.1, Carbs 4.3, Protein 7.2

Chives Fritters

Prep time: 10 minutes
Cook time: 10 minutes
Servings: 2
Ingredients:
- 1 cup broccoli, shredded
- 1 tablespoon chives
- 1 egg, beaten
- 1 teaspoon ground black pepper
- 1/3 cup almond flour
- 1 tablespoon avocado oil

Method:
1. Mix broccoli with chives, egg, ground black pepper, and almond flour.
2. Preheat the avocado oil in the skillet.
3. Make the fritters from the chives mixture and roast them in hot oil for 3 minutes per side.

Nutritional info per serve: Calories 86, Fat 5.6, Fiber 2.3, Carbs 5.3, Protein 5.3

Sprouts Salad

Prep time: 10 minutes
Cook time: 0 minutes
Servings: 4
Ingredients:
- 2 cups Brussel sprouts, boiled
- 1 pecan, chopped
- 1/4 cup plain yogurt
- 1 tablespoon fresh dill, chopped
- 1 tablespoon lemon juice

Method:
1. Mix all ingredients in a salad bowl.
2. Stir the salad.

Nutritional info per serve: Calories 57, Fat 2.9, Fiber 2.2, Carbs 6.1, Protein 2.9

Cabbage Balls

Prep time: 10 minutes
Cook time: 10 minutes
Servings: 3
Ingredients:
- 1 cup white cabbage, shredded
- 1 tablespoon hemp seeds
- 1 teaspoon ground coriander
- ¼ cup plain yogurt
- ½ cup coconut flour
- 1 tablespoon coconut oil
- ½ teaspoon salt

Method:
1. In the mixing bowl, mix cabbage, hemp seeds, ground coriander, yogurt, coconut flour, and salt.
2. Make the balls from the cabbage mixture and put them in the hot skillet.
3. Add coconut oil and roast the cabbage balls for 4 minutes per side or until they are golden brown.

Nutritional info per serve: Calories 71, Fat 5.2, Fiber 1.6, Carbs 4.4, Protein 1.9

Turmeric Radishes

Prep time: 10 minutes
Cook time: 15 minutes
Servings: 2
Ingredients:

- 2 cups radishes, halved
- 2 tablespoons coconut oil
- 1 teaspoon ground turmeric
- 1 teaspoon salt

Method:
1. Mix the radishes with coconut oil, ground turmeric, and salt.
2. Put the mixture in the baking tray and roast it for 15 minutes in the oven at 365F.

Nutritional info per serve: Calories 140, Fat 13.8, Fiber 2.1, Carbs 4.7, Protein 0.9

Jicama Noodles

Prep time: 15 minutes
Cook time: 8 minutes
Servings: 6
Ingredients:
- 1-pound jicama, peeled
- 2 tablespoons coconut cream
- 1 teaspoon sesame oil
- ½ teaspoon dried cilantro

Method:
1. Spiralize the jicama with the help of the spiralizer.
2. Then preheat the sesame oil in the skillet.
3. Add jicama noodles, dried cilantro, and coconut cream.
4. Stir the mixture and cook it on medium heat for 5 minutes.

Nutritional info per serve: Calories 47, Fat 2, Fiber 3.8, Carbs 7, Protein 0.7

Rosemary Radish

Prep time: 10 minutes
Cook time: 10 minutes
Servings: 4
Ingredients:
- 1-pound radish, sliced
- 1 teaspoon dried rosemary
- 1 tablespoon butter

Method:
1. Melt the butter in the skillet.
2. Then add radish and dried rosemary.
3. Roast the radish for 10 minutes. Stir the meal from time to time.

Nutritional info per serve: Calories 45, Fat 3, Fiber 1.9, Carbs 4.1, Protein 0.8

Broccoli Slaw

Prep time: 15 minutes
Cook time: 5 minutes
Servings: 4
Ingredients:
- 1 cup broccoli, shredded
- 1 tablespoon plain yogurt
- 1 teaspoon sesame oil
- 1 teaspoon sesame seeds
- 1 tablespoon lime juice
- 1 teaspoon butter
- 1 cup white cabbage, shredded

Method:
1. Roast the shredded broccoli with butter for 5 minutes. Stir it from time to time.
2. Then mix cooked broccoli with plain yogurt, sesame oil, sesame seeds, lime juice, and white cabbage.
3. Carefully mix the meal.

Nutritional info per serve: Calories 39, Fat 2.6, Fiber 1.2, Carbs 3.5, Protein 1.2

Coated Radish

Prep time: 10 minutes
Cook time: 10 minutes
Servings: 4
Ingredients:
- 2 eggs, beaten
- 1 cup radish, trimmed
- 1 tablespoon coconut oil
- 3 tablespoons coconut flour

Method:
1. Dip the radish in the eggs and then coat in the coconut flour.
2. Preheat the coconut oil well.
3. Add the coated radishes in the hot coconut oil and roast for 2-3 minutes or until radishes are golden brown.

Nutritional info per serve: Calories 88, Fat 6.4, Fiber 2.3, Carbs 4.2, Protein 3.7

White Mushrooms Saute

Prep time: 10 minutes
Cook time: 35 minutes
Servings: 4
Ingredients:
- 1-pound white mushrooms, chopped
- 1 tablespoon coconut oil
- 1 cup of coconut milk
- 1 teaspoon dried thyme
- 1 teaspoon ground cumin
- 1 spring onion, sliced

Method:
1. Mix mushrooms with coconut oil and cook in the saucepan for 10 minutes. Stir them from time to time.
2. Then add coconut milk, dried thyme, and ground cumin. Add spring onion.
3. Stir the mixture and close the lid.
4. Cook the saute on medium heat for 25 minutes.

Nutritional info per serve: Calories 200, Fat 18.2, Fiber 2.9, Carbs 8.7, Protein 5.2

Radish in Bacon Sauce

Prep time: 10 minutes
Cook time: 15 minutes
Servings: 2
Ingredients:
- 7 ounces radishes, cut in half
- 1 oz bacon, chopped, cooked
- 1 cup heavy cream
- 1 teaspoon curry powder
- 1 teaspoon butter

Method:
1. Melt butter in the saucepan.
2. Add curry powder, bacon, and heavy cream.
3. Bring the mixture to boil and add radishes.

4.	Close the lid and simmer the meal for 10 minutes.
Nutritional info per serve: Calories 320, Fat 30.3, Fiber 1.9, Carbs 5.8, Protein 7.3

Sesame Broccoli
Prep time: 10 minutes
Cook time: 10 minutes
Servings: 6
Ingredients:
- 4 cups broccoli, chopped
- 2 cups of water
- ¼ cup apple cider vinegar
- 1 teaspoon sesame oil
- 1 teaspoon sesame seeds
- 1 teaspoon chili flakes

Method:
1.	Boil the broccoli in the water for 10 minutes.
2.	Then drain water and add apple cider vinegar, sesame oil, sesame seeds, and chili flakes.
3.	Shake the broccoli and transfer it in the serving bowl.
Nutritional info per serve: Calories 32, Fat 1.2, Fiber 1.6, Carbs 4.3, Protein 1.8

Garlic Soup
Prep time: 10 minutes
Cook time: 20 minutes
Servings: 4
Ingredients:
- 1 cup radish, chopped
- 6 cups chicken stock
- 2 oz leek, chopped
- 3 tablespoons olive oil
- 1 teaspoon minced garlic
- 1 teaspoon dried parsley

Method:
1.	Roast the leek with olive oil for 2-3 minutes.
2.	Then add minced garlic, dried parsley, and radish.
3.	Add chicken stock and close the lid.
4.	Simmer the soup on medium heat for 10 minutes.
Nutritional info per serve: Calories 119, Fat 11.4, Fiber 0.7, Carbs 4.4, Protein 1.5

Cheese Mushrooms
Prep time: 10 minutes
Cook time: 15 minutes
Servings: 6
Ingredients:
- 2-pound mushroom caps
- 1 cup Cheddar cheese, shredded
- 1 teaspoon dried rosemary
- 1 tablespoon sesame oil
- ½ teaspoon salt

Method:
1.	Brush the tray with sesame oil.
2.	Put the mushrooms caps in the tray in one layer.
3.	Sprinkle them with dried rosemary and salt.
4.	Top the mushrooms with cheese and bake in the oven at 360F for 25 minutes.
Nutritional info per serve: Calories 129, Fat 9, Fiber 1.6, Carbs 5.3, Protein 9.5

Cilantro and Cabbage Salad
Prep time: 10 minutes
Cook time: 0 minutes
Servings: 4
Ingredients:
- 2 cups white cabbage, shredded
- ¼ cup fresh cilantro, chopped
- 2 tablespoons coconut milk
- 1 teaspoon lemon juice
- 1 teaspoon minced garlic
- ½ teaspoon dried dill

Method:
1.	Mix white cabbage with cilantro, coconut milk, minced garlic, and dried dill.
2.	Stir the salad and add lemon juice.
Nutritional info per serve: Calories 28, Fat 1.9, Fiber 1.1, Carbs 2.8, Protein 0.7

Cauliflower Pizza with Greens
Prep time: 15 minutes
Cook time: 20 minutes
Servings: 6
Ingredients:
- 2 cups cauliflower, chopped
- 2 oz provolone cheese, shredded
- 2 tablespoons almond flour
- 1 teaspoon dried dill
- 1 teaspoon dried cilantro
- 1 tablespoon coconut oil
- 1 egg, beaten

Method:
1.	Mix almond flour with dried dill, cilantro, egg, and coconut oil. Knead the dough.
2.	Then put the dough in the baking pan and flatten in the shape of pizza crust.
3.	Bake it for 5 minutes at 365F.
4.	Then top the pizza crust with chopped cauliflower and Provolone cheese.
5.	Bake the pizza for 15 minutes at 365F more.
Nutritional info per serve: Calories 81, Fat 5.6, Fiber 0.9, Carbs 4.1, Protein 4.3

Mustard Salad
Prep time: 10 minutes
Cook time: 0 minutes
Servings: 4
Ingredients:
- 4 cups mixed lettuce leaves, torn
- 1 cup arugula, chopped
- 1 tablespoon mustard
- 1 tablespoon coconut milk
- 1 egg yolk, hard-boiled
- 1 teaspoon smoked paprika

Method:
1.	Mix egg yolk with coconut milk, smoked paprika, and mustard. The mustard dressing is cooked.

2. Then mix lettuce and arugula.
3. Sprinkle the greens mixture with mustard dressing.
Nutritional info per serve: Calories 46, Fat 3, Fiber 1.1, Carbs 3.5, Protein 1.9

Zucchini Ravioli

Prep time: 20 minutes
Cook time: 30 minutes
Servings: 4
Ingredients:
- 1 zucchini, trimmed
- 2 tablespoons cream cheese
- ¼ cup fresh parsley, chopped
- 1 teaspoon butter, softened
- ½ teaspoon smoked paprika

Method:
1. Slice the zucchini lengthwise.
2. Then mix cream cheese with parsley and smoked paprika.
3. Fill the zucchini slices with cream cheese mixture and roll into the shape of ravioli.
4. Grease the baking pan with butter and put the ravioli inside.
5. Bake the meal at 360F for 30 minutes.
Nutritional info per serve: Calories 36, Fat 2.9, Fiber 0.8, Carbs 2.2, Protein 1.1

Lemon Salad

Prep time: 10 minutes
Cook time: 0 minutes
Servings: 4
Ingredients:
- 1 avocado, pitted, peeled, chopped
- 1 teaspoon lemon zest, grated
- 1 tablespoon lemon juice
- 1 cup fresh spinach, chopped
- 1 cup lettuce, chopped
- 1 teaspoon sesame oil

Method:
1. Mix all ingredients in the salad bowl.
2. Shake the salad well.
Nutritional info per serve: Calories 117, Fat 11, Fiber 3.7, Carbs 5.2, Protein 1.3

Broccoli Crackers

Prep time: 20 minutes
Cook time: 15 minutes
Servings: 4
Ingredients:
- 1 cup cauliflower, shredded
- 1 tablespoon flax seeds
- 1 tablespoon coconut flour
- 1 teaspoon ground coriander
- 1 teaspoon salt
- 1 egg, beaten
- 1 teaspoon coconut oil

Method:
1. Mix shredded cauliflower with flax seeds, coconut flour, ground coriander, salt, egg, and coconut oil.
2. Knead the dough.
3. Then line the baking tray with baking paper.
4. Roll up the dough and cut into small pieces (crackers).
5. Put the crackers in the lined baking tray and bake at 365F for 15 minutes.
Nutritional info per serve: Calories 56, Fat 3.3, Fiber 2.4, Carbs 3.9, Protein 2.7

Avocado Spread

Prep time: 10 minutes
Cook time: 0 minutes
Servings: 4
Ingredients:
- 1 avocado, peeled, pitted, chopped
- 1 garlic clove, diced
- ½ teaspoon ground nutmeg
- 1 teaspoon dried dill
- 2 tablespoons cream cheese

Method:
1. Mash the avocado until smooth.
2. Add garlic, ground nutmeg, dill, and cream cheese.
3. Stir the mixture until smooth.
Nutritional info per serve: Calories 123, Fat 11.7, Fiber 3.5, Carbs 5, Protein 1.5

Paprika Okra

Prep time: 10 minutes
Cook time: 30 minutes
Servings: 2
Ingredients:
- 1 cup okra, roughly sliced
- 1 teaspoon smoked paprika
- 1 tablespoon sesame oil
- ½ teaspoon salt

Method:
1. Mix okra with smoked paprika, sesame oil, and salt.
2. Put the mixture in the baking tray and bake in the oven at 365F for 30 minutes. Stir the vegetables during the cooking from time to time to avoid burning.
Nutritional info per serve: Calories 83, Fat 7, Fiber 2, Carbs 4.3, Protein 1.1

Spinach Soup

Prep time: 10 minutes
Cook time: 20 minutes
Servings: 4
Ingredients:
- 4 cups chicken broth
- 2 cups fresh spinach, chopped
- 1 teaspoon ground black pepper
- 1 teaspoon sesame oil
- 1 spring onion, diced
- 1 teaspoon dried sage

Method:
1. Roast the spring onion with sesame oil in the saucepan until it is light brown.
2. Then add sage, ground black pepper, and spinach.

3. Add Chicken broth and cook the soup for 10 minutes.
Nutritional info per serve: Calories 59, Fat 2.6, Fiber 0.8, Carbs 3.2, Protein 5.5

Lettuce and Mozzarella Salad
Prep time: 10 minutes
Servings: 6
Ingredients:
- 5 cups lettuce, chopped
- 1 cup Mozzarella, shredded
- 1 tablespoon sesame oil
- 1 teaspoon cumin seeds
- 1 tablespoon lemon juice
- 1 teaspoon mustard seeds

Method:
1. In the mixing bowl, mix mustard seeds with lemon juice, cumin seeds, and sesame oil.
2. Then mix shredded mozzarella with lettuce in the salad bowl.
3. Top the salad with shredded Mozzarella mixture.

Nutritional info per serve: Calories 43, Fat 3.4, Fiber 0.4, Carbs 1.8, Protein 1.7

Thai Soup
Prep time: 10 minutes
Cook time: 20 minutes
Servings: 4
Ingredients:
- 1 cup organic almond milk
- 1 teaspoon curry paste
- 2 cups fresh spinach, chopped
- ½ cup turnip, chopped
- 4 cups chicken broth
- 1 teaspoon salt

Method:
1. Pour almond milk in the saucepan and bring to boil.
2. Add curry paste, turnip, chicken broth, and salt.
3. Simmer the liquid for 10 minutes.
4. Then add spinach and boil the soup for 5 minutes.

Nutritional info per serve: Calories 193, Fat 16.5, Fiber 1.9, Carbs 6.2, Protein 6.9

Basil Bake
Prep time: 15 minutes
Cook time: 20 minutes
Servings: 4
Ingredients:
- 1 tablespoon dried basil
- 2 cups cauliflower, chopped
- 1 cup of coconut milk
- 1 teaspoon butter

Method:
1. Mix cauliflower with dried basil and coconut milk.
2. Grease the baking ramekins with butter and put cauliflower mixture inside.
3. Bake the meal at 360F for 20 minutes.

Nutritional info per serve: Calories 159, Fat 15.3, Fiber 2.6, Carbs 6, Protein 2.4

Marinated Broccoli Salad
Prep time: 10 minutes
Cook time: 0 minutes
Servings: 4
Ingredients:
- 1 cup broccoli, chopped, boiled
- 2 tablespoons apple cider vinegar
- 1 teaspoon sesame oil
- 1 cup lettuce, chopped
- 1 teaspoon chili flakes

Method:
1. Mix broccoli with apple cider vinegar, sesame oil, and chili flakes.
2. Then add lettuce and carefully mix the salad.

Nutritional info per serve: Calories 21, Fat 1.2, Fiber 0.7, Carbs 2, Protein 0.7

Sesame Bok Choy
Prep time: 10 minutes
Cook time: 10 minutes
Servings: 2
Ingredients:
- 8 oz bok choy
- 1 teaspoon sesame seeds
- 1 tablespoon sesame oil
- 1 teaspoon ground black pepper

Method:
1. Roast the bok choy in sesame oil for 2 minutes per side.
2. Then sprinkle it with ground black pepper and sesame seeds.
3. Stir the meal and cook it for 3 minutes more.

Nutritional info per serve: Calories 86, Fat 7.8, Fiber 1.6, Carbs 3.5, Protein 2.1

Scallions Soup
Prep time: 5 minutes
Cook time: 15 minutes
Servings: 6
Ingredients:
- 6 cups chicken broth
- 2 cups broccoli, chopped
- 2 oz scallions, chopped
- 1 teaspoon chili powder
- ½ teaspoon salt

Method:
1. Mix all ingredients from the list above in the saucepan and bring it to boil.
2. Simmer the soup for 10 minutes on medium heat.

Nutritional info per serve: Calories 53, Fat 1.6, Fiber 1.2, Carbs 3.9, Protein 5.9

Eggplant Puree
Prep time: 15 minutes
Cook time: 0 minutes
Servings: 4
Ingredients:
- 1 large eggplant, peeled, grilled

- 1 tablespoon cream cheese
- 1 teaspoon minced garlic
- 1 teaspoon chili powder
- ¼ cup coconut cream

Method:
1. Blend the eggplant until smooth and mix it with cream cheese, minced garlic, chili powder, and coconut cream.
2. Carefully mix the meal.

Nutritional info per serve: Calories 75, Fat 4.8, Fiber 4.6, Carbs 8.2, Protein 1.8

Cumin Soup

Prep time: 5 minutes
Cook time: 25 minutes
Servings: 4
Ingredients:
- 2 scallions, diced
- 1 carrot, diced
- 1 oz turnip, chopped
- 1 teaspoon cumin seeds
- 1 teaspoon sesame oil
- 1 teaspoon salt
- 1 teaspoon cayenne pepper
- 5 cups chicken broth

Method:
1. Roast the carrot with turnip and sesame oil in the saucepan for 6 minutes. Stir the vegetables.
2. Then add scallions, cumin seeds, salt, cayenne pepper, and chicken broth.
3. Boil the soup on medium heat for 15 minutes.

Nutritional info per serve: Calories 81, Fat 3.1, Fiber 1.3, Carbs 6.2, Protein 6.7

Oregano Fennel

Prep time: 10 minutes
Cook time: 30 minutes
Servings: 4
Ingredients:
- 1-pound fennel bulb
- 1 teaspoon dried oregano
- 1 tablespoon sesame oil
- 1 teaspoon ground black pepper

Method:
1. Chop the fennel bulb roughly and sprinkle with dried oregano, sesame oil, and ground black pepper.
2. Then put the fennel bulb in the lined with baking paper tray and roast in the oven at 365F for 30 minutes.

Nutritional info per serve: Calories 68, Fat 3.7, Fiber 3.8, Carbs 8.9, Protein 1.5

Zucchini Cream Soup

Prep time: 10 minutes
Cook time: 25 minutes
Servings: 4
Ingredients:
- 1 cup heavy cream
- 2 cups of water
- 1 cup zucchini, chopped
- 1 teaspoon onion powder
- 1 teaspoon dried dill
- 1 teaspoon salt

Method:
1. Pour water in the saucepan.
2. Add zucchini, onion powder, dried dill, and salt. Bring the mixture to boil and simmer it for 10 minutes.
3. After this, blend the mixture until smooth and add heavy cream.
4. Simmer the soup for 5 minutes more.

Nutritional info per serve: Calories 111, Fat 11.2, Fiber 0.4, Carbs 2.4, Protein 1.1

Mushroom Bake

Prep time: 10 minutes
Cook time: 40 minutes
Servings: 5
Ingredients:
- 2-pounds cremini mushrooms, chopped
- 1 oz Parmesan, grated
- 1 tablespoon butter
- 1 teaspoon dried thyme
- 1 teaspoon ground coriander

Method:
1. Line the baking tray with baking paper and put the cremini mushrooms inside.
2. Sprinkle them with butter, thyme, and ground coriander.
3. Then mix the mushrooms and bake them in the oven at 360F for 40 minutes.

Nutritional info per serve: Calories 88, Fat 3.7, Fiber 1.2, Carbs 7.8, Protein 6.4

Ginger Cream Soup

Prep time: 10 minutes
Cook time: 25 minutes
Servings: 4
Ingredients:
- 1 zucchini, chopped
- 1 cup radish, chopped
- 1 teaspoon ginger powder
- 3 cups of water
- 1 cup heavy cream
- 1 teaspoon white pepper

Method:
1. Mix heavy cream, water, and white pepper in the saucepan. Bring the liquid to boil.
2. Add ginger powder, radish, and zucchini.
3. Boil the soup for 10 minutes.
4. Then blend the soup with the help of the immersion blender until smooth.
5. Simmer the soup for 10 minutes more.

Nutritional info per serve: Calories 119, Fat 11.3, Fiber 1.2, Carbs 4.1, Protein 1.5

Butter Zucchini Pasta

Prep time: 10 minutes
Cook time: 5 minutes
Servings: 4
Ingredients:
- 2 zucchini, sliced lengthwise
- 1 oz Parmesan, grated
- 2 teaspoons butter

- 1 teaspoon dried basil
- ½ teaspoon chili flakes

Method:
1. Melt the butter in the skillet.
2. Add sliced zucchini, dried basil, and chili flakes.
3. Roast the zucchinis for 2-3 minutes.
4. Add grated Parmesan and carefully mix the pasta.

Nutritional info per serve: Calories 55, Fat 3.6, Fiber 1.1, Carbs 3.6, Protein 3.5

Mozzarella Swiss Chard

Prep time: 10 minutes
Cook time: 10 minutes
Servings: 4
Ingredients:
- 2 cups swiss chard, chopped
- 1 cup Mozzarella, shredded
- 1 tablespoon butter, softened
- 1 teaspoon ground turmeric

Method:
1. Mix swiss chard with butter and saute the mixture for 5 minutes on low heat.
2. Add ground turmeric and Mozzarella and close the lid.
3. Cook the swiss chard on medium heat for 5 minutes more.

Nutritional info per serve: Calories 51, Fat 4.2, Fiber 0.4, Carbs 1.3, Protein 2.4

Blue Cheese Cauliflower

Prep time: 10 minutes
Cook time: 15 minutes
Servings: 5
Ingredients:
- 2 cups cauliflower florets
- 1 cup heavy cream
- 3 oz Blue cheese, crumbled
- 1 teaspoon white pepper
- ½ teaspoon dried sage

Method:
1. Mix cauliflower florets with heavy cream, crumbled cheese, white pepper, and dried sage.
2. Bring the mixture to boil and simmer the cauliflower for 15 minutes on low heat.
3. Cool the cooked cauliflower till the room temperature and transfer in the serving bowls.

Nutritional info per serve: Calories 154, Fat 13.8, Fiber 1.1, Carbs 3.5, Protein 5

Chard Salad

Prep time: 10 minutes
Cook time: 0 minutes
Servings: 4
Ingredients:
- 1 cup Swiss chard, cut into strips
- 1 cup arugula, chopped
- 1 zucchini, chopped, grilled
- 1 oz Parmesan, grated
- 1 tablespoon avocado oil
- ½ teaspoon salt

Method:
1. Mix Swiss chard with arugula, zucchini, avocado oil, and salt.
2. Then add grated Parmesan and stir the salad well.

Nutritional info per serve: Calories 38, Fat 2.1, Fiber 0.9, Carbs 2.6, Protein 3.2

Flax Seeds Spinach

Prep time: 10 minutes
Servings: 4
Ingredients:
- 2 cups fresh spinach
- 1 tablespoon flax seeds
- ½ teaspoon chia seeds
- 1 tablespoon lemon juice
- 1 teaspoon avocado oil

Method:
1. Chop the spinach roughly and put it in the bowl.
2. Add flax seeds, chis seeds, lemon juice, and avocado oil.
3. Stir the salad well.

Nutritional info per serve: Calories 24, Fat 1.3, Fiber 1.5, Carbs 1.9, Protein 1.1

Oregano Chard Salad

Prep time: 10 minutes
Cook time: 0 minutes
Servings: 4
Ingredients:
- 2 cups Swiss chard, chopped
- 1 teaspoon dried oregano
- 1 tablespoon lime juice
- 1 avocado, chopped

Method:
1. Sprinkle the Swiss chard with dried oregano, lime juice, and shake gently.
2. Top the swiss chard with avocado.

Nutritional info per serve: Calories 109, Fat 9.9, Fiber 3.9, Carbs 5.8, Protein 1.3

Baked Broccoli

Prep time: 10 minutes
Cook time: 25 minutes
Servings: 4
Ingredients:
- 2 cups broccoli, chopped
- 2 oz Parmesan, grated
- 1 teaspoon ground black pepper
- 1 teaspoon avocado oil

Method:
1. Sprinkle the broccoli with avocado oil and put it in the baking tray. Flatten it in one layer.
2. Sprinkle the broccoli with grated Parmesan and ground black pepper.
3. Bake the broccoli at 360F for 25 minutes.

Nutritional info per serve: Calories 64, Fat 3.4, Fiber 1.4, Carbs 3.9, Protein 5.9

Apple Cider Vinegar Lettuce

Prep time: 10 minutes
Cook time: 0 minutes
Servings: 4

Ingredients:
- 4 cups lettuce, chopped
- 2 tablespoons apple cider vinegar
- 1 teaspoon chia seeds

Method:
1. Put the lettuce in the salad bowl and sprinkle with apple cider vinegar and chia seeds.
2. Shake the lettuce well.

Nutritional info per serve: Calories 21, Fat 0.8, Fiber 1.2, Carbs 2.7, Protein 0.6

Coconut Bok Choy

Prep time: 10 minutes
Cook time: 12 minutes
Servings: 1
Ingredients:
- 6 oz bok choy, sliced
- 1 tablespoon coconut flour
- 1 teaspoon coconut shred
- 1 egg, beaten
- 1 tablespoon avocado oil

Method:
1. Mix coconut flour with coconut shred.
2. Then dip the bok choy in the egg and coat in the coconut mixture.
3. Preheat the avocado oil well.
4. Put the coated bok choy in the hot oil and roast for 3 minutes per side or until the bok choy is light brown.

Nutritional info per serve: Calories 145, Fat 8.6, Fiber 5, Carbs 9.3, Protein 9.4

Mushroom Cream Soup

Prep time: 10 minutes
Cook time: 20 minutes
Servings: 4
Ingredients:
- 1 cup mushrooms, chopped
- 1 tablespoon coconut oil
- 2 tablespoons cream cheese
- 3 cups of water
- 1 teaspoon salt
- 1 oz celery stalk, chopped

Method:
1. Put all ingredients in the saucepan. Stir the mixture until homogenous.
2. Boil the soup on medium heat for 20 minutes.
3. Then blend the soup until you get the creamy texture.

Nutritional info per serve: Calories 52, Fat 5.2, Fiber 0.3, Carbs 0.9, Protein 1

Parmesan Pancake

Prep time: 10 minutes
Cook time: 16 minutes
Servings: 4
Ingredients:
- 3 eggs, beaten
- 1 cup coconut flour
- ¼ cup of coconut milk
- 1 oz Parmesan, grated
- 1 teaspoon baking powder
- 1 teaspoon apple cider vinegar
- 1 tablespoon avocado oil

Method:
1. Mix eggs with coconut flour, coconut milk, Parmesan, baking powder, and apple cider vinegar.
2. Stir the batter until it is homogenous.
3. Then preheat the avocado oil in the skillet well.
4. Pour the small amount of the pancake mixture (a batter) in the hot oil and flatten it in the shape of the pancake.
5. Roast the pancake on medium heat for 2 minutes per side.
6. Repeat the same steps with the remaining pancake batter.

Nutritional info per serve: Calories 231, Fat 12.8, Fiber 10.5, Carbs 18.1, Protein 10.8

Brussel Sprouts Soup

Prep time: 10 minutes
Cook time: 30 minutes
Servings: 7
Ingredients:
- 1 cup Brussel sprouts
- 2 oz bacon, chopped, roasted
- 1 teaspoon butter
- 1 spring onion, diced
- 6 cups chicken broth
- 1 teaspoon dried rosemary

Method:
1. Roast the spring onion in the butter until it is light brown.
2. Then transfer the onion in the saucepan.
3. Add bacon, Brussel sprouts, chicken broth, and dried rosemary.
4. Close the lid and cook the soup on medium heat for 25 minutes.

Nutritional info per serve: Calories 91, Fat 5.2, Fiber 0.7, Carbs 2.9, Protein 7.7

Baked Asparagus

Prep time: 10 minutes
Cook time: 30 minutes
Servings: 3
Ingredients:
- 1-pound asparagus
- 1 teaspoon lime juice
- 1 teaspoon butter

Method:
1. Line the baking tray with baking paper.
2. Put the asparagus in the baking tray, flatten it gently and sprinkle with butter and lime juice.
3. Bake the asparagus at 360F for 30 minutes.

Nutritional info per serve: Calories 42, Fat 1.5, Fiber 3.2, Carbs 6.1, Protein 3.4

Keto Soup

Prep time: 10 minutes
Cook time: 20 minutes
Servings: 4
Ingredients:
- 1 jalapeño pepper, chopped
- 1 cup spinach, chopped

- 1 cup broccoli, chopped
- ½ cup of coconut milk
- 3 cups of water
- 1 teaspoon allspices

Method:
1. Put all ingredients in the saucepan.
2. Boil the soup on medium heat for 20 minutes.

Nutritional info per serve: Calories 81, Fat 7.3, Fiber 1.6, Carbs 4, Protein 1.6

Grilled Mushrooms

Prep time: 10 minutes
Cook time: 25 minutes
Servings: 2
Ingredients:
- 4 Portobello mushrooms
- 1 tablespoon sesame oil
- ½ teaspoon salt

Method:
1. Put the mushrooms in the baking tray and sprinkle with sesame oil and salt.
2. Bake the mushrooms at 360F for 25 minutes.

Nutritional info per serve: Calories 100, Fat 6.8, Fiber 2, Carbs 6, Protein 6

Grilled Garlic Eggplants

Prep time: 10 minutes
Cook time: 10 minutes
Servings: 4
Ingredients:
- 2 eggplants, sliced lengthwise
- 1 teaspoon minced garlic
- 1 teaspoon salt
- 2 teaspoons sesame oil

Method:
1. Rub the slices eggplants with minced garlic, salt, and sesame oil.
2. Then preheat grill to 390F.
3. Put the eggplants in the grill and roast them for 2 minutes per side.

Nutritional info per serve: Calories 90, Fat 2.8, Fiber 9.7, Carbs 16.3, Protein 2.7

Parmesan Brussel Sprouts

Prep time: 10 minutes
Cook time: 25 minutes
Servings: 4
Ingredients:
- 10 oz Brussel sprouts
- 2 oz Parmesan, grated
- 1 teaspoon coconut oil
- 1 teaspoon chili flakes

Method:
1. Grease the baking tray with coconut oil and put the Brussel sprouts inside in one layer.
2. Sprinkle them with chili flakes and bake in the oven at 360F for 20 minutes.
3. Then stir the vegetables and top them with parmesan.
4. Bake the meal for 5 minutes more.

Nutritional info per serve: Calories 86, Fat 4.4, Fiber 2.7, Carbs 7, Protein 7

Eggplant Saute

Prep time: 10 minutes
Cook time: 50 minutes
Servings: 4
Ingredients:
- 1 bell pepper, chopped
- 1 eggplant, chopped
- ¼ cup tomatoes, rushed
- 1 tablespoon butter
- 1 chili pepper, chopped
- ¼ cup of water

Method:
1. Put all ingredients in the pot and close the lid.
2. Preheat the oven to 360F.
3. Put the pot with the vegetable mixture in the preheated oven and cook for 50 minutes.

Nutritional info per serve: Calories 66, Fat 3.2, Fiber 4.6, Carbs 9.5, Protein 1.6

Cabbage Pancake

Prep time: 10 minutes
Cook time: 10 minutes
Servings: 4
Ingredients:
- 2 cups white cabbage, shredded
- 4 eggs, beaten
- 1 teaspoon salt
- 1 tablespoon avocado oil

Method:
1. Mix shredded cabbage with eggs and salt.
2. Then preheat the avocado oil in the skillet well.
3. Make the small pancakes from the cabbage mixture and roast them in the hot oil for 5 minutes per side or until the pancakes are light brown.

Nutritional info per serve: Calories 76, Fat 4.9, Fiber 1, Carbs 2.6, Protein 6

Vegetable Soup

Prep time: 10 minutes
Cook time: 20 minutes
Servings: 6
Ingredients:
- 2 cups bell pepper, chopped
- 1 carrot, chopped
- 1 teaspoon dried rosemary
- 5 cups chicken broth
- 1 cup of water
- 1 teaspoon ground black pepper
- 1 teaspoon coconut oil

Method:
1. Melt the coconut oil in the saucepan and add the carrot. Roast the carrot for 5 minutes.
2. Then stir it and add bell pepper, dried rosemary, chicken broth, water, and ground black pepper.
3. Close the lid and cook the soup on medium heat for 15 minutes.

Nutritional info per serve: Calories 57, Fat 2, Fiber 1, Carbs 5.1, Protein 4.6

Celery Root Puree

Prep time: 15 minutes
Cook time: 15 minutes
Servings: 4
Ingredients:
- 2 cups celery root, chopped
- 1 cup of water
- 1 tablespoon butter
- 1 teaspoon salt

Method:
1. Put the celery in the saucepan. Add water and boil it for 15 minutes.
2. Then drain water and mash the celery root with the help of the potato masher.
3. Add butter and salt. Stir the puree well.

Nutritional info per serve: Calories 58, Fat 3.1, Fiber 1.4, Carbs 7.2, Protein 1.2

Green Cabbage Soup

Prep time: 10 minutes
Cook time: 15 minutes
Servings: 4
Ingredients:
- 1 cup green cabbage, shredded
- 1 carrot, diced
- 1 zucchini, spiralized
- 4 cups of water
- ½ cup heavy cream
- 1 teaspoon salt

Method:
1. Pour water in the saucepan and bring it to boil.
2. Add diced carrot, heavy cream, salt, and green cabbage.
3. Simmer the mixture for 5 minutes.
4. After this, add zucchini and cook the soup for 5 minutes more.

Nutritional info per serve: Calories 70, Fat 5.7, Fiber 1.4, Carbs 4.6, Protein 1.3

Kale Soup

Prep time: 10 minutes
Cook time: 20 minutes
Servings: 5
Ingredients:
- ½ cup Cheddar cheese, shredded
- 3 cups kale, chopped
- 1 oz prosciutto, chopped
- 1 teaspoon sesame oil
- ½ teaspoon fennel seeds
- ½ cup heavy cream
- 1 teaspoon salt

Method:
1. Pour sesame oil in the saucepan and preheat it.
2. Add prosciutto and roast it for 2-3 minutes.
3. Then add kale, fennel seeds, salt, and heavy cream.
4. Bring the soup to boil and add Cheddar cheese.
5. Cook the soup for 3-4 minutes more or until the cheese is melted.

Nutritional info per serve: Calories 124, Fat 9.4, Fiber 0.7, Carbs 4.9, Protein 5.5

KETOGENIC DESSERT RECIPES

Butter Truffles

Prep time: 10 minutes
Cook time: 5 minutes
Servings: 10
Ingredients:
- 3 oz dark chocolate, chopped
- 2 tablespoons butter
- ⅔ cup coconut cream
- 2 tablespoons Erythritol
- ¼ teaspoon vanilla extract
- 1 teaspoon of cocoa powder

Method:
1. Melt the chocolate and mix it with butter.
2. Add coconut cream, Erythritol, and vanilla extract.
3. Then make the small balls (truffles) and coat them in the cocoa powder.
4. Refrigerate the dessert for 10-15 minutes before serving.

Nutritional info per serve: Calories 103, Fat 8.7, Fiber 0.7, Carbs 6.1, Protein 1.1

Pecan Brownies

Prep time: 15 minutes
Cook time: 25 minutes
Servings: 4
Ingredients:
- 3 eggs, beaten
- 2 tablespoons cocoa powder
- 2 teaspoons Erythritol
- ½ cup coconut flour
- 2 pecans, chopped
- ½ cup of coconut milk

Method:
1. In the mixing bowl, mix eggs with cocoa powder, Erythritol, coconut flour, pecans, and coconut milk.
2. Stir the mixture until smooth and pour it in the brownie mold. Flatten the surface of the brownie batter if needed.
3. Bake it at 360F for 25 minutes.
4. When the brownie is cooked, cut it into bars.

Nutritional info per serve: Calories 178, Fat 16, Fiber 2.8, Carbs 5.4, Protein 6.3

Flaxseeds Doughnuts

Prep time: 20 minutes
Cook time: 12 minutes
Servings: 24
Ingredients:
- ¼ cup erythritol
- ¼ cup flaxseed meal
- ¾ cup coconut flour
- 1 teaspoon baking powder
- 1 teaspoon vanilla extract
- 2 eggs, beaten
- 3 tablespoons butter
- ¼ cup heavy cream

Method:
1. In the mixing bowl, mix erythritol, flaxseed meal, coconut flour, baking powder, vanilla extract, eggs, butter, and cream.
2. Knead the soft dough and roll up it.
3. Cut the dough into doughnuts with the help of the cutter and put in the lined with a baking paper baking tray.
4. Bake the doughnuts in the preheated to 365F oven for 12 minutes or until the dessert is light brown.

Nutritional info per serve: Calories 44, Fat 3, Fiber 1.8, Carbs 3, Protein 1.2

Jelly Bears

Prep time: 20 minutes
Cook time: 10 minutes
Servings: 7
Ingredients:
- 1 cup of water
- 2 oz strawberries, mashed
- 1 tablespoon gelatin
- 1 teaspoon Erythritol

Method:
1. Mix water with mashed strawberries and Erythritol.
2. Bring the liquid to boil and chill for 10 minutes.
3. Then add gelatin and stir the liquid until it is smooth.
4. Pour it in the silicon molds with the shape of bears and refrigerate until solid.

Nutritional info per serve: Calories 6, Fat 0, Fiber 0.6, Carbs 0.6, Protein 0.9

Pecan Candies

Prep time: 10 minutes
Cook time: 0 minutes
Servings: 6
Ingredients:
- 5 tablespoons butter, softened
- 4 pecans, chopped
- 1 tablespoon Erythritol
- 1 tablespoon coconut shred

Method:
1. Mix butter with pecans, Erythritol, and coconut shred.
2. Make the small balls from the pecan mixture and refrigerate until solid.

Nutritional info per serve: Calories 155, Fat 16.8, Fiber 1.1, Carbs 1.6, Protein 1.2

Cocoa Pie

Prep time: 10 minutes
Cook time: 40 minutes
Servings: 5
Ingredients:
- 1 teaspoon baking powder
- 1 teaspoon vanilla extract
- 2 eggs, beaten
- 4 tablespoons cocoa powder
- 2 tablespoons swerve
- 8 tablespoons coconut cream

- 4 teaspoon coconut flour
- 1 teaspoon avocado oil

Method:
1. In the mixing bowl, mix baking powder with vanilla extract, eggs, cocoa powder, swerve, coconut cream, and coconut flour.
2. Stir the mixture until you get a smooth batter.
3. Then brush the baking pan with avocado oil and pour the pie batter inside.
4. Bake the pie at 360F for 40 minutes.

Nutritional info per serve: Calories 105, Fat 8.4, Fiber 2.6, Carbs 6.3, Protein 3.8

Cream Jelly

Prep time: 2 hours
Cook time: 1 minute
Servings: 5
Ingredients:
- 2 tablespoons Erythritol
- 1 teaspoon vanilla extract
- 2 cups heavy cream
- 2 tablespoons gelatin

Method:
1. Mix gelatin with ¼ cup of cream and microwave for 1 minute.
2. Then mix gelatin mixture with remaining heavy cream, vanilla extract, and Erythritol. Stir the liquid carefully.
3. Pour it in the silicone molds and refrigerate.
4. When the jelly is solid, the dessert is cooked.

Nutritional info per serve: Calories 177, Fat 17.8, Fiber 0, Carbs 1.5, Protein 3.4

Vanilla Mousse

Prep time: 7 minutes
Cook time: 7 minutes
Servings: 3
Ingredients:
- 2 blackberries, halved
- 1 cup heavy cream
- ½ teaspoon vanilla extract
- 2 teaspoon swerve
- 4 tablespoons butter

Method:
1. Whip the heavy cream and mix it with butter, swerve, and vanilla extract.
2. Whisk the mousse until homogenous.
3. Then transfer it in the serving cups and top with blackberries.

Nutritional info per serve: Calories 276, Fat 30.2, Fiber 0, Carbs 1.4, Protein 1

Cheese Pie

Prep time: 10 minutes
Cook time: 40 minutes
Servings: 12
Ingredients:
- 1 cup coconut, shredded
- 2 tablespoons flax seeds
- ¼ cup of coconut oil
- ½ cup heavy cream
- 1 cup cream cheese
- 3 tablespoons Erythritol
- 1 teaspoon vanilla extract
- 1 tablespoon gelatin

Method:
1. Mix the shredded coconut with flax seeds, coconut oil, heavy cream, cream cheese, Erythritol, and vanilla extract.
2. Whisk the mixture until smooth and add gelatin.
3. Start to preheat the liquid until gelatin is melted.
4. Then transfer the pie in the baking mold and refrigerate for 40 minutes.

Nutritional info per serve: Calories 157, Fat 15.7, Fiber 0.9, Carbs 2, Protein 2.5

Avocado Mousse

Prep time: 15 minutes
Cook time: 0 minutes
Servings: 4
Ingredients:
- 1 avocado, peeled, pitted, chopped
- 1/3 cup coconut cream
- 1 tablespoon Erythritol
- 1 teaspoon vanilla extract

Method:
1. Blend the avocado until smooth.
2. Then add coconut cream, Erythritol, and vanilla extract.
3. Carefully stir the cooked mousse and transfer it in the serving bowl.

Nutritional info per serve: Calories 152, Fat 14.6, Fiber 3.8, Carbs 5.6, Protein 1.4

Chocolate Pie

Prep time: 10 minutes
Cook time: 30 minutes
Servings: 8
Ingredients:
- 3 tablespoons butter, softened
- ½ cup heavy cream
- 1 teaspoon baking powder
- 1 cup coconut flour
- 1 oz dark chocolate, chopped

Method:
1. Mix butter with baking powder, coconut flour, and heavy cream.
2. Then transfer the mixture in the non-stick baking pan. Flatten the surface of the pie with the help of the spatula and top with chopped chocolate.
3. Bake the pie at 360F for 30 minutes.

Nutritional info per serve: Calories 91, Fat 8.4, Fiber 0.8, Carbs 3.6, Protein 0.7

Coconut Panna Cotta

Prep time: 40 minutes
Cook time: 10 minutes
Servings: 2
Ingredients:
- 1 cup coconut cream
- 1 teaspoon vanilla extract
- 2 teaspoons Erythritol
- 2 teaspoon coconut shred

- 1 tablespoon gelatin powder

Method:
1. Mix coconut cream with gelatin powder, vanilla extract, and Erythritol and preheat for 4 minutes.
2. Whisk the mixture until gelatin is dissolved and pour it in the serving cups.
3. Top every cup with coconut shred and refrigerate for 40 minutes.

Nutritional info per serve: Calories 310, Fat 30.3, Fiber 3, Carbs 7.6, Protein 5.8

No-Baked Cheesecake

Prep time: 45 minutes
Cook time: 1 minute
Servings: 8
Ingredients:
- 1 cup cream cheese
- 3 tablespoons Erythritol
- 1 tablespoon gelatin
- 5 tablespoons water

Method:
1. Mix gelatin with water and leave for 10 minutes. Then microwave the mixture for 1 minute or until it is liquid.
2. After this, mix cream cheese with liquid gelatin and Erythritol.
3. Pour the cheesecake mixture in the cheesecake mold and refrigerate for 30-40 minutes or until the cheesecake is solid.

Nutritional info per serve: Calories 104, Fat 10.1, Fiber 0, Carbs 0.8, Protein 2.9

Coconut Cookies

Prep time: 15 minutes
Cook time: 13 minutes
Servings: 6
Ingredients:
- ½ cup coconut flour
- 2 teaspoons coconut oil
- ¾ teaspoon coconut shred
- 1 teaspoon Erythritol
- 3 tablespoons coconut milk

Method:
1. In the mixing bowl, mix coconut flour with coconut oil, coconut shred, and Erythritol.
2. Add coconut milk and knead the dough.
3. Then make 6 balls from the dough and press them gently in the shape of the cookies.
4. Bake the cooked at 360F for 13 minutes.

Nutritional info per serve: Calories 37, Fat 3.7, Fiber 0.6, Carbs 1.2, Protein 0.3

Blackberries Bars

Prep time: 10 minutes
Cook time: 15 minutes
Servings: 12
Ingredients:
- ½ cup butter
- 2 oz blackberries, chopped
- 2 tablespoons Erythritol
- 2 tablespoons coconut flour
- ½ cup coconut, shredded

Method:
1. Mix butter with coconut flour and coconut shred and knead the dough.
2. Then put the mixture in the baking pan and flatten in the shape of the pie crust.
3. After this, mix blackberries with Erythritol.
4. Top the pie crust with blackberries mixture and bake in the oven at 360F for 15 minutes.
5. Cut the cooked meal into bars.

Nutritional info per serve: Calories 87, Fat 9, Fiber 1.1, Carbs 1.7, Protein 0.5

Cheesecake Bars

Prep time: 25 minutes
Cook time: 10 minutes
Servings: 8
Ingredients:
- 1 cup cream cheese
- 3 egg, beaten
- ¼ cup of coconut milk
- 3 tablespoons Erythritol
- 1 teaspoon vanilla extract
- ¼ cup coconut flour
- 1 tablespoon butter
- 1 tablespoon flax meal

Method:
1. In the mixing bowl, mix eggs with coconut milk, Erythritol, vanilla extract, coconut flour, butter, and flax meal.
2. Put the mixture in the baking pan and flatten in the shape of the pie crust.
3. Then bake it at 360F for 10 minutes.
4. Chill the cooked pie crust well and spread it with cream cheese.
5. Cut the meal into bars.

Nutritional info per serve: Calories 162, Fat 15.4, Fiber 0.6, Carbs 1.9, Protein 4.7

Cocoa Muffins

Prep time: 30 minutes
Cook time: 12 minutes
Servings: 6
Ingredients:
- 6 teaspoons butter
- 1 egg, beaten
- 2 tablespoons Erythritol
- 2 teaspoons cocoa powder
- 1 cup coconut flour

Method:
1. Put all ingredients in the mixing bowl and whisk until you get a smooth batter.
2. After this, pour the batter in the muffin molds (fill ½ part of every mold) and bake at 365F for 12 minutes.
3. Cool the cooked muffins and remove them from the molds.

Nutritional info per serve: Calories 126, Fat 6.6, Fiber 8.2, Carbs 13.7, Protein 3.7

Coconut Pudding

Prep time: 20 minutes
Cook time: 10 minutes
Servings: 2

Ingredients:
- ½ cup coconut cream
- 2 eggs, beaten
- 1 teaspoon coconut flour
- 2 tablespoons Erythritol
- 1 teaspoon vanilla extract

Method:
1. Mix all ingredients in the saucepan and stir until smooth.
2. Bring the liquid to boil and remove from the heat.
3. Transfer it in the serving cups and refrigerate for 15-20 minutes.

Nutritional info per serve: Calories 212, Fat 18.8, Fiber 1.7, Carbs 4.6, Protein 7.1

Cream Cheese Mousse

Prep time: 10 minutes
Cook time: 0 minutes
Servings: 2
Ingredients:
- ½ cup coconut cream
- 3 tablespoons cream cheese
- 1 tablespoon Erythritol
- 1 tablespoon coconut shred

Method:
1. Mix coconut cream with coconut shred, Erythritol, and cream cheese.
2. Whisk the mixture until it is soft and fluffy.
3. Transfer the mousse in the serving cups.

Nutritional info per serve: Calories 238, Fat 23.8, Fiber 2.3, Carbs 5.7, Protein 3

Chocolate Bacon Strips

Prep time: 30 minutes
Cook time: 5 minutes
Servings: 6
Ingredients:
- 6 bacon sliced, cooked
- 2 oz dark chocolate
- 1 tablespoon coconut oil
- ¼ teaspoon dried mint

Method:
1. Freeze the bacon slices for 15-20 minutes in the freezer.
2. Meanwhile, melt chocolate and mix it with coconut oil and dried mint.
3. Then dip every bacon slice in the chocolate mixture and refrigerate for 10-15 minutes.

Nutritional info per serve: Calories 173, Fat 13, Fiber 0.3, Carbs 5.9, Protein 7.8

Cocoa Fudge

Prep time: 10 minutes
Cook time: 30 minutes
Servings: 4
Ingredients:
- 4 tablespoons coconut oil
- ¼ cup of coconut milk
- ½ teaspoon vanilla extract
- 2 teaspoons Erythritol
- 3 tablespoons cocoa powder

Method:
1. Melt the coconut oil and mix it with cocoa powder, Erythritol, vanilla extract, and coconut milk. Stir the mixture until homogenous.
2. Then line the baking mold with baking paper.
3. Pour the fudge mixture inside, flatten it and refrigerate for 30 minutes.
4. Cut the fudge into bars.

Nutritional info per serve: Calories 162, Fat 17.7, Fiber 1.5, Carbs 3.1, Protein 1.1

Coconut Cookies

Prep time: 15 minutes
Cook time: 10 minutes
Servings: 6
Ingredients:
- 2 tablespoons coconut shred
- 1 teaspoon vanilla extract
- 3 tablespoons coconut oil
- ½ cup coconut flour
- 1 tablespoon Erythritol

Method:
1. Put all ingredients in the mixing bowl and, mix and knead the dough.
2. Make 6 coconut cookies by using a cutter.
3. Bake the cookies at 360F for 10 minutes.

Nutritional info per serve: Calories 108, Fat 11.8, Fiber 1, Carbs 3.4, Protein 0.7

Sweet Mousse

Prep time: 10 minutes
Cook time: 10 minutes
Servings: 5
Ingredients:
- 1 cup heavy cream
- 1 tablespoon Erythritol
- 5 teaspoons cream cheese
- 1 tablespoon coconut flour

Method:
1. Bring the heavy cream to boil and add coconut flour and Erythritol.
2. Simmer the cream mixture for 30 seconds.
3. Then add cream cheese and whisk the mousse until it is smooth.
4. Transfer it in the serving cups.

Nutritional info per serve: Calories 100, Fat 10.2, Fiber 0.5, Carbs 4.6, Protein 0.9

Lemon Pie

Prep time: 15 minutes
Cook time: 25 minutes
Servings: 6
Ingredients:
- ½ lemon, chopped
- 1 cup almond flour
- ¼ cup of coconut oil
- ¼ cup of coconut milk
- 1 teaspoon baking powder
- 3 tablespoons Erythritol

Method:
1. Mix almond flour with coconut oil, coconut milk, baking powder, and Erythritol.

2. Transfer the mixture in the non-stick baking pan and top with chopped lemon.
3. Bake the pie at 360F for 25 minutes.
4. Then cool the pie well and cut into servings.
Nutritional info per serve: Calories 130, Fat 13.8, Fiber 0.9, Carbs 9.9, Protein 1.3

2-Ingredients Ice Cream
Prep time: 10 minutes
Cook time: 0 minutes
Servings: 2
Ingredients:
- 2 raspberries, frozen
- 2 blackberries, frozen

Method:
1. Put the raspberries and blackberries in the food processor and blend until smooth.
2. Transfer the mixture in the serving glasses.
Nutritional info per serve: Calories 10, Fat 0.1, Fiber 1.3, Carbs 2.4, Protein 0.2

Berry Muffins
Prep time: 10 minutes
Cook time: 14 minutes
Servings: 8
Ingredients:
- 1/3 cup coconut oil
- 1 teaspoon vanilla extract
- 2 tablespoons Erythritol
- 1 cup coconut flour
- 1 oz raspberries
- 1 egg, beaten
- 1 teaspoon baking powder

Method:
1. Put all ingredients except raspberries in the mixing bowl and mix until smooth.
2. Then add raspberries and carefully mix the muffin batter with the help of the spoon.
3. Transfer the mixture in the muffin molds (fill ½ part of every mold) and bake at 365F for 14 minutes.
Nutritional info per serve: Calories 150, Fat 11.2, Fiber 6.2, Carbs 14.6, Protein 2.7

Cocoa Squares
Prep time: 10 minutes
Cook time: 21 minutes
Servings: 9
Ingredients:
- 4 tablespoons butter, softened
- ½ teaspoon baking powder
- 4 tablespoons Erythritol
- 1 teaspoon vanilla extract
- 4 ounces cream cheese
- 6 eggs, beaten
- 3 tablespoons cocoa powder

Method:
1. Mix butter with baking powder, Erythritol, vanilla extract, cream cheese, eggs, and cocoa powder.
2. When the mixture is homogenous, transfer it in the baking pan and bake for 21 minutes at 360F.
Nutritional info per serve: Calories 137, Fat 12.7, Fiber 0.6, Carbs 8.4, Protein 5

Avocado Pie
Prep time: 10 minutes
Cook time: 30 minutes
Servings: 6
Ingredients:
- 1 avocado, pitted, peeled, sliced
- 1 cup heavy cream
- 1 ½ cup coconut flour
- 1 teaspoon baking powder
- 3 tablespoons Erythritol
- 1 tablespoon butter

Method:
1. Mix coconut flour with heavy cream, baking powder, Erythritol, and butter.
2. Make the smooth mixture and pour it in the non-stick baking pan.
3. Top the batter with avocado and bake at 360F for 30 minutes.
Nutritional info per serve: Calories 275, Fat 18.9, Fiber 14.3, Carbs 23.8, Protein 5.1

Mint Brownies
Prep time: 10 minutes
Cook time: 35 minutes
Servings: 12
Ingredients:
- 1 cup butter
- 6 eggs, beaten
- 3 tablespoons cocoa powder
- 1 teaspoon vanilla extract
- ½ teaspoon baking powder
- ½ cup coconut cream
- ½ cup coconut flour
- 1 teaspoon dried mint

Method:
1. Mix butter with eggs, cocoa powder, vanilla extract, baking powder, coconut cream, coconut flour, and dried mint.
2. When the mixture is smooth, pour it in the non-sticky brownie mold and bake at 360F for 35 minutes.
3. Cut the brownie into bars when they are cooked.
Nutritional info per serve: Calories 214, Fat 20.6, Fiber 2.6, Carbs 5, Protein 4.1

Almond Bars
Prep time: 15 minutes
Cook time: 12 minutes
Servings: 4
Ingredients:
- ½ cup almond flour
- 2 oz almonds, chopped
- 3 tablespoons butter
- 1 tablespoon Erythritol
- 1 teaspoon vanilla extract
- ½ teaspoon baking powder

Method:
1. Mix almond flour with butter, Erythritol, vanilla extract, and baking powder.
2. Then add almond and knead the dough.
3. Put the dough in the lined with the baking paper tray and cut into bars.

4. Bake the dessert for 12 minutes at 360F.
Nutritional info per serve: Calories 643, Fat 61.8, Fiber 7.9, Carbs 14.9, Protein 12.2

Coconut Chia Pudding

Cook time: 30 minutes
Servings: 2
Ingredients:
- 1 cup of coconut milk
- 1 tablespoon coconut shred
- 3 tablespoons chia seeds

Method:
1. Mix coconut milk with coconut shred and chia seeds.
2. Transfer the mixture in the servings glasses and leave for 25 minutes to rest.
Nutritional info per serve: Calories 404, Fat 37.6, Fiber 10.4, Carbs 16.6, Protein 6.3

Matcha Muffins

Prep time: 10 minutes
Cook time: 14 minutes
Servings: 5
Ingredients:
- 1 teaspoon matcha tea
- 1 teaspoon baking powder
- 1 cup of coconut milk
- 1 cup coconut flour
- 1 teaspoon vanilla extract
- 1 tablespoon butter, melted

Method:
1. In the mixing bowl, mix matcha tea with baking powder, coconut milk, coconut flour, vanilla extract, and butter.
2. Stir the mixture until you get a smooth batter and pour it in the muffin molds.
3. Bake the muffins at 360F for 14 minutes.
Nutritional info per serve: Calories 231, Fat 16.1, Fiber 10.7, Carbs 19.4, Protein 4.3

Coconut Parfaits

Prep time: 10 minutes
Cook time: 0 minutes
Servings: 6
Ingredients:
- 2 cups of coconut milk
- 1 teaspoon vanilla extract
- 2 tablespoons Erythritol
- 4 strawberries, chopped
- 4 pecans, chopped

Method:
1. Mix coconut milk with vanilla extract and Erythritol.
2. The put strawberries in every serving glass.
3. Top them with coconut milk and pecans.
Nutritional info per serve: Calories 254, Fat 25.8, Fiber 2.9, Carbs 11.5, Protein 2.9

Vanilla Shake

Prep time: 5 minutes
Cook time: 3 minutes
Servings: 4
Ingredients:
- 2 cups of coconut milk
- 1 avocado, pitted, peeled, chopped
- 1 teaspoon vanilla extract
- 1 tablespoon Erythritol

Method:
1. Put all ingredients in the food processor and blend for 3 minutes.
2. Pour the vanilla shake in the glasses.
Nutritional info per serve: Calories 382, Fat 38.4, Fiber 6, Carbs 14.9, Protein 3.7

Lemon Pudding

Prep time: 10 minutes
Cook time: 10 minutes
Servings: 4
Ingredients:
- 2 cups of coconut milk
- 1 teaspoon lemon zest
- 1 teaspoon vanilla extract
- 3 egg yolks
- 1 tablespoon Erythritol

Method:
1. Mix coconut milk with egg yolks and vanilla extract.
2. Bring the liquid to boil. Stir it constantly.
3. Then add Erythritol and lemon zest.
4. Whisk the pudding and transfer it in the serving glasses. Chill the pudding to the room temperature.
Nutritional info per serve: Calories 320, Fat 32, Fiber 2.7, Carbs 11.1, Protein 4.8

Almond Biscotti

Prep time: 10 minutes
Cook time: 30 minutes
Servings: 7
Ingredients:
- 1 cup almond flour
- 1 teaspoon baking powder
- 1/3 teaspoon ground clove
- 1 teaspoon vanilla extract
- 2 tablespoons coconut oil
- 1 egg, beaten
- 1 tablespoon Erythritol
- ¼ cup almonds, chopped

Method:
1. Mix almond flour with baking powder, ground clove, vanilla extract, coconut oil, egg, and Erythritol. Add almonds.
2. Knead the dough and make the shape of loaf from it.
3. Then put it in the preheated to 365F oven and bake for 20 minutes.
4. Then slice the cooked loaf into pieces and return in the oven. Put the sliced loaf in one layer.
5. Cook the dessert at 360F for 10 minutes more.
6. Chill the cooked biscotti well.
Nutritional info per serve: Calories 156, Fat 14.2, Fiber 2.2, Carbs 6.8, Protein 5

Peppermint Cream

Prep time: 20 minutes

Cook time: 0 minutes
Servings: 3
Ingredients:
- ½ cup butter softened
- 1 tablespoon Erythritol
- 1 tablespoon cocoa powder
- 1 avocado, pitted, peeled, chopped
- 2 tablespoons ricotta cheese

Method:
1. Mix butter with cocoa powder.
2. Then add Erythritol, avocado, and ricotta cheese.
3. Blend the mixture until you get smooth and soft cream.

Nutritional info per serve: Calories 426, Fat 44.8, Fiber 5, Carbs 12.3, Protein 3.1

Zucchini Pudding

Prep time: 15 minutes
Cook time: 10 minutes
Servings: 6
Ingredients:
- 1 zucchini, grated
- 2 eggs, whisked
- ½ teaspoon baking powder
- ½ cup coconut cream
- 1 cup coconut flour
- 2 tablespoons Erythritol
- ½ teaspoon vanilla extract
- ¾ teaspoon ground cardamom

Method:
1. Put all ingredients in the food processor and blend until smooth.
2. Then transfer the mixture in the saucepan and simmer for 5 minutes.
3. Cool the cooked pudding and transfer it in the serving glasses.

Nutritional info per serve: Calories 154, Fat 8.3, Fiber 8.9, Carbs 21.1, Protein 5.4

Egg Pudding

Prep time: 10 minutes
Cook time: 10 minutes
Servings: 6
Ingredients:
- 1 ⅔ cups of coconut milk
- 5 eggs, beaten
- 5 tablespoons Erythritol
- 1 teaspoon vanilla extract

Method:
1. Mix eggs with coconut milk, Erythritol, and vanilla extract.
2. Pour the liquid in the saucepan and simmer it for 10 minutes on low heat.
3. Chill the pudding and put it in the serving bowls.

Nutritional info per serve: Calories 208, Fat 19.5, Fiber 1.5, Carbs 6.6, Protein 6.1

Basil Cookies

Prep time: 15 minutes
Cook time: 15 minutes
Servings: 6
Ingredients:
- 1 tablespoon dried basil
- 2 tablespoons Erythritol
- 1 tablespoon coconut oil, softened
- ½ cup coconut flour
- 3 tablespoons almond meal
- 2 tablespoons avocado oil

Method:
1. In the mixing bowl, mix dried basil, Erythritol, coconut oil, coconut flour, and almond meal.
2. Knead the dough and roll it up with the help of the rolling pin.
3. Then make the cookies with the help of the cutter.
4. Brush the baking tray with avocado oil.
5. Put the cookies inside and bake them for 15 minutes at 355F.

Nutritional info per serve: Calories 83, Fat 5.4, Fiber 4.6, Carbs 12.6, Protein 2

Clove Pudding

Prep time: 20 minutes
Cook time: 10 minutes
Servings: 2
Ingredients:
- 4 teaspoons gelatin
- ¼ teaspoon Erythritol
- 1 cup organic almond milk
- 1 teaspoon ground clove
- ¼ teaspoon ground cinnamon

Method:
1. Mix gelatin with almond milk and leave for 10 minutes.
2. Then stir the liquid, add ground clove, cinnamon, and Erythritol.
3. Bring the liquid to boil and remove from the heat.
4. Cool the pudding and pour it in the serving glasses.

Nutritional info per serve: Calories 327, Fat 28.8, Fiber 3.2, Carbs 8.2, Protein 14.8

Sweet Paprika Bars

Prep time: 20 minutes
Cook time: 15 minutes
Servings: 4
Ingredients:
- 1 teaspoon pumpkin puree
- 1 egg, beaten
- ½ teaspoon vanilla extract
- ½ cup coconut flour
- ¼ teaspoon ground paprika
- 1 tablespoon ricotta cheese
- 1 tablespoon Erythritol

Method:
1. Mix pumpkin puree with egg, vanilla extract, coconut flour, ground paprika, ricotta cheese, and Erythritol.
2. Then transfer the mixture in the lined with the baking paper tray and flatten it if needed.
3. Bake the meal in the oven for 15 minutes at 360F.

4. Then remove the meal from the oven, cut into bars, and chill well.
Nutritional info per serve: Calories 83, Fat 2.9, Fiber 6.1, Carbs 14.3, Protein 3.9

Chia and Cocoa Biscuits

Prep time: 10 minutes
Cook time: 12 minutes
Servings: 8
Ingredients:
- 2 tablespoons chia seeds
- 2 cups coconut flour
- 1 egg, beaten
- ¼ cup butter, softened
- 2 tablespoons coconut, shredded
- 2 tablespoons Erythritol
- 1 tablespoon cocoa powder
- 1 teaspoon baking soda

Method:
1. Put all ingredients in the mixing bowl and knead the dough.
2. Then cut the dough into pieces and roll into balls.
3. Press the balls gently and put in the baking tray.
4. Bake the biscuits for 12 minutes at 365F.
Nutritional info per serve: Calories 219, Fat 12, Fiber 14.8, Carbs 27.3, Protein 6.1

Pecan Fudge

Prep time: 30 minutes
Cook time: 0 minutes
Servings: 2
Ingredients:
- 1 oz dark chocolate (keto)
- ½ teaspoon of cocoa powder
- 2 tablespoons coconut oil
- 1 pecan, chopped

Method:
1. Melt the chocolate and mix it with coconut oil, cocoa powder, and pecan.
2. Whisk the mixture until smooth. Preheat it a little bit if needed.
3. Then pour the mixture in the silicone mold, flatten well and refrigerate for 20 minutes.
4. Cut the pecan fudge into pieces.
Nutritional info per serve: Calories 239, Fat 23.4, Fiber 1.9, Carbs 9.8, Protein 1.9

Walnut Brownies

Prep time: 20 minutes
Cook time: 25 minutes
Servings: 6
Ingredients:
- 1 egg, beaten
- ⅓ cup of cocoa powder
- 2 tablespoons erythritol
- 7 tablespoons coconut oil
- ½ teaspoon ground cinnamon
- ¼ cup coconut flour
- 2 oz walnuts, chopped
- ½ teaspoon baking powder

Method:
1. Put all ingredients in the food processor and blend until homogenous.
2. Then line the baking pan with baking paper and pour the brownie batter inside. Flatten the brownie dough and bake it at 360F for 25 minutes.
3. Then cool the cooked dessert and cut into bars.
Nutritional info per serve: Calories 237, Fat 23.3, Fiber 4.2, Carbs 12.3, Protein 4.7

Cream Cheese Bombs

Prep time: 20 minutes
Cook time: 0 minutes
Servings: 5
Ingredients:
- 5 tablespoons cream cheese
- 1 teaspoon vanilla extract
- 2 eggs, boiled, chopped
- 2 tablespoons Erythritol
- ¾ teaspoon lemon zest, grated
- 1 tablespoon coconut shred

Method:
1. Put all ingredients in the mixing bowl and mix.
2. Then make the bombs with the help of the ice cream scopper.
3. Refrigerate the cream cheese bombs for 10-15 minutes before serving.
Nutritional info per serve: Calories 73, Fat 6.2, Fiber 0.2, Carbs 7, Protein 3

Blueberries Scones

Prep time: 15 minutes
Cook time: 30 minutes
Servings: 10
Ingredients:
- ½ cup almond flour
- 1 cup blueberries
- 2 eggs, beaten
- ½ cup coconut cream
- ½ cup of coconut oil
- 5 tablespoons Erythritol
- 2 teaspoons vanilla extract
- 2 teaspoons baking powder

Method:
1. Blend all ingredients in the food processor until you get a smooth batter.
2. Pour the batter in the silicone mold and bake at 360F for 30 minutes.
3. Chill the cooked dessert well and cut into scones.
Nutritional info per serve: Calories 179, Fat 17.3, Fiber 1.2, Carbs 12.1, Protein 2.7

Vanilla Donuts

Prep time: 15 minutes
Cook time: 20 minutes
Servings: 6
Ingredients:
- 4 tablespoons coconut flour
- 2 tablespoons almond meal
- 1 teaspoon vanilla extract

- 2 tablespoons Erythritol
- 2 eggs, beaten
- 2 tablespoons heavy cream
- 1 teaspoon coconut oil, softened

Method:
1. Mix coconut flour with almond meal, vanilla extract, Erythritol, eggs, heavy cream, and coconut oil.
2. Knead the soft and non-sticky dough.
3. Then roll it up and make the donuts with the help of the donut cutter.
4. Bake the donuts at 360F for 20 minutes.

Nutritional info per serve: Calories 98, Fat 6.4, Fiber 3.6, Carbs 11.1, Protein 3.7

Tender Cookies

Prep time: 10 minutes
Cook time: 13 minutes
Servings: 12
Ingredients:
- 1 teaspoon vanilla extract
- ½ cup of coconut oil
- 2 eggs, beaten
- 2 tablespoons Erythritol
- 2 cups coconut flour
- 1 oz dark chocolate, chopped

Method:
1. In the mixing bowl, mix the vanilla extract with coconut oil, eggs, Erythritol, coconut flour.
2. When the mixture is homogenous, add chopped chocolate and stir it.
3. Make the small balls from the dough and put them in the baking tray.
4. Bake the cookies at 360F for 13 minutes.

Nutritional info per serve: Calories 182, Fat 12.5, Fiber 8.1, Carbs 17.4, Protein 3.8

Keto Caramel

Prep time: 10 minutes
Cook time: 10 minutes
Servings: 4
Ingredients:
- 4 teaspoons coconut oil
- ½ cup Erythritol
- ½ teaspoon vanilla extract
- 1 pecan, chopped

Method:
1. Melt the coconut oil in the saucepan.
2. Add Erythritol and vanilla extract. Melt the mixture.
3. Then remove it from the heat, add pecan, and pour the caramel in the glass jar.

Nutritional info per serve: Calories 150, Fat 16.5, Fiber 0.4, Carbs 3.6, Protein 0.4

Crustless Yogurt Cake

Prep time: 20 minutes
Cook time: 40 minutes
Servings: 12
Ingredients:
- 2 cups plain yogurt
- 2 strawberries, chopped
- 1 teaspoon vanilla extract
- 2 tablespoons gelatin
- 2 tablespoons Erythritol
- 10 tablespoons water

Method:
1. Mix water with gelatin and leave the mixture for 10 minutes.
2. Then microwave it until liquid and mix it with plain yogurt. Whisk the mixture until smooth.
3. After this, add vanilla extract, strawberries, and Erythritol.
4. Pour the yogurt mixture in the silicone mold and freeze for 30-40 minutes.

Nutritional info per serve: Calories 35, Fat 0.5, Fiber 0, Carbs 5.6, Protein 3.3

Almond Mousse

Prep time: 10 minutes
Servings: 2
Ingredients:
- 4 tablespoons cream cheese
- 4 tablespoons organic almond milk
- 1 teaspoon Erythritol

Method:
1. Blend cream cheese with almond milk and Erythritol.
2. When the mixture is smooth and fluffy, transfer it in the serving glasses.

Nutritional info per serve: Calories 139, Fat 14.1, Fiber 0.7, Carbs 4.7, Protein 2.2

Cocoa Paste

Prep time: 10 minutes
Cook time: 0 minutes
Servings: 6
Ingredients:
- 2 oz butter, softened
- 4 tablespoons cocoa powder
- 1 teaspoon ground cinnamon

Method:
1. Whisk the butter with cocoa powder until fluffy and transfer in the serving bowl.
2. Top the paste with ground cinnamon.

Nutritional info per serve: Calories 7.7, Fat 8.1, Fiber 1.3, Carbs 2.3, Protein 0.8

Ricotta Bars

Prep time: 25 minutes
Cook time: 0 minutes
Servings: 6
Ingredients:
- 6 tablespoons coconut oil, softened
- 6 tablespoons ricotta cheese
- 1 teaspoon vanilla extract
- 3 tablespoons Erythritol

Method:
1. Mix ricotta cheese with coconut oil.
2. When the mixture is smooth, add vanilla extract and Erythritol.
3. Stir the mixture and transfer in the baking tray. Flatten the mixture and freeze for 20 minutes.
4. Cut the cooked meal into the bars.

Nutritional info per serve: Calories 141, Fat 14.8, Fiber 0, Carbs 8.4, Protein 1.8

Stevia Pie

Prep time: 10 minutes
Cook time: 30 minutes
Servings: 4
Ingredients:
- 1 cup of coconut milk
- 1 cup almond flour
- 1 teaspoon baking powder
- 3 eggs, beaten
- 2 tablespoons liquid stevia
- 1 teaspoon vanilla extract
- Cooking spray

Method:
1. Mix coconut milk with almond flour, baking powder, eggs, liquid stevia, and vanilla extract.
2. Spray the baking pan with cooking spray from inside.
3. Pour the coconut mixture in the baking pan and bake at 350F for 30 minutes.

Nutritional info per serve: Calories 349, Fat 31.6, Fiber 4.4, Carbs 10.3, Protein 11.5

Lime Meringue

Prep time: 15 minutes
Cook time: 2.5 hours
Servings: 5
Ingredients:
- 2 egg whites,
- 5 teaspoons Erythritol
- 1 teaspoon lime juice
- 1 tablespoon coconut flour

Method:
1. Whisk the egg whites until you get the sift peaks.
2. Then add Erythritol, lime juice, and coconut flour. Whisk the egg whites for 1 minute more.
3. Then line the baking tray with baking paper.
4. Make the small meringues from the egg white mixture (use the spoon) and bake them at 340F for 2.5 hours.

Nutritional info per serve: Calories 13, Fat 0.2, Fiber 0.6, Carbs 6.2, Protein 1.7

Cinnamon Buns

Prep time: 20 minutes
Cook time: 25 minutes
Servings: 8
Ingredients:
- ½ cup coconut flour
- ½ cup almond meal
- 1 teaspoon baking powder
- 1 tablespoon Erythritol
- 1 tablespoon ground cinnamon
- 2 tablespoons butter, softened
- ¼ cup of coconut milk

Method:
1. In the mixing bowl, mix coconut flour with almond meal, baking powder, Erythritol, and knead the dough.
2. Then roll it up and spread with softened butter.
3. After this, sprinkle the dough with ground cinnamon and roll it.
4. Cut the roll into buns and put in the non-stick baking pan in one layer.
5. Bake the dessert at 355F for 25 minutes or until the buns are light brown.

Nutritional info per serve: Calories 110, Fat 8.4, Fiber 4.4, Carbs 9.6, Protein 2.5

Coconut Pie

Prep time: 10 minutes
Cook time: 30 minutes
Servings: 10
Ingredients:
- ½ cup coconut flour
- 1 tablespoon butter
- 1 egg, beaten
- ¾ teaspoon salt
- ½ cup ricotta cheese
- ½ cup coconut cream
- 4 tablespoons Erythritol
- 1 teaspoon vanilla extract
- 1 tablespoon coconut oil

Method:
1. Put all ingredients in the mixing bowl and stir until smooth.
2. Then transfer the prepared batter in the non-stick baking pan and flatten it if needed.
3. Bake the pie at 360F for 30 minutes.
4. Then chill the cooked dessert well and cut into servings.

Nutritional info per serve: Calories 98, Fat 7.4, Fiber 2.7, Carbs 11.4, Protein 3

Coconut Custard

Prep time: 10 minutes
Cook time: 15 minutes
Servings: 8
Ingredients:
- 1⅓ cup of coconut milk
- 4 tablespoons lime zest
- 6 eggs, beaten
- 5 tablespoons Erythritol
- 1 teaspoon lime juice

Method:
1. Mix coconut milk with lime zest, eggs, and Erythritol.
2. Bring the mixture to boil. Stir it constantly.
3. Then pour the custard in the serving glasses and cool to the room temperature.
4. Sprinkle the dessert with lime juice.

Nutritional info per serve: Calories 302, Fat 29.5, Fiber 2.8, Carbs 16.3, Protein 6.7

Almond Bun

Prep time: 15 minutes
Cook time: 35 minutes
Servings: 6
Ingredients:
- 3 tablespoons coconut oil
- 1 cup almond flour

- 1 oz almonds, chopped
- ½ teaspoon baking powder
- ½ teaspoon apple cider vinegar
- 1 tablespoon Erythritol
- 2 tablespoons almond meal
- 1 tablespoon ricotta cheese

Method:
1. In the mixing bowl, mix coconut oil with almond flour, baking powder, apple cider vinegar, and almond meal. Knead the dough.
2. Then roll up the dough.
3. In the separated bowl, mix ricotta cheese, Erythritol, and almonds.
4. Spread the ricotta mixture over the dough. Roll the dough into roll.
5. Cut the roll into 6 buns and bake at 360F for 35 minutes.

Nutritional info per serve: Calories 202, Fat 18.2, Fiber 2.6, Carbs 7.8, Protein 5.3

Vanilla Topping

Prep time: 15 minute
Cook time: 10 minutes
Servings: 6
Ingredients:
- ½ cup heavy cream
- 2 tablespoons Erythritol
- 1 teaspoon vanilla extract

Method:
1. Being the heavy cream to boil. Add Erythritol and vanilla extract.
2. Simmer the mixture for 5 minutes.
3. After this, chill the cooked topping and store it in the fridge for up to 4 days.

Nutritional info per serve: Calories 202, Fat 18.2, Fiber 2.6, Carbs 7.8, Protein 5.3

Vanilla Flan

Prep time: 10 minutes
Cook time: 75 minutes
Servings: 4
Ingredients:
- 4 teaspoons Erythritol
- 1 tablespoon coconut oil
- 4 tablespoons coconut milk
- 1 teaspoon vanilla extract
- 4 eggs, beaten
- 1 cup organic almond milk

Method:
1. Grease the baking pan with coconut oil.
2. Then top the baking pan with Erythritol.
3. After this, mix coconut milk with vanilla extract, eggs, and almond milk. Whisk the mixture.
4. Pour ti over the Erythritol.
5. Bake the flan at 350F for 75 minutes.
6. Then turn the flan down and transfer in the serving plate.

Nutritional info per serve: Calories 145, Fat 12, Fiber 0.6, Carbs 8.3, Protein 6.1

Raspberry Cream

Prep time: 30 minutes
Cook time: 0 minutes
Servings: 4
Ingredients:
- 2 cups coconut cream
- 2 oz raspberries
- 2 tablespoons Erythritol
- 1 tablespoon coconut shred

Method:
1. Put all ingredients in the food processor and blend until smooth.
2. Then transfer the mixture in the serving bowl and refrigerate for 20 minutes.

Nutritional info per serve: Calories 197, Fat 20, Fiber 2.5, Carbs 10.9, Protein 1.9

Vanilla Pancake Pie

Prep time: 15 minutes
Cook time: 15 minutes
Servings: 6
Ingredients:
- 1 tablespoon vanilla extract
- 1 cup coconut flour
- 1 teaspoon baking powder
- ¼ cup heavy cream
- 1 tablespoon Erythritol
- 1 teaspoon sesame oil
- 4 tablespoons ricotta cheese
- 1 teaspoon plain yogurt

Method:
1. Mix all ingredients except ricotta cheese, Erythritol, and plain yogurt, and whisk until you get a smooth batter.
2. Then preheat the non-stick baking pan and pour the small amount of batter inside.
3. Flatten it in the shape of pancake and roast for 1 minute per side. Repeat the same steps with all remaining batter.
4. Then mix plain yogurt with ricotta cheese and Erythritol.
5. Spread every pancake with the ricotta cheese mixture and put them one-on-one in the shape of the pie.

Nutritional info per serve: Calories 126, Fat 5.4, Fiber 8, Carbs 17.2, Protein 4

Frozen Ice

Prep time: 40 minutes
Cook time: 0 minutes
Servings: 2
Ingredients:
- ½ cup heavy cream
- ¼ cup of orange juice

Method:
1. Blend the heavy cream with orange juice.
2. Then pour the liquid in the ice cubes molds and freeze until they are solid.

Nutritional info per serve: Calories 118, Fat 11.2, Fiber 0.1, Carbs 4.1, Protein 0.8

Nutmeg Pies

Prep time: 15 minutes
Cook time: 25 minutes
Servings: 7
Ingredients:

- 1 tablespoon pumpkin pie spices
- 1 teaspoon ground nutmeg
- 2 tablespoons coconut oil
- 1 cup almond flour
- 3 tablespoons coconut cream
- 1 tablespoon butter
- 1 teaspoon baking powder
- 3 tablespoons Erythritol
- Cooking spray

Method:
1. Spray the baking pan with cooking spray.
2. Then mix all remaining ingredients in the mixing bowl. Knead the dough and cut it into small pieces.
3. Put the pieces of dough in the prepared baking pan and bake them at 355F for 25 minutes.

Nutritional info per serve: Calories 164, Fat 14.9, Fiber 2.1, Carbs 11.3, Protein 3.7

Coconut Mascarpone

Prep time: 10 minutes
Cook time: 0 minutes
Servings: 5
Ingredients:
- 2 tablespoons Erythritol
- 2 cups mascarpone
- 1 teaspoon vanilla extract
- 3 tablespoons coconut shred

Method:
1. Whisk the mascarpone with Erythritol and vanilla extract.
2. Then transfer the meal in the serving plates and top with coconut shred.

Nutritional info per serve: Calories 205, Fat 15.9, Fiber 0.6, Carbs 10.3, Protein 11.2

Seeds Bars

Prep time: 30 minutes
Cook time: 0 minutes
Servings: 4
Ingredients:
- 4 pecans, chopped
- 1 oz walnuts, chopped
- 1 tablespoon sunflower seeds
- 2 tablespoons coconut oil
- 1 tablespoon Erythritol
- 1 teaspoon flax seeds

Method:
1. Mix pecans with walnuts, sunflower seeds, coconut oil, Erythritol, and flax seeds.
2. When the mixture is homogenous, transfer it in the lined with the baking paper tray and flatten well.
3. Cut the mixture into the bars and refrigerate for 10-15 minutes.

Nutritional info per serve: Calories 207, Fat 21.5, Fiber 2.2, Carbs 6, Protein 3.5

Lime Cheese

Prep time: 10 minutes
Cook time: 0 minutes
Servings: 4
Ingredients:
- 1 cup cream cheese
- 1 teaspoon lime zest, grated
- 1 tablespoon lime juice
- 1 teaspoon vanilla extract
- 1 tablespoon Erythritol
- 1 oz walnuts, chopped

Method:
1. Put all ingredients in the food processor and blend the mixture.
2. Store the lime cheese in the freezer for up to 3 days.

Nutritional info per serve: Calories 250, Fat 24.4, Fiber 0.5, Carbs 6.2, Protein 6.1

Egg Cake

Prep time: 10 minutes
Cook time: 40 minutes
Servings: 8
Ingredients:
- 1 cup heavy cream
- 6 eggs, beaten
- 1 cup coconut flour
- 1 teaspoon vanilla extract
- 3 tablespoons Erythritol
- 1 tablespoon butter

Method:
1. Put all ingredients in the food processor and blend the mixture until you get a smooth batter.
2. Then pour the batter in the non-stick baking pan and bake at 360F for 40 minutes.

Nutritional info per serve: Calories 173, Fat 11.8, Fiber 6, Carbs 16.4, Protein 6.5

Sorbet

Prep time: 50 minutes
Cook time: 0 minutes
Servings: 4
Ingredients:
- 3 oz strawberries, chopped
- 1 cup of water

Method:
1. Blend the strawberries with water and pour in the silicone mold.
2. Freeze the mixture for 40 minutes.
3. After this, blend it again with the help of the food processor and transfer in the serving bowls.

Nutritional info per serve: Calories 7, Fat 0.1, Fiber 0.4, Carbs 1.6, Protein 0.1

Swerve Cookies

Prep time: 15 minutes
Cook time: 15 minutes
Servings: 5
Ingredients:
- ½ teaspoon baking powder
- ¼ teaspoon lemon juice
- 2 tablespoons swerve
- 1 cup coconut flour
- 2 tablespoons coconut oil
- 1 tablespoon ground nutmeg

Method:
1. Mix all ingredients in the mixing bowl, knead the dough.

2. Then cut the dough into small pieces and roll into balls.
3. Put the dough balls in the baking pan and bake at 360F for 15 minutes or until the cookies are light brown.
Nutritional info per serve: Calories 151, Fat 8.4, Fiber 9.9, Carbs 16.9, Protein 3.3

Vanilla Custard

Prep time: 10 minutes
Cook time: 10 minutes
Servings: 2
Ingredients:
- ½ cup heavy cream
- 3 egg yolks
- 1 teaspoon vanilla extract
- 1 teaspoon liquid stevia

Method:
1. Whisk the egg yolks with heavy cream and simmer the mixture for 5 minutes. Stir it constantly.
2. Then add vanilla extract and liquid stevia. Stir the mixture and cool to room temperature.
Nutritional info per serve: Calories 190, Fat 17.9, Fiber 0, Carbs 2, Protein 4.7

Cardamom Shortcakes

Prep time: 10 minutes
Cook time: 3 minutes
Servings: 8
Ingredients:
- 2 eggs, beaten
- 1 cup coconut flour
- 2 tablespoons Erythritol
- 1 teaspoon baking powder
- ¾ cup raspberries
- 1 teaspoon coconut oil, softened
- ½ cup coconut cream

Method:
1. Mix eggs with coconut flour, Erythritol, baking powder, coconut oil, and coconut cream.
2. When the mixture is homogenous, pour it in the lined with a baking paper baking tray.
3. Top the mixture with raspberries and bake at 355F for 30 minutes.
4. Cut the cooked dessert into servings.
Nutritional info per serve: Calories 122, Fat 6.8, Fiber 7.1, Carbs 16.3, Protein 3.9

Nutmeg Balls

Prep time: 25 minutes
Cook time: 0 minutes
Servings: 6
Ingredients:
- ½ cup of coconut oil
- 3 tablespoons almond flour
- 3 tablespoons heavy cream
- 1 teaspoon ground nutmeg
- 3 tablespoons Erythritol

Method:
1. In the mixing bowl, mix coconut oil with almond flour, heavy cream, ground nutmeg, and Erythritol.
2. Make a smooth mixture.
3. Make the balls from the mixture and refrigerate for 10-15 minutes before serving.
Nutritional info per serve: Calories 205, Fat 22.7, Fiber 0.5, Carbs 8.6, Protein 0.9

Lime Cookies

Prep time: 15 minutes
Cook time: 14 minutes
Servings: 6
Ingredients:
- ¼ tablespoon Psyllium husk
- ½ cup coconut flour
- ½ teaspoon vanilla extract
- ¼ teaspoon baking powder
- ½ teaspoon lime juice
- 2 tablespoons coconut oil, softened
- 1 egg, beaten
- 1 teaspoon lime zest, grated
- 2 tablespoons Erythritol

Method:
1. Mix all ingredients in the mixing bowl. Knead the dough.
2. Then roll up the dough with the help of the rolling pin.
3. Cut the dough into the cookies with the help of the cutter and put it in the tray.
4. Bake the cookies at 360F for 14 minutes or until they are light brown.
Nutritional info per serve: Calories 95, Fat 6.3, Fiber 5.2, Carbs 13.4, Protein 2.3

Coffee Mousse

Prep time: 30 minutes
Cook time: 15 minutes
Servings: 5
Ingredients:
- ½ cup coffee, brewed
- 1 cup cream cheese
- 2 tablespoons gelatin
- 1½ teaspoon vanilla extract
- 1 teaspoon Erythritol
- ½ cup coconut cream

Method:
1. Mix coconut cream with gelatin and preheat the liquid until gelatin is dissolved.
2. Then add cream cheese, coffee, vanilla extract, and Erythritol.
3. Whisk the mixture for 3-4 minutes and pour in the serving glasses.
4. Refrigerate the mousse for at least 10-15 minutes before serving.
Nutritional info per serve: Calories 240, Fat 21.9, Fiber 0.5, Carbs 4.1, Protein 6.5

Butter Cookies

Prep time: 15 minutes
Cook time: 12 minutes
Servings: 10
Ingredients:
- 1 cup coconut flour
- ½ teaspoon Psyllium husk
- 2 tablespoons Erythritol
- 1 tablespoon coconut shred

- 1 teaspoon baking powder
- ½ cup butter, softened
- 1 teaspoon vanilla extract

Method:
1. Put all ingredients in the mixing bowl and knead the dough.
2. Cut the dough into 10 pieces and make the balls.
3. Bake the dough balls for 12 minutes at 360F.

Nutritional info per serve: Calories 137, Fat 10.9, Fiber 5.4, Carbs 11.5, Protein 1.7

Pecan Granola

Prep time: 10 minutes
Cook time: 30 minutes
Servings: 6
Ingredients:
- 1 cup coconut shredded
- 3 pecans, chopped
- 1 oz almonds, chopped
- 2 tablespoons Erythritol
- 2 tablespoons chia seeds
- 2 tablespoons butter
- 1 teaspoon allspices

Method:
1. Put all ingredients in the bowl and mix.
2. Then transfer the mixture in the lined with the baking paper tray and flatten it.
3. Bake the granola for 30 minutes at 345F.
4. Then cool it well and crush roughly.

Nutritional info per serve: Calories 256, Fat 25.3, Fiber 4.9, Carbs 13.6, Protein 2.2

Sweet Bacon Bombs

Prep time: 30 minutes
Cook time: 0 minutes
Servings: 4
Ingredients:
- 1 tablespoon Erythritol
- 1 teaspoon ground clove
- 1 teaspoon vanilla extract
- 4 tablespoons cream cheese
- 1 tablespoon coconut shred
- 1 oz bacon, chopped, roasted

Method:
1. Put all ingredients in the mixing bowl and stir with the help of the spoon until homogenous.
2. Then make the balls from the mixture and refrigerate them for 25 minutes.

Nutritional info per serve: Calories 86, Fat 7.4, Fiber 0.4, Carbs 4.9, Protein 3.5

Almond Pudding

Prep time: 30 minutes
Cook time: 0 minutes
Servings: 4
Ingredients:
- 1 tablespoon chia seeds
- 1 cup organic almond milk
- 1 oz almonds, chopped
- 1 teaspoon Erythritol

Method:
1. Mix almond milk with chia seeds, Erythritol, and almonds.
2. Transfer the mixture in the serving glasses and leave to rest for 20 minutes.

Nutritional info per serve: Calories 81, Fat 6.3, Fiber 2.1, Carbs 4.5, Protein 2.5

Egg Clouds

Prep time: 15 minutes
Cook time: 1.5 hour
Servings: 7
Ingredients:
- 4 egg whites
- 4 tablespoons Erythritol

Method:
1. Whisk the egg whites until you get soft peaks.
2. Then mix egg white mixture with Erythritol, carefully mix the mixture.
3. Line the baking tray with baking paper.
4. Make the egg white clouds from the mixture with the help of the spoon and put them in the baking tray.
5. Bake the dessert at 345F for 1.5 hours.

Nutritional info per serve: Calories 10, Fat 0, Fiber 0, Carbs 8.7, Protein 2.1

Matcha Custard

Prep time: 20 minutes
Cook time: 10 minutes
Servings: 4
Ingredients:
- 1 cup coconut cream
- 1 tablespoon matcha tea
- 2 tablespoons Erythritol
- 1 teaspoon vanilla extract
- 4 eggs, beaten

Method:
1. Mix coconut cream with eggs, matcha tea, Erythritol, and vanilla extract.
2. Bring the mixture to boil and remove from the heat.
3. Chill the cooked custard and transfer in the serving glasses.

Nutritional info per serve: Calories 206, Fat 18.7, Fiber 1.3, Carbs 11.9, Protein 6.9

Milk Sorbet

Prep time: 40 minutes
Cook time: 0 minutes
Servings: 3
Ingredients:
- 1 cup of coconut milk
- ½ cup of water
- 1 tablespoon liquid stevia
- 1 teaspoon vanilla extract

Method:
1. Put all ingredients in the mixing bowl and mix.
2. Then pour the mixture in the silicone mold and freeze until solid.
3. Transfer the frozen mixture in the food processor and blend until smooth.

4. Pour the cooked sorbet in the serving bowls.
Nutritional info per serve: Calories 188, Fat 19.1, Fiber 1.8, Carbs 4.6, Protein 1.8

Salty Cookies
Prep time: 10 minutes
Cook time: 13 minutes
Servings: 6
Ingredients:
- 1 teaspoon salt
- 2 tablespoons Erythritol
- ¼ cup heavy cream
- ¼ cup butter
- 2 tablespoons cocoa powder
- 3 tablespoons coconut shred
- ½ teaspoon vanilla extract
- ¼ cup coconut flour

Method:
1. Mix all ingredients except salt in the mixing bowl and knead the dough.
2. Make the cookies from the dough and sprinkle them with salt.
3. Bake the cookies at 360F for 13 minutes.
Nutritional info per serve: Calories 127, Fat 11.9, Fiber 2.9, Carbs 10.2, Protein 1.4

Fluffy Cookies
Prep time: 10 minutes
Cook time: 15 minutes
Servings: 6
Ingredients:
- 1 teaspoon ground clove
- 2 tablespoon coconut shred
- 1 cup almond flour
- 2 eggs, beaten
- 5 tablespoons heavy cream
- 2 tablespoons Erythritol
- 1 teaspoon baking powder

Method:
1. Mix all ingredients from the list above in the mixing bowl.
2. Knead the dough and make 6 cookies.
3. Put the cookies in the baking tray and bake them at 360F for 15 minutes.
Nutritional info per serve: Calories 109, Fat 10.2, Fiber 1, Carbs 7.7, Protein 3.1

Vanilla Butter Bars
Prep time: 30 minutes
Cook time: 0 minutes
Servings: 6
Ingredients:
- 4 tablespoons butter, softened
- 4 ounces of cocoa powder
- 2 tablespoons Erythritol
- 1 tablespoon vanilla extract

Method:
1. Mix all ingredients and put them in the silicone mold.
2. Refrigerate the mixture until solid.
3. Cut the dessert into bars.
Nutritional info per serve: Calories 116, Fat 10.2, Fiber 5.6, Carbs 15.6, Protein 3.5

Peppermint Cookies
Prep time: 15 minutes
Cook time: 14 minutes
Servings: 12
Ingredients:
- 1 teaspoon peppermint extract
- ½ cup coconut cream
- 1 ½ cup coconut flour
- 1 teaspoon coconut oil
- 1 teaspoon baking powder
- ¼ teaspoon apple cider vinegar
- ¼ cup Truvia

Method:
1. Put all ingredients in the mixing bowl and mix until homogenous. Knead the dough.
2. Then cut the dough into 12 pieces and roll them in the cookies.
3. Bake the cookies at 360F for 14 minutes.
Nutritional info per serve: Calories 88, Fat 4.3, Fiber 6.2, Carbs 10.8, Protein 2.2

Cinnamon Marshmallows
Prep time: 10 minutes
Cook time: 10 minutes
Servings: 6
Ingredients:
- 2 tablespoons gelatin
- 5 tablespoons Erythritol
- 1 cup hot water
- 2 teaspoons ground cinnamon

Method:
1. Mix water with Erythritol and ground cinnamon.
2. Then add gelatin and whisk the mixture until it is dissolved.
3. After this, whisk the liquid with the help of the hand mixer until the mixture will turn into white.
4. Transfer the cooked marshmallow in the lined with the baking paper tray and flatten well.
5. Cut the cooked dessert into bars.
Nutritional info per serve: Calories 10, Fat 0, Fiber 0.4, Carbs 13.1, Protein 2

Orange Ice Cream
Prep time: 8 hours
Cook time: 10 minutes
Servings: 3
Ingredients:
- 1 cup heavy cream
- 2 egg yolks
- 1 tablespoon Erythritol
- 1 teaspoon orange zest, grated
- 2 tablespoons orange juice

Method:
1. Mix heavy cream with egg yolks, Erythritol, orange zest, and orange juice.
2. Whisk the mixture until smooth and preheat for 10 minutes. Stir it constantly.

3. Then pour the mixture in the ice cream maker and cook the ice cream according to the ice cream maker directions.
Nutritional info per serve: Calories 179, Fat 17.8, Fiber 0.1, Carbs 7.8, Protein 2.7

Yogurt Pudding

Prep time: 15 minutes
Cook time: 0 minutes
Servings: 3
Ingredients:
- 2 cups yogurt
- 5 tablespoons Erythritol
- 3 tablespoons coconut shred

Method:
1. Mix yogurt with Erythritol and coconut shred.
2. Pour the pudding in the glasses.

Nutritional info per serve: Calories 150, Fat 10.3, Fiber 1, Carbs 8.2, Protein 5.7

Cream Popsicle

Prep time: 2 hours
Cook time: 0 minutes
Servings: 5
Ingredients:
- 1 avocado, pitted
- 1 tablespoon lemon juice
- 3 cups of coconut milk

Method:
1. Blend the avocado until smooth and mix with lemon juice and coconut milk.
2. Pour the liquid in the popsicle molds and freeze until solid.

Nutritional info per serve: Calories 414, Fat 42.2, Fiber 5.9, Carbs 11.5, Protein 4.1

Keto Smoothie

Prep time: 5 minutes
Cook time: 0 minutes
Servings: 4
Ingredients:
- ½ cup of coconut milk
- 2 peaches, chopped
- 1 cup fresh basil

Method:
1. Put all ingredients in the food processor and blend until smooth.
2. Pour the smoothie in the serving glasses.

Nutritional info per serve: Calories 100, Fat 7.4, Fiber 1.9, Carbs 8.8, Protein 1.6

Watermelon Sorbet

Prep time: 1 hour
Cook time: 0 minutes
Servings: 4
Ingredients:
- 2 cups watermelon
- 1 teaspoon fresh mint, chopped

Method:
1. Blend the watermelon until smooth and freeze it for 1 hour.
2. Then blend the frozen watermelon and mix it with fresh mint.

Nutritional info per serve: Calories 23, Fat 0.1, Fiber 0.3, Carbs 5.8, Protein 0.5

Sweet Ice Cubes

Prep time: 60 minutes
Cook time: 0 minutes
Servings: 4
Ingredients:
- 2 cups of water
- 3 tablespoons lemon juice
- 1 cup watermelon, chopped

Method:
1. Mix water with lemon juice and watermelon.
2. Transfer the mixture in the ice cube molds and freeze them for 50 minutes.
3. Remove the cooked dessert from the ice cube molds.

Nutritional info per serve: Calories 14, Fat 0.1, Fiber 0.2, Carbs 3.1, Protein 0.3

Peach Ice Cream

Prep time: 40 minutes
Cook time: 10 minutes
Servings: 2
Ingredients:
- ½ cup of coconut milk
- 1 peach, pitted, chopped
- 1 teaspoon vanilla extract

Method:
1. Blend the peach until smooth and mix it with coconut cream and vanilla extract.
2. Pour the mixture in the silicone mold and freeze for 40 minutes.

Nutritional info per serve: Calories 174, Fat 14.5, Fiber 2.5, Carbs 10.6, Protein 2.1

Strawberry Popsicles

Prep time: 1 hour
Cook time: 0 minutes
Servings: 4
Ingredients:
- 1½ cups strawberries
- 2 cups of water

Method:
1. Blend the strawberries until smooth, mix them with water.
2. Pour the liquid in the popsicle molds and freeze for 50 minutes.

Nutritional info per serve: Calories 63, Fat 0.6, Fiber 4, Carbs 15.2, Protein 1.3

Cantaloupe Sorbet

Prep time: 75 minutes
Cook time: 0 minutes
Servings: 4
Ingredients:
- 2 cups cantaloupe, chopped
- ½ cup of water

Method:
1. Blend the cantaloupe until smooth.

2. Add water and pour the mixture in the silicone mold.
3. Freeze the mixture for 1 hour.
4. Then put the frozen mixture in the blender and blend until smooth.
Nutritional info per serve: Calories 27, Fat 0.2, Fiber 0.7, Carbs 6.4, Protein 0.7

Carambola Jelly
Prep time: 60 minutes
Cook time: 15 minutes
Servings: 3
Ingredients:
- 3 oz carambola, sliced
- 1 cup of water
- 2 tablespoons Erythritol
- 1 tablespoon gelatin

Method:
1. Mix gelatin with water and Erythritol.
2. Bring the liquid to boil and remove from the heat.
3. Pour the liquid in the silicone molds and top with sliced carambola.
4. Refrigerate the jelly for 60 minutes.
Nutritional info per serve: Calories 13, Fat 0.1, Fiber 0.8, Carbs 11.9, Protein 2.3

Blueberry Ice Cream
Prep time: 40 minutes
Cook time: 0 minutes
Servings: 4
Ingredients:
- 2 cups Plain yogurt
- ½ cup blueberries

Method:
1. Mash the blueberries and mix them with yogurt.
2. Pour the mixture in the silicone mold and freeze for 30 minutes.
3. Transfer the cooked ice cream in the serving bowls/glasses.
Nutritional info per serve: Calories 98, Fat 11.6, Fiber 0.4, Carbs 11.3, Protein 7.1

APPENDIX : RECIPES INDEX

2-Ingredients Ice Cream 173
2-Meat Stew 137

A

Allspice Pork 151
Almond Bars 173
Almond Bars 83
Almond Biscotti 174
Almond Bowl 39
Almond Bun 178
Almond Chicken 113
Almond Meatballs 139
Almond Mousse 177
Almond Pork 134
Almond Porridge 26
Almond Pudding 182
Almond Squid 107
Almond Zucchini 83
Anise Beef 150
Apple Cider Vinegar Kale 69
Apple Cider Vinegar Lettuce 165
Aromatic Cumin Chicken 130
Artichoke and Mushrooms Mix 55
Artichoke Bake 66
Artichoke Dip 91
Arugula and Halloumi Salad 55
Arugula Chicken 119
Arugula Salad 48
Asparagus Chips 87
Asparagus Eggs 22
Asparagus Masala 159
Asparagus Pockets 53
Asparagus Soup 157
Avocado and Chicken Salad 40
Avocado and Meat Salad 149
Avocado and Walnut Bowl 158
Avocado Boats 22
Avocado Mix 66
Avocado Mousse 170
Avocado Pie 173
Avocado Spread 162

B

Bacon and Eggs Rolls 22
Bacon and Oregano Broccoli 68
Bacon Beef 139
Bacon Broccoli Mash 153
Bacon Brussels Sprouts 59
Bacon Chicken 131
Bacon Eggs 80
Bacon Mix 31
Bacon Muffins 21
Bacon Okra 61
Bacon Pancakes 34
Bacon Peppers 83
Bacon Salad 51
Bacon Wraps 80
Bacon Zucchini Noodles 52
Bacon-Wrapped Chicken 122
Baked Asparagus 166
Baked Broccoli 165

Baked Coconut Eggs 88
Baked Eggplant 66
Baked Kale 156
Baked Okra 76
Baked Parmesan Broccoli 63
Baked Radishes 67
Baked Rutabaga 154
Baked Zucchini 63
Basil Bake 163
Basil Bites 86
Basil Chicken 122
Basil Clam Chowder 110
Basil Cookies 175
Basil Crackers 90
Basil Meatloaf 146
Basil Scotch Eggs 32
Basil Scramble 24
Basil Shrimp 104
Basil Shrimp Noodles 52
Basil Tomato Mix 65
BBQ Pork Ribs 148
BBQ Shredded Chicken 132
Beef and Broccoli Stew 142
Beef and Chili 148
Beef and Eggplant Stew 142
Beef and Vegetables Stew 133
Beef and Zucchini Muffins 138
Beef Bowl 20
Beef Burgers 42
Beef Casserole 30
Beef Lasagna 136
Beef Loin in Parmesan Sauce 148
Beef Rolls 142
Beef Salad 52
Beef Sauce with Broccoli 139
Beef Saute 141
Beef Soup with Spinach 152
Beef Stew 55
Beef Stuffed Avocado 138
Beef Tacos 40
Beef with Noodles 141
Beef with Pickled Chilies 139
Bergamot Pork 149
Berry Cubes 89
Berry Muffins 173
Blackberries Bars 171
Blackberry Granola 27
Blue Cheese Cauliflower 165
Blue Cheese Quiche 36
Blueberries Scones 176
Blueberry Ice Cream 185
Boiled Crab Legs 106
Bok Choy Pan 23
Breakfast Beef Mix 37
Broccoli and Bacon Bowls 40
Broccoli and Cucumber Bowl 56
Broccoli and Spinach Bowl 74
Broccoli Biscuits 82
Broccoli Crackers 162

Broccoli Curry 156
Broccoli Puree 71
Broccoli Slaw 160
Broccoli Spread 155
Brussel Sprouts Fritters 155
Brussel Sprouts Soup 166
Brussel Sprouts with Eggs 29
Brussels Sprout Bake 51
Butter Asparagus 58
Butter Beef 149
Butter Cauliflower Puree 72
Butter Chicken 122
Butter Cookies 181
Butter Eggs 20
Butter Pork 134
Butter Truffles 169
Butter Waffles 35
Butter Zucchini Pasta 164
Buttered Onion 156
Butternut Squash Spaghetti with Salami 26

C

Cabbage and Arugula Salad 69
Cabbage Balls 159
Cabbage Mix 58
Cabbage Pancake 167
Cabbage Stew 72
Cajun Chicken 120
Cajun Pork 148
Cajun Zucchini 70
Cajun Zucchini Noodles 70
Calamari Salad 104
Cantaloupe Sorbet 184
Carambola Jelly 185
Cardamom Chicken 124
Cardamom Chicken Cubes 54
Cardamom Eggplant 68
Cardamom Sausages 140
Cardamom Shortcakes 181
Cardamom Shrimp 109
Carrot Chips 87
Carrot Lamb Roast 144
Cauli Bowl 27
Cauli Soup 45
Cauliflower Bowl 25
Cauliflower Bread 28
Cauliflower Cakes 22
Cauliflower Cream 155
Cauliflower Cream 50
Cauliflower Cupcakes 27
Cauliflower Florets in Cheese 87
Cauliflower Mix 64
Cauliflower Pizza 40
Cauliflower Pizza with Greens 161
Cauliflower Polenta 74
Cauliflower Puree 58
Cauliflower Puree 63
Cauliflower Risotto 47
Cauliflower Sauce 77
Cauliflower Tortillas 61
Cauliflower Tots 75

Cayenne Green Beans 61
Cayenne Mahi Mahi 99
Cayenne Muffins 29
Cayenne Shrimp 84
Celery Boats 84
Celery Cream Soup 154
Celery Cream Soup 155
Celery Root Puree 168
Celery Skewers 90
Chai Pancakes 34
Chard Salad 165
Cheddar Chicken Thighs 115
Cheddar Green Beans 58
Cheddar Jalapenos 72
Cheddar Kale 69
Cheddar Peppers 79
Cheddar Pizza 41
Cheddar Pollock 95
Cheddar Salad 56
Cheddar Tilapia 92
Cheese and Peppers Bowl 74
Cheese and Pork Casserole 133
Cheese and Spinach Cream 155
Cheese Baked Eggs 22
Cheese Chicken Casserole 113
Cheese Cubes 86
Cheese Edamame Beans 157
Cheese Meatloaf 38
Cheese Mushrooms 161
Cheese Pie 170
Cheese Pizza 117
Cheese Plate 79
Cheese Ramekins 75
Cheese Wrapped Chicken Wings 119
Cheese Zucchini Noodle 43
Cheesecake Bars 171
Cheesy Broccoli 63
Cheesy Cauliflower Florets 69
Cheesy Fritatta 24
Cheesy Tuna Bake 96
Chia and Broccoli Soup 53
Chia and Cocoa Biscuits 176
Chia Bowls 31
Chia Crackers 81
Chia Drink 31
Chia Oatmeal 32
Chia Smoothie 29
Chicken and Broccoli Casserole 121
Chicken and Cream 119
Chicken and Leek Stew 131
Chicken Calzone 127
Chicken Caps 79
Chicken Cream Soup 127
Chicken Curry 118
Chicken Frittata 37
Chicken in Avocado 130
Chicken in Parmesan Sauce 124
Chicken Lettuce Wraps 130
Chicken Meatballs 112
Chicken Meatballs 38

Chicken Meatballs with Turmeric 121
Chicken Meatloaf 123
Chicken Pancakes 121
Chicken Pie 114
Chicken Pockets 49
Chicken Relish 43
Chicken Roast 128
Chicken Scramble 30
Chicken Soup with Basil 47
Chicken Spread 126
Chicken Stir-Fry 40
Chicken Tortillas 118
Chicken Tortillas 41
Chicken under Onion Blanket 125
Chicken with Asparagus Blanket 131
Chicken with Crumbled Cheese 129
Chicken with Olives 115
Chicken with Peppers 114
Chicken with Sauce 120
Chicken Wraps 88
Chili Asparagus 52
Chili Avocado 60
Chili Biscuits 77
Chili Bok Choy 59
Chili Burger 42
Chili Caps 86
Chili Chicken 118
Chili Chicken Ground 129
Chili Cod 99
Chili Collard Greens 62
Chili Drumsticks 112
Chili Ground Pork 137
Chili Mussel Stew 110
Chili Pork Skewers 136
Chili Zucchini Rounds 75
Chipotle Cream 50
Chipotle Lamb Ribs 143
Chives and Bacon Muffins 29
Chives Fritters 159
Chocolate Bacon 87
Chocolate Bacon Strips 172
Chocolate Pecans 90
Chocolate Pie 170
Chocolate Smoothie 35
Chorizo Dip 77
Chorizo Eggs 23
Chorizo Muffins 80
Chorizo Pizza 25
Chorizo Tacos 81
Chorizo Wrap 54
Cilantro and Cabbage Salad 161
Cilantro Asparagus 158
Cilantro Cauliflower Rice 60
Cilantro Chicken 130
Cilantro Cod 109
Cilantro Crackers 77
Cilantro Jalapenos 72
Cilantro Salmon 95
Cilantro Smoothie 36
Cilantro Steak 49

Cilantro Turnip Bake 67
Cinnamon Beef Stew 142
Cinnamon Buns 178
Cinnamon Chicken Drumsticks 126
Cinnamon Eggs 22
Cinnamon Hake 94
Cinnamon Marshmallows 183
Cinnamon Porridge 32
Cinnamon Rutabaga 65
Clam Soup 52
Clam Soup with Pancetta 102
Clam Stew 96
Clams and Bacon 107
Clove Carrots 68
Clove Chicken 116
Clove Lamb 144
Clove Pudding 175
Coated Chicken 127
Coated Radish 160
Coated Shrimps 108
Coated Zucchinis 83
Cocoa Fudge 172
Cocoa Mix 36
Cocoa Muffins 171
Cocoa Pancakes 34
Cocoa Paste 177
Cocoa Pie 169
Cocoa Squares 173
Coconut Bok Choy 166
Coconut Bread 72
Coconut Broccoli 62
Coconut Chia 27
Coconut Chia Pudding 174
Coconut Chicken 113
Coconut Chicken 121
Coconut Chicken Fillets 114
Coconut Chicken Wings 53
Coconut Cookies 171
Coconut Cookies 172
Coconut Custard 178
Coconut Eggs 25
Coconut Lamb Shoulder 145
Coconut Mascarpone 180
Coconut Mushroom Cream Soup 153
Coconut Mushroom Soup 56
Coconut Pancakes 24
Coconut Panna Cotta 170
Coconut Parfaits 174
Coconut Pie 178
Coconut Pork Bowl 148
Coconut Pudding 171
Coconut Smoothie 20
Coconut Souffle 37
Coconut Tilapia 105
Cod Casserole 106
Cod Curry 94
Cod in Sauce 93
Cod Packets 102
Cod Sticks 104
Cod Sticks 97

Cod with Chives 93
Coffee Cubes 91
Coffee Mousse 181
Coffee Porridge 32
Cordon Bleu Chicken 117
Coriander Chicken 123
Coriander Cod 97
Coriander Eggplant Slices 62
Crab Dip 78
Crab Fritters 98
Crab Meatballs 46
Crab Spread 85
Cream Cauliflower Mix 66
Cream Cheese Bombs 176
Cream Cheese Chicken 128
Cream Cheese Dip 79
Cream Cheese Eggs 28
Cream Cheese Mousse 172
Cream Cheese Rolls 49
Cream Jelly 170
Cream Muffins 28
Cream Pancakes 33
Cream Popsicle 184
Creamy Cabbage 64
Creamy Cod 100
Creamy Halibut 103
Creamy Omelet Roll 21
Creamy Pork Skewers 151
Creamy Ramekins 29
Creamy Spinach 60
Creamy Turkey 117
Cremini Mushrooms Muffins 46
Crispy Bites 87
Crunchy Chicken Wings 128
Crustless Chicken Pie 123
Crustless Yogurt Cake 177
Cucumber Bites 85
Cucumber Salad 65
Cumin Green Beans 75
Cumin Meatballs 135
Cumin Pork Casserole 47
Cumin Seabass 104
Cumin Soup 164
Cumin Stew 117
Curry Cod 101
Curry Crabs 111
Curry Meatballs 135
Curry Soup 50
Curry Tofu 67

D
Dijon Brussel Sprouts 71
Dijon Chicken 119
Dill Beef Patties 141
Dill Bell Peppers 68
Dill Bowls 44
Dill Cabbage Mix 60
Dill Cauliflower 60
Dill Chicken Muffins 129
Dill Chicken Soup 121
Dill Crab Cakes 108

Dill Eggs 23
Dill Lamb Shank 145
Dill Pickled Zucchini 71
Dill Tomatoes 65
Duck Casserole 130
Duck Salad 116
Duck Spread 126
Duck with Zucchinis 115

E
Egg Balls 31
Egg Balls 77
Egg Burrito 31
Egg Cake 180
Egg Casserole 24
Egg Clouds 182
Egg Halves 90
Egg Hash 33
Egg Pudding 175
Egg Sandwich 89
Eggplant Chips 87
Eggplant Puree 163
Eggplant Sauce 75
Eggplant Saute 167
Eggs and Beef Pie 23
Eggs Bake 20
Eggs in Rings 21
Eggs Salad 89
Enchilada Mix 44
Endive Salad 66
Energy Bars 80
Escargot Ramekins 86

F
Fajita Chicken 120
Fajita Pork 135
Fennel Chicken 131
Fennel Mussels 109
Fennel Salad 66
Fennel Seabass 96
Fenugreek Celery Stalks 154
Feta Pie 34
Fish Pancakes 84
Fish Soup 57
Flax Meal Granola 35
Flax Seeds Spinach 165
Flax Seeds Zucchini Bread 37
Flaxseeds Doughnuts 169
Fluffy Cookies 183
Fluffy Eggs 32
Fried Halloumi 80
Frozen Ice 179

G
Garam Masala Bake 33
Garlic and Avocado Spread 81
Garlic and Curry Chicken 116
Garlic and Dill Chicken 113
Garlic Artichokes 57
Garlic Bake 39
Garlic Catfish 101
Garlic Cauliflower Fritters 153
Garlic Chicken 112

Garlic Duck Bites 124
Garlic Mackerel 105
Garlic Mash 156
Garlic Oysters 103
Garlic Pork Loin 134
Garlic Pork Ribs 150
Garlic Pork Ribs 152
Garlic Pork Salad 53
Garlic Radicchio 73
Garlic Rinds 88
Garlic Soup 161
Garlic Swiss Chard 64
Garlic Turnips Sticks 72
Garlic Zucchini Boats 43
Garlic Zucchini Noodles 60
Ginger and Parsley Smoothie 36
Ginger Cod 98
Ginger Cream Soup 164
Ginger Lamb Chops 144
Goat Cheese Pancakes 49
Greek-Style Tuna 110
Green Bean Salad 50
Green Cabbage Soup 168
Greens and Chicken Bowl 128
Greens and Coconut Soup 56
Greens Omelette 159
Greens Soup 157
Grilled Chicken Sausages 119
Grilled Garlic Eggplants 167
Grilled Mushrooms 167
Grilled Pork Sausage 151
Ground Beef Salad 41
Ground Pork Pie 133
Guacamole Sandwich 28

H

Halibut and Spinach 97
Halibut with Mushrooms 108
Halloumi Salad 41
Halloumi Salad 48
Ham Bites 81
Ham Bites 84
Ham Terrine 90
Harissa Turnip 76
Hemp Bites 32
Herbed Eggs 23
Herbed Ginger Chicken 131
Herbed Muffins 78
Herbed Oysters 94
Herbed Spaghetti Squash 61
Hot Salmon 106
Hot Sauce Lamb 143
Hot Sauce Sausage 151

I

Indian Style Chicken 128
Italian Spices Seabass 95
Italian Sticks 87
Italian Style Chicken 114
Italian Style Mushrooms 58
Italian Style Wings 86

J

Jalapeno Bake 26
Jalapeño Bites 88
Jalapeno Chicken 127
Jalapeno Chicken Chowder 122
Jalapeno Chicken with Cream Cheese 131
Jalapeno Pork Chops 136
Jalapeno Salad 90
Jalapeno Sauce 67
Jalapeno Stuffed Eggs 77
Jalapeno Tilapia 100
Jelly Bears 169
Jerky 84
Jicama Noodles 160

K

Kalamata Snack 82
Kale Bake 27
Kale Chips 85
Kale Soup 168
Keto Bake 25
Keto Beef 149
Keto Caramel 177
Keto Coffee 23
Keto Pesto 65
Keto Pie 147
Keto Smoothie 184
Keto Soup 166
Keto Tomato Salad 45
Keto Tomatoes 156

L

Lamb and Celery Casserole 144
Lamb and Pecan Salad 143
Lamb in Almond Sauce 144
Lamb Meatballs 49
Lamb Saute with Mint and Lemon 146
Lavender Lamb 145
Leek Chicken 129
Leek Stuffed Beef 134
Lemon Bell Peppers 153
Lemon Cauliflower Shred 70
Lemon Chicken 113
Lemon Chicken Breast 120
Lemon Chips 91
Lemon Duck Breast 115
Lemon Flounder 102
Lemon Greens 155
Lemon Octopus 102
Lemon Pie 172
Lemon Pork Belly 133
Lemon Pudding 174
Lemon Salad 162
Lemon Spinach 63
Lemon Stuffed Pork 133
Lemon Zucchini 66
Lemongrass Soup 47
Lettuce and Cod Salad 105
Lettuce and Mozzarella Salad 163
Lettuce Salad 56
Lettuce Sandwich 154
Lettuce Tacos 50
Lime Beef 57

Lime Cabbage Mix 64
Lime Cheese 180
Lime Chicken Wings 112
Lime Cookies 181
Lime Green Beans 156
Lime Haddock 92
Lime Lamb 146
Lime Meringue 178
Lime Mussels 101
Lime Ribs 143
Lime Salad 74
Lime Shrimp 98
Lime Trout 93
Lime Waffles 35
Lobster Soup 55

M

Macadamia Bowls 33
Macadamia Chicken 126
Marinara Bites 88
Marinara Chicken Tart 45
Marinated Broccoli 153
Marinated Broccoli Salad 163
Marinated Garlic 76
Marinated Pork 133
Marjoram Chicken Breast 125
Marjoram Pork Tenderloin 141
Marjoram Seabass 105
Masala Chicken Thighs 115
Masala Fennel 68
Masala Ground Pork 143
Matcha Bombs 39
Matcha Custard 182
Matcha Muffins 174
Mayo Salad 51
Meatballs in Coconut Sauce 140
Meatballs Soup 46
Mexican Lamb Chops 145
Milk Sorbet 182
Mint Brownies 173
Mint Lamb Chops 142
Mint Sauce 67
Monterey Jack Cheese Asparagus 159
Monterey Jack Cheese Chicken 122
Monterey Jack Cheese Rolls 90
Monterey Jack Cheese Sauce 71
Monterey Jack Muffins 30
Mozzarella Bites 83
Mozzarella Burgers 43
Mozzarella Chicken 120
Mozzarella Chicken 130
Mozzarella Eggplant 62
Mozzarella Frittata 21
Mozzarella Pancakes 26
Mozzarella Salad 65
Mozzarella Swiss Chard 165
Mug Bread 27
Mushroom Bake 164
Mushroom Caps 38
Mushroom Chicken 119
Mushroom Cream Soup 166

Mushroom Pan 74
Mushroom Scramble 21
Mushroom Shrimps 100
Mushrooms Omelette 36
Mushrooms with Shrimps 85
Mustard Asparagus 156
Mustard Cod 95
Mustard Greens Soup 157
Mustard Lamb Chops 143
Mustard Salad 161
Mustard Salad 45
Mustard Tilapia 108

N

No-Baked Cheesecake 171
Noodle Soup 48
Nutmeg Balls 181
Nutmeg Balls 85
Nutmeg Lamb 147
Nutmeg Mushroom Mix 64
Nutmeg Mushrooms 75
Nutmeg Pies 179
Nutmeg Pork Chops 136

O

Oil and Herbs Lamb 150
Onion and Chicken Bake 45
Onion Beef Roast 147
Onion Chicken 113
Onion Cookies 29
Onion Edamame 61
Onion Mahi Mahi 103
Onion Mushroom and Spinach 61
Onion Salmon 95
Onion Spinach 70
Orange Chicken 123
Orange Ice Cream 183
Oregano and Basil Scallops 109
Oregano Chard Salad 165
Oregano Chicken Wings 112
Oregano Duck 125
Oregano Eggplants 158
Oregano Fennel 164
Oregano Frittata 29
Oregano Meatballs 116
Oregano Mushroom Caps 78
Oregano Olives 70
Oregano Pork Chops 135
Oregano Salmon 94
Oysters Stir-Fry 110

P

Pancakes Pie 49
Pancetta Lamb 146
Paprika Beef Jerky 84
Paprika Beef Steaks 143
Paprika Cauliflower Rice 62
Paprika Chicken Fillet 114
Paprika Chicken Wings 112
Paprika Cod 105
Paprika Okra 162
Paprika Pork Strips 136
Paprika Wings 79

Parmesan Artichokes 157
Parmesan Bake 51
Parmesan Broccoli Mix 59
Parmesan Brussel Sprouts 167
Parmesan Chicken Thighs 126
Parmesan Chips 81
Parmesan Cod 94
Parmesan Lamb 144
Parmesan Pancake 166
Parmesan Rings 33
Parmesan Tilapia Bites 100
Parsley Asparagus 153
Parsley Chicken 115
Parsley Cod 102
Parsley Dip 85
Parsley Eggs 26
Parsley Kohlrabi 71
Parsley Pilaf 73
Parsley Sea Bass 96
Parsley Taco Beef 140
Parsley Tuna Fritters 96
Peach Ice Cream 184
Pecan Brownies 169
Pecan Candies 169
Pecan Fudge 176
Pecan Granola 182
Pepper and Chicken Soup 44
Pepper Brussels Sprouts 59
Pepper Cabbage 69
Pepper Cucumbers 88
Pepper Shrimp 99
Pepper Tuna Cakes 107
Peppermint Cookies 183
Peppermint Cream 174
Pepperoni Balls 79
Peppers Kebabs 89
Peppers Nachos 83
Pesto Fritatta 38
Poached Eggs 25
Pomegranate Scallops 107
Pork and Cream Cheese Rolls 134
Pork and Mushrooms Roast 137
Pork and Vegetable Meatballs 137
Pork Balls Bake 138
Pork Cakes 25
Pork Dumplings 48
Pork Kebabs 77
Pork Muffins 79
Pork Pan 24
Pork Rinds Balls 78
Pork Rolls 140
Pork with Gouda Cheese 151
Portobello Skewers 54
Prosciutto Salad 64
Provolone Cream 51
Provolone Kale 62
Pumpkin Bowls 89

R

Radish Hash 31
Radish in Bacon Sauce 160

Radish Salad 67
Raspberries Bowl 38
Raspberry Cream 179
Red Chard Stew 68
Ricotta Bars 177
Ricotta Cabbage 71
Ricotta Chicken Salad 44
Ricotta Omelette 38
Roasted Bok Choy 154
Roasted Cauliflower Florets 82
Roasted Sea Eel 94
Rosemary Chicken 118
Rosemary Clams 105
Rosemary Grilled Peppers 154
Rosemary Pork Tenderloin 136
Rosemary Radish 160
Rosemary Tomatoes 90
Rosemary Zucchini Mix 68
Rutabaga Cakes 157
Rutabaga Pan 34

S

Saffron Duck 124
Sage Beef 150
Sage Chicken 123
Sage Chicken Wings 112
Sage Cod Fillets 94
Sage Pâte 47
Sage Pork Chops 138
Salmon and Radish Stew 109
Salmon Boats 92
Salmon Bowl 40
Salmon Burger 109
Salmon Eggs 21
Salmon Kababs 92
Salmon Kababs 101
Salmon Meatballs 93
Salmon Quesadillas 103
Salmon Sauce 106
Salmon Soup 57
Salty Cookies 183
Sardine Salad 105
Sardines Stuffed Avocado 45
Sausage and Asparagus Bowl 152
Sausage Casserole 147
Sausage Sandwich 20
Sausage Side Dish 73
Sausage Stew with Turnip 148
Sauteed Collard Greens 158
Savory Cauliflower Salad 42
Scallions and Provolone Pork Pie 46
Scallions Beef Meatloaf 139
Scallions Chicken 123
Scallions Green Beans 70
Scallions Muffins 28
Scallions Salmon Cakes 97
Scallions Salmon Spread 98
Scallions Sandwich 91
Scallions Soup 163
Seafood Mix 23
Seasoned Chicken 124

Seaweed Chips 89
Seeds Bars 180
Seeds Chips 78
Seeds Granola 37
Seitan Salad 55
Sesame Bok Choy 163
Sesame Broccoli 161
Sesame Brussel Sprouts 58
Shredded Chicken Pancakes 127
Shrimp and Avocado Salad 42
Shrimp and Spinach Mix 56
Shrimp and Turnip Stew 100
Shrimp Bites 82
Shrimp Bowl 99
Shrimp Chowder 95
Shrimp Salad 103
Shrimp Soup 100
Shrimps Pan 30
Smoked Paprika Pork 141
Smoked Paprika Sausage Soup 152
Soft Trout 92
Sorbet 180
Sour Cod 96
Sour Duck Breast 124
Spearmint Veal 150
Spicy Bake 37
Spicy Beef 149
Spicy Ground Beef Casserole 140
Spicy Marjoram Oysters 107
Spicy Risotto 76
Spicy Salmon 103
Spicy Salmon 93
Spinach Dip 78
Spinach Eggplant Sandwich 43
Spinach Fritters 158
Spinach Mash 59
Spinach Sauce 59
Spinach Soup 162
Spinach Wraps 85
Spring Onion Cubes 137
Sprouts Salad 159
Sriracha Calamari 101
Sriracha Chicken 128
Sriracha Slaw 74
Steak Salad 44
Stevia Pie 178
Strawberries Chicken 125
Strawberry Popsicles 184
Strawberry Pudding 31
Stuffed Avocado 26
Stuffed Bell Peppers 42
Stuffed Calamari with Herbs 110
Stuffed Chicken 118
Stuffed Chicken with Olives 129
Stuffed Cucumber 88
Stuffed Eggplants 54
Stuffed Salmon with Spinach 108
Sumac Shakshuka 36
Sweet Bacon 87
Sweet Bacon Bombs 182

Sweet Cauliflower Salad 76
Sweet Chicken Wings 124
Sweet Cranberry Sauce 75
Sweet Ice Cubes 184
Sweet Lamb with Oregano 146
Sweet Leg of Lamb 145
Sweet Mousse 172
Sweet Paprika Bars 175
Sweet Pork 135
Sweet Pork Belly 141
Sweet Porridge 33
Sweet Salmon Steaks 99
Sweet Swordfish 110
Swerve Cookies 180

T

Taco Jicama 73
Taco Tilapia 107
Tarragon Chicken 115
Tarragon Mushrooms 59
Tarragon Seabass 107
Tender Catfish 99
Tender Chicken Fillets 122
Tender Cookies 177
Tender Indian Pork 149
Tender Lamb Stew 146
Tender Onions 63
Tender Veal 150
Thai Soup 163
Thai Style Pork 137
Thyme Beef 147
Thyme Cupcakes 81
Thyme Halloumi 86
Thyme Muffins 30
Thyme Pork Chops 135
Thyme Sausages 125
Tilapia Bowl 93
Tilapia with Olives 97
Tomato and Thyme Shrimps 98
Tomato Beef Bake 151
Tomato Chicken 126
Tomato Cream 47
Tomato Cream Soup 54
Tomato Cups 43
Tomato Lamb Ribs 152
Tomato Mackerel 108
Tomato Pan 41
Tomato Pork Ribs 138
Tomato Pulled Pork 139
Tomato Sea Bass 98
Tomatoes Salad 39
Tortilla Bake 53
Tuna Bowls 39
Tuna Meatballs 102
Tuna Pie 92
Tuna Salad 106
Tuna Skewers 104
Tuna Tartare 51
Turkey Bake 116
Turkey Burgers 117
Turkey Meatballs 86

Turkey Salad 118
Turkey Soup 117
Turmeric Beef Tenders 138
Turmeric Calamari 101
Turmeric Chicken 48
Turmeric Chicken Skin 125
Turmeric Eggplant 65
Turmeric Eggs 80
Turmeric Pie 46
Turmeric Radishes 159
Turmeric Salmon Balls 104
Turmeric Sausages 82
Turnip Soup 55

V

Vanilla Butter Bars 183
Vanilla Chai 26
Vanilla Custard 181
Vanilla Donuts 176
Vanilla Flan 179
Vanilla Mousse 170
Vanilla Pancake Pie 179
Vanilla Pancakes 20
Vanilla Shake 174
Vanilla Toast 35
Vanilla Topping 179
Veal and Cabbage Salad 147
Veal and Sorrel Saute 150
Vegetable Soup 167
Vinegar Chicken 120
Vinegar Salmon 106

W

Walnut Bowls 27
Walnut Brownies 176
Walnut Salad 73
Watercress Soup 153
Watermelon Sorbet 184
White Beef Soup 140
White Fish Stew 98
White Mushrooms Saute 160
Wrapped Ham Bites 149
Wrapped Scallops 92

Y

Yogurt Asparagus 158
Yogurt Chicken 129
Yogurt Pudding 184

Z

Zucchini and Pancetta Mix 72
Zucchini Baked Bars 54
Zucchini Cakes 70
Zucchini Chips 83
Zucchini Cream Soup 164
Zucchini Latkes 28
Zucchini Noodle Salad 73
Zucchini Pudding 175
Zucchini Ravioli 162
Zucchini Rolls 82
Zucchini Rolls 89
Zucchini Sandwich 42
Zucchini Sauce 84
Zucchini Sticks 69
Zucchini Stuffed Peppers 53

CPSIA information can be obtained
at www.ICGtesting.com
Printed in the USA
LVHW012121200521
687980LV00003B/28